The Incredible Internet Guide™ to
DIETS &
NUTRITION

By Marc Dauphinais

Cover Art by Robin Fox & Associates

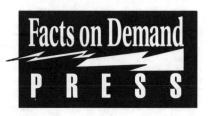

©2000 By Marc Dauphinais &
Facts on Demand Press
1971 E Fifth Street, Suite 101
Tempe, AZ 85281
(800) 929-3811
www.brbpub.com/iig

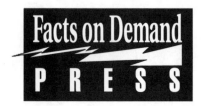

The Incredible Internet Guide™ to Diets & Nutrition

©2000 By Marc Dauphinais and Facts on Demand Press
1971 E Fifth Street, Suite 101
Tempe, AZ 85281
(800) 929-3811

ISBN 1-889150-14-2
Graphic Design by Robin Fox & Associates
Edited by James R Flowers Jr.

Cataloging-in-Publication Data

784.D38 Dauphinais, Marc
DAU   The incredible Internet guide to diets &
           nutrition / by Marc Dauphinais. -- 1st ed.
                   236 p. cm. -- (Incredible Internet guides)
                   ISBN: 1-889150-14-2

                   1.Nutrition--Computer network resources.
           2. Dietetics--Computer network resources.   3. Diet
           therapy--Computer network resources. I. Title.

           RA784.D38 2000   025.06'6132
                                          QBI99-1761

To Rita Dauphinais . . .
The little old lady I know as Mom.
Because of her, I know that there are angels in our midst.

CONTENTS

Fitness & High Performance 105

Issues in Food Safety 129

Combating Fraud Online 141

Diets & Nutrition Site Profiles 163

Find out more about some of the sites listed in this book, including whether or not they offer chat rooms, message boards, mailing lists, and more!

Introduction

I am not a dietician nor am I a nutritionist. I am not a personal trainer nor am I an exercise physiologist. I am certainly not a diet doctor with claims of having the keys to eradicate obesity and disease for all humankind.

I am merely a consumer who, along with millions of others, has searched the libraries, bookstores, and Internet for simple solutions to help me achieve good health and longevity.

Recently, I was rendered inactive for four months due to an athletic injury. I knew I wasn't going to be burning many calories for a while, and I feared that I would balloon outward while left alone in the kitchen with the family away at school and work. So, I went online to see if the World Wide Web could help me hold my weight steady or even help me lose a few pounds.

What I found was a morass, a quagmire, of tens of thousands of web sites offering programs, philosophies, and products to "help" me in my quest for a diet. There were huge and impressive sites from universities, medical groups, governments, the food industry, and dieticians. There were countless sites posted by individuals, some consisting of personal weight loss journals, and there were many sources of support for those battling the effects of obesity and disease. Of course, I found many sites hawking their own versions of magic bullets, snake oils, and elixirs all trying to get me to type in my credit card number.

I found myself lost in lists provided by search engines that often led me to dead ends, outdated sites, or useless information. Occasionally I would wander into an excellent site with hundreds of pages of good information and with links to other worthwhile sites. There were also times when I thought that I was getting good information, but my instinct told me that there seemed to be a bias.

I learned that an effective online search takes lots of time and patience. That is the basis for the *Incredible Internet Guide to Diets & Nutrition* -- to save you time and help you find what you are looking for fast.

From web sites in Canada, across the ocean to the United Kingdom, down under to Australia and into India I found a common thread that is woven through the fabric of achieving a healthy lifestyle. The mantra of "variety, balance, and moderation" is that thread, and it courses throughout the *Incredible Internet Guide to Diets & Nutrition*.

As you browse through the *Incredible Internet Guide to Diets & Nutrition*, you will notice that it begins with a chapter on nutrition basics, which lays the groundwork for understanding much about what we eat. From there, we have developed a logical progression to discussing weight loss principles and onto developing a strategy for adopting a healthy lifestyle. Alternative diets such as vegetarian, vegan, and fruitarian diets are discussed as well as disease prevention and food safety. The final chapter on consumer awareness is last but of utmost importance. Checking those credentials of both web sites and of people who hope to profit from you can be of great benefit to the consumer.

With this book in your hand, you can verify the credentials of medical professionals, discover new exercises, acquire new recipes, and go directly to health information online. We're organized so that you don't have to be.

What changes did my family and I make?

Writing this book (and using its resources) has caused my own family to make changes. First, we began to add one or two meatless meals to our family's menu each week. We logged on to the huge resource, www.vegsource.com/recipe, to find some new entrees. The old wok came out of the attic, and is used regularly for stir fry dinners and soups. Surprisingly, the children accepted the change with enthusiasm. We now regularly visit our local organic food store, and we try new adventures in wholesome eating. Visit www.wholefoods.com for your own culinary adventure.

Second, we have become much more conscious of issues in food safety. Our kitchen is better equipped thanks to sites such as the government's Center for Food Safety (www.fsis.usda.gov/OA/pubs/consumerpubs.html), and the Center for Science in the Public Interest (www.cspinet.org), the Ralph Naderesque government watchdog group. We're washing and scrubbing our hands, our produce, our counters, our cutting boards, and our refrigerator like never before. Our handling of meat and poultry is much more cautious, and our food choices in the deli section have diminished greatly. A spray bottle with a bleach solution is always handy.

And finally, my weight did not balloon after all. In addition to the other sites in this book, I found great resources for a healthy lifestyle at Cyberdiet (www.cyberdiet.com) and Dr. C. Everett Koop's web site, www.drkoop.com.

Using this Book is as Easy as 1 - 2 - 3

1

First, decide what you are looking for. Then, search the table of contents to find a chapter and section to look in. For example,

➢ *If you want to verify that your doctor is licensed to practice, go to the chapter called "Combating Fraud Online" and look up the state in which you live.*

> ➤ *If you're looking for sites to help you start running, go to the chapter named Fitness & High Performance and then view the list called Running.*

> ➤ *If you're searching for a weight loss program, go to the chapter called Weight Loss Programs: The Good, The Bad & The Ugly.*

2

Once you find the page number for a section that interests you, turn to that section and read through the list of sites and their descriptions. Or simply browse them all.

3

To get more information on a site, look it up in the back half of the book (where web sites are listed in alphabetical order, like a dictionary)

~Or~

Go online and type in the URL of the site you want to view.

If you are new on the Web, you'll soon discover that there's one basic truth about the Internet clickstream: there are a lot of different things that can be found on a web site. So, in **the second half** of the *Incredible Internet Guide to Diets & Nutrition* you'll find an alphabetical listing of sites that merit additional description – over 1100 of them. Here, each site has its URL, a description of what's on that site, and icons to show you at a glance what the site has to offer. So, if you want to know ahead of time what to expect at a site, read the site's profile.

I can't find a page -- what's wrong?

There are a number of things you should be aware of, which this book has no control over. First, some web sites simply "die" off – disappear. Also, web sites do change addresses – they move around. Generally, the webmaster will set up a link that takes you to the new location, but not always.

Some sites are only accessible through their main page. One way to try to find a site that won't open is to "truncate" the URL. This is accomplished by deleting the last section of the address. For example, if <u>www.brbpub.com/iig/diet</u> would not open for you, then try using only <u>www.brbpub.com/iig</u> as the address. Once you are at the "main page" or an "index page," you should then be able to use links to navigate to the specific page you need.

How to save something off a web site

There are a number of ways to save something online for viewing offline.

To copy/paste text, use your mouse to simply highlight the area you want. Then, choose copy from the Edit menu of your browser, and then choose paste from the Edit menu of your word processing program.

To save a web page's text and/or links, choose "Save file as . . ." from your browser's File menu. You can save the page as plain text (which will eliminate all graphics and links), or you can save it as HTML (which will retain the links if you open it in a program capable of viewing HTML files).

To download an item, simply right click (using your right mouse button) on the link to the file. Then choose "Save target as. . ."

Remember, too, that when you find a site you like and you want to return to it later, use the "Bookmarks" (on Netscape Navigator) or "Favorites" (on Internet Explorer) to remember the site location for you. We suggest that you create an exclusive Dieting folder in your Bookmarks or Favorites just for your Dieting sites.

How do you write to us?

We'd certainly like to hear from you, and we'd be especially interested in hearing about anything new or original regarding diets, nutrition and the Internet. We're not too excited about web pages that consist mainly of links to other sites. There are plenty of those already. Additionally, if you find an error in this edition of the *Incredible Internet Guide to Diets & Nutrition,* feel free to e-mail us a correction.

Our e-mail address is mdauphin@gateway.net.

Sorry, we cannot respond to all e-mail, but we especially like to hear good ideas and good words about diets, nutrition and our book.

Visit the *Incredible Internet Guides* online

Visit the web site for the *Incredible Internet Guide Series* at www.brbpub.com/iig. You will find a chat room, message boards, free e-mail addresses as well as information on other titles in the series, including the *Incredible Internet Guide to Star Wars.*

Understanding Nutrition

In the beginning, there were four basic food groups. That's all there was to it. We didn't need to know anything further about nutrition. My own mother never gave us a vitamin pill while we were growing up. She would say, "You don't need vitamins if you're eating right!" Then came the Food Pyramid, which laypeople could digest easily enough. But the pyramid was followed by Linus Pauling and Vitamin C, fiber and cancer, fat and heart disease, artificial sweeteners and cancer, cholesterol and heart disease, antioxidants and free radicals, and more in a list of "nutrition" items that seems to grow everyday.

Just what do we really need to know, and how much do we need to know in order to achieve and maintain the healthy lifestyle we want for ourselves and for our children? Is it necessary to take vitamins and supplements if in fact we do strive for that goal of variety, balance, and moderation in our diets each day? The sites in this chapter lead us to everything we need to know about what we eat. They give us a solid foundation on which to build our healthy eating plans, whether we plan to lose weight, gain weight, try a vegetarian lifestyle, or focus on preventive nutrition. Begin with the food pyramid and dive as deep as you like into these sites.

Understanding the Food Pyramid

The food pyramid with all its food groups should be a simple concept, but there is obviously some confusion among us; after all, if we really understood it and followed it wouldn't we all be a lot healthier? Some of these sites come from the food industry, while others originate from the UDSA. They all have something good to offer.

5 A Day
www.5aday.com

American Dietetic Association: Whole - Grain Goodness
www.eatright.org/nfs/nfs30.html

CSPI: Rate Your Diet Quiz
www.cspinet.org/quiz/quiz_diet1.html

Dole 5 A Day
www.dole5aday.com

Family Food Zone: Food Guide Pyramid
www.familyfoodzone.com/pyramid/index.html

Food Guide Pyramid
www.nal.usda.gov:8001/py/pmap.htm

Fruit: Some Nutrition Facts
www.islandnet.com/~arton/fruitbl.html

Idaho Potato
www.idahopotato.com/index.html

Kids Food CyberClub: Food Guide Pyramid
www.kidsfood.org/f_pyramid/pyramid.html

Mayo Clinic Health Oasis: Carbohydrates: Their Role in Your Diet
www.mayohealth.org/mayo/9903/htm/carbohyd.htm

NCI/CDC 5 A Day Online Tracking Chart
http://5aday.nci.nih.gov

Understanding The Food Guide Pyramid
www.4meridia.com/consumer/archive/pyramid.cfm

Understanding the Food Label

Every food item we buy is supposed to have a food label on the package. Find out just what information you can garner from reading (before eating)your groceries. .

Cyberdiet's Vitamins & Minerals
www.cyberdiet.com/foodfact/vitmins/vitmins.html

Cyerdiet's Fast Food Quest
www.cyberdiet.com/ffq/index.html

Dietsite.com: Food Label Terms
www.dietsite.com/nutritionfacts/FoodLabels/Food%20label%20Descr
iptors

Dietsite.com: **How to Read A Food Label**
www.dietsite.com/nutritionfacts/FoodLabels/How%20to%20Read%20a%
20Label.htm

How to Read a Food Label
www.4meridia.com/consumer/archive/label.cfm

IFIC: Backgrounder - Food Labeling
http://ificinfo.health.org/backgrnd/bkgr5.htm

All About Additives

What do alpha tocopherol, cirtus red #2, sodium ascorbate, and ferrous gluconate all have in common? They are classified as "additives." Are they safe? Do we really need them? Why are they in our food to begin with? What do they do? These sites help us wade through the confusing, and sometimes scary world of food additives.

CSPI: Additives to Avoid
www.cspinet.org/reports/food.htm

CSPI: All About Additives
www.cspinet.org/additives

CSPI: Caffeine Content of Foods & Drugs
www.cspinet.org/new/cafchart.htm

Dietsite.com: Food Additive Labeling Terms
www.dietsite.com/NutritionFacts/FoodAdditives/Labeling/Labeling
%20content.htm

Dietsite.com: Food Additives
www.dietsite.com/nutritionfacts/FoodAdditives/index.htm

Dietsite.com: Major Functions of Food Additives
www.dietsite.com/NutritionFacts/FoodAdditives/MajorFunctions/Ma
jor%20functions%20content.htm

IFIC Review: Caffeine & Health: Clarifying the Controversies
http://ificinfo.health.org/review/ir-caffh.htm

IFIC: Food Additives
http://ificinfo.health.org/backgrnd/bkgr9.htm

Antioxidants: A Primer

Oxygen radicals are not some type of new militant leftist organization. What damage can they do? What's their relationship to heart disease? What are good sources of antioxidants in our food supply, and do we need to use supplements to get enough? Try these sites.

American Dietetic Association: Antioxidant Vitamins for Optimal Health
www.eatright.org/nfs/nfs84.html

American Dietetic Association:
Nutrition & Health for Older Americans: Antioxidants
www.eatright.org/olderamericans/antioxidants.html

American Dietetic Association: The Proof Is In The Tea Leaves
www.eatright.org/nfs/nfs87.html

IFIC Insight: Antioxidants: Working Toward A Definition
http://ificinfo.health.org/insight/NovDec98/antioxidants.htm

Mayo Clinic Health Oasis: Antioxidants
www.mayohealth.org/mayo/9308/htm/antioxid.htm

Calculators & Tools

Are you counting calories in or calories out? Are you keeping track of grams of fat, carbohydrates, or protein? Try a handy calculator from one of these sites to keep track of your own statistics.

American Medical Association Health Insight: Interactive Health
www.ama-assn.org/consumer/interact.htm

Cyberdiet's Daily Food Planner
www.cyberdiet.com/dfl

Cyberdiet's Eating Right
www.cyberdiet.com/ni/htdocs

Cyberdiet's Nutritional Profile
www.cyberdiet.com/profile/profile.cgi

Diet Analysis Web Page
http://dawp.anet.com

Dietsite.com: Diet & Recipe Analysis
www.dietsite.com/nutr/index.htm

FitBody 3.0
www.darwin326.com/fitbody

Food Finder
www.olen.com/food

InteliHealth: Home to John Hopkins Health Information: Gadgets & Quizzes
www.intelihealth.com/IH/ihtIH?t=20705&c=225043&p=~br,IHW|~st,14
220|~r,WSIHW000|~b,*|&d=dmtContent

Men's Health: Caloric Calculator
www.menshealth.com/features/eat_this/sports/index.html

Nutritional Analysis Tool
www.ag.uiuc.edu/~food-lab/nat/mainnat.html

PHYS: Portion Finder
www.phys.com/b_nutrition/02solutions/05portion/game.htm

Discussing Good Nutrition

These sites have lots of tips and suggestions about adopting and maintaining healthy eating habits. From food shopping ideas to recipes to the basics of nutrition, you'll no doubt find some thoughts to chew on.

American Council on Science & Health: Nutrition & Fitness
www.acsh.org/nutrition/index.html

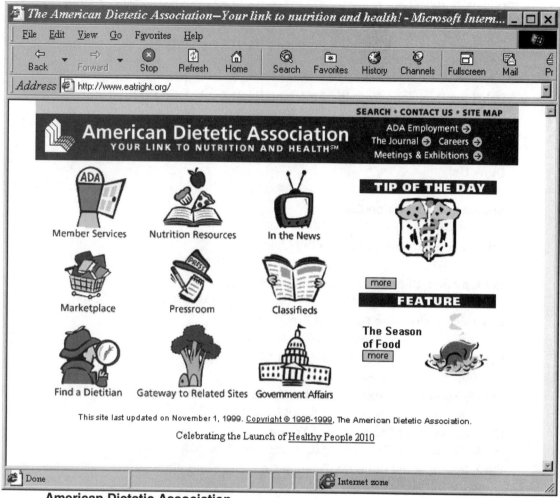

American Dietetic Association
www.eatright.org

American Dietetic Association: Search Daily Tips
www.eatright.org/cgi/searchtemp.cgi?dir=erm&template=searcherm.htm

American Dietetic Association: Tip of the Day
www.eatright.org/erm.html

American Medical Association Health Insight: Interactive Health
www.ama-assn.org/consumer/interact.htm

American Medical Association Health Insight: Interactive Health: Personal Nutritionist
www.ama-assn.org/insight/yourhlth/pernutri/pernutri.htm

Ask the Dietician
www.dietitian.com

Colorado State University Cooperative Extension: Osteoporosis
www.colostate.edu/depts/CoopExt/PUBS/FOODNUT/09359.html

Colorado State University Cooperative Extension: Women's Health Issues
www.colostate.edu/depts/CoopExt/PUBS/FOODNUT/09360.html

Cyberdiet's Food Facts
www.cyberdiet.com/foodfact/f_food.html

Delicious Decisions from the American Heart Association: Enjoy Eating
www.deliciousdecisions.org/ee/index.html

**Delicious Decisions from the American Heart Association:
Heart Healthy Chef's Tour**
www.deliciousdecisions.org/cb/hhc.html

Delicious Decisions from the American Heart Association: Out & About
www.deliciousdecisions.org/oa/index.html

Dietsite.com
www.dietsite.com

Drink Up!
http://primusweb.com/fitnesspartner/library/nutrition/fluids.htm

drkoop.com: Nutrition Center
www.drkoop.com/wellness/nutrition

drkoop.com: Nutrition for Healthy Living
www.drkoop.com/wellness/nutrition/healthyliving

drkoop.com: Submit Your Nutrition Questions
www.drkoop.com/wellness/fitness/expert/howard.asp

Duke University: The Rice Diet Program
www.ricediet.com/us/index1.html

Eat Well, Live Well Research & Information Centre
www.healthyeating.org

Family Food Zone: Pantry Tips for Meals in Minutes
www.familyfoodzone.com/shop/index2.html

IFIC: Glossary of Food-Related Terms
http://ificinfo.health.org/glossary.htm

IFIC: International Food Information Council Foundation
http://ificinfo.health.org

International Food Information Council: Ten Tips To Healthy Eating
http://ificinfo.health.org/brochure/adult10.htm

Jean Frermont's Food & Nutrition on the Web
www.sfu.ca/~jfremont

La Leche League International
www.lalecheleague.org

Mayo Clinic - Subscribe to Nutrition Update
www.mayohealth.org/cgi-bin/apps/list_mailer2?list=nutrition

Mayo Clinic Diet Center
www.mayohealth.org/mayo/common/htm/dietpage.htm

MotherNature.com: Library
www.mothernature.com/library/default.asp

PHYS: The Personal Nutritionist
http://www4.phys.com/b_nutrition/01self_analysis/06pyramid/pyramid.html

Stayhealthy.com
www.stayhealthy.com/centers/nutrition.cfm

You Are What You Eat: A Guide to Good Nutrition
http://library.advanced.org/11163/gather/cgi-bin/wookie.cgi

E-Zines

There's good reading in an E-zine, and the news they offer is usually "new." They're often loaded with graphics and have interactive quizzes and calculators. Plus, if an article peaks your curiousity there are typically links to begin further exploration of that topic.

Delicious! Online: Your Guide to Natural Living
www.delicious-online.com

eNutrition
www.enutrition.com

Healthy Eating
http://bewell.com/healthy/eating/index.asp

PHYS: The Place for Health, Fitness, Nutrition, Wellness, Weight Loss Exercise, Diet, & More
www.phys.com

FAQs

The questions never cease when it comes to nutrition. Try these sites for some answers.

American Dietetic Association: Questions Men Ask About Nutrition & Fitness
www.eatright.org/nfs/nfs51.html

Ask the Dietician
www.dietitian.com

Babies Today Online: Breastfeeding Articles & Resources
http://216.167.1.124/breastfeeding//

drkoop.com: Submit Your Nutrition Questions
www.drkoop.com/wellness/fitness/expert/howard.asp

FDA/CFSAN: Food, Nutrition, & Cosmetics Q&As
http://vm.cfsan.fda.gov/~dms/qa-top.html

Go Ask Alice Home Page
www.goaskalice.columbia.edu

Go Ask Alice: Fitness & Nutrition
www.goaskalice.columbia.edu/Cat3.html

La Leche League International: FAQs About Breastfeeding
www.lalecheleague.org/FAQ/FAQMain.html

Talk With The Experts: Ask the Mayo Dietician
www.mayohealth.org/mayo/expert/htm/ask2.htm

Infant Nutrition

There is no food pyramid for infants; they're off the hook. But they're not quite ready for chocolate yet. It turns out that they're food pyramid is a pure reflection of Mom's. These sites lend unequivocal support to breastfeeding your child.

American Dietetic Association: Position Paper: Promotion of Breastfeeding
www.eatright.org/adap0697.html

Babies Today Online: Breastfeeding Articles & Resources
http://216.167.1.124/breastfeeding//

drkoop.com: Nutrition For Infants
www.drkoop.com/wellness/nutrition/healthyliving/index.asp?id=33

InteliHealth: Home to John Hopkins Health Information: Feeding Your Baby
www.intelihealth.com/IH/ihtIH?t=3481&p=~br,IHW|~st,7165|~r,WSIH
W000|~b,*|&st=3324

InteliHealth: Home to John Hopkins Health Information: Nutrition for Mom
www.intelihealth.com/IH/ihtIH?t=4461&p=~br,IHW|~st,3324|~r,WSIH
W000|~b,*|&

La Leche League International
www.lalecheleague.org

La Leche League International: Breastfeeding Chats
www.lalecheleague.org/Chat/chat.html

La Leche League International: FAQs About Breastfeeding
www.lalecheleague.org/FAQ/FAQMain.html

La Leche League International: Useful Links
www.lalecheleague.org/links.html

Natural Child Project
www.naturalchild.com/home

Just the Fats, Please

There's fatty acids, trans fats, fat replacers, and oils. There's good fat, bad fat, and fake fat. Sort out the fat facts with these sites.

American Dietetic Association: Fat Replacers
www.eatright.org/adap0498.html

American Dietetic Association: Fat: One of Life's Essentials
www.eatright.org/nfs/nfs90.html

American Dietetic Association: Fats & Oils in the Diet - The Great Debate
www.eatright.org/nfs/nfs82.html

American Dietetic Association: What Are Triglycerides?
www.eatright.org/nfs/nfs13.html

American Dietetic Association: What Is Olestra?
www.eatright.org/nfs/nfs18.html

American Dietetic Association: The ABCs of Fats, Oils, & Cholesterols
www.eatright.org/nfs/nfs2.html

American Heart Association: Trans Fatty Acids
www.americanheart.org/Heart_and_Stroke_A_Z_Guide/tfa.html

Ask the Dietician: Fatty Acids & Trans Fat
www.dietitian.com/fattyaci.html

Ask the Dietician: Triglycerides
www.dietitian.com/triglyce.html

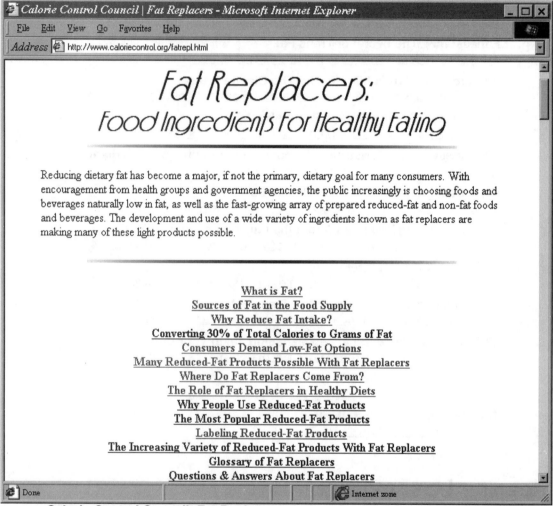

Calorie Control Council: Fat Replacers
www.caloriecontrol.org/fatrepl.html

Center for Science in the Public Interest: Problems With Olestra
www.cspinet.org/olestra/11cons.html

Colorado State University Cooperative Extension: Cholesterol & Fats
www.colostate.edu/depts/CoopExt/PUBS/FOODNUT/09319.html

CSPI: A Brief History of Olestra
www.cspinet.org/olestra/history.html

CSPI: Fat or Fiction Quiz
www.cspinet.org/cgi-bin/quiz.cgi

CSPI: Olestra Adverse Effects Report Form
www.cspinet.org/olestraform

CSPI: Olestra Quiz
www.cspinet.org/olestra/oquiz.html

CSPI: The Facts About Olestra
www.cspinet.org/olestra/index.html

Fake-fat Olestra Sickens Thousands
www.cspinet.org/new/olestra/olestra_12_22_98.htm

FDA Backgrounder: Olestra & Other Fat Substitutes
http://vm.cfsan.fda.gov/~dms/bgolestr.html

FitnessLink: The Secret of Trans Fat
www.fitnesslink.com/food/transfat.htm

Harvard School of Public Health: The Olestra Project
www.hsph.harvard.edu/Academics/nutr/olestra/olestra.html

IFIC Review: Sorting Out the Facts About Fat
http://ificinfo.health.org/review/ir-fat.htm

IFIC Review: Uses & Nutritional Impact of Fat Reduction Ingredients
http://ificinfo.health.org/review/fatr.htm

IFIC: Backgrounder: Fat & Fat Replacers
http://ificinfo.health.org/backgrnd/bkgr7.htm

IFIC: Everything You Need About the Function of Fats in Foods
http://ificinfo.health.org/brochure/functfat.htm

IFIC: Fats & Fat Replacers
http://ificinfo.health.org/press/fatmyths.htm

IFIC: Questions & Answers About Trans Fats
http://ificinfo.health.org/qanda/transqa.htm

IFIC: The Benefits of Balance: Managing Fat in Your Diet
http://ificinfo.health.org/brochure/balance.htm

Nutrition Action Healthletter: Trans Fat
www.cspinet.org/nah/6_99/transfat3.html

Trans Fat Info Web: Introduction
www.enig.com/0001t10.html

Keeping Up-To-Date

These sites can help keep us up to date on the latest thinking and research in the world of nutrition. Some of them can send them via your e-mail free of charge, while others report the nutrition news from around the world. They are worth a try.

American Dietetic Association: Journal Highlights
www.eatright.org/pr/highlights.html

Children's Nutrition Research Center
www.bcm.tmc.edu/cnrc/newsletter/spr99let.html

Cyberdiet's E-mail Newsletter
www.cyberdiet.com/subscribe

Cyberdiet's Food Facts
www.cyberdiet.com/foodfact/f_food.html

drkoop.com: Nutrition Center
www.drkoop.com/wellness/nutrition

drkoop.com: Nutrition News
www.drkoop.com/wellness/nutrition/news

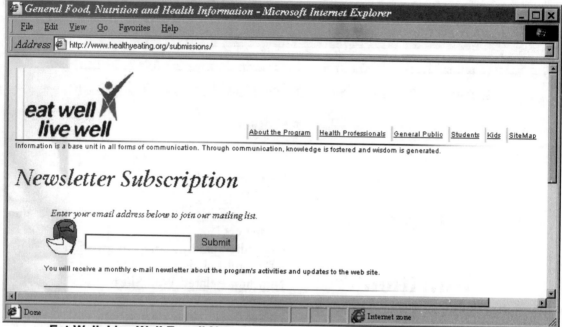

Eat Well, Live Well E-mail Newsletter
www.healthyeating.org/submissions

Eat Well, Live Well Newsletter Archive
www.healthyeating.org/newsletters

Feeding Kids Newsletter
www.nutritionforkids.com/Feeding_Kids.htm

Feeding Kids Newsletter: Subscribe
www.nutritionforkids.com/Subscribe2.htm

Food & Health Communications, Inc.
www.foodandhealth.com

InteliHealth: Home to John Hopkins Health Information: Nutrition Headlines
www.intelihealth.com/IH/ihtIH?t=8015&p=~br,IHW|~st,9103|~r,WSIH
W000|~b,*|

Mayo Clinic - Subscribe to Nutrition Update
www.mayohealth.org/cgi-bin/apps/list_mailer2?list=nutrition

MotherNature.com: News & Views
www.mothernature.com/news/default.asp

Nutrition Action Healthletter: Index
www.cspinet.org/nah/index.htm

Nutrition Action Healthletter: Subscribe
https://vs.cais.com/cspi/join4.html

Stayhealthy.com
www.stayhealthy.com/centers/nutrition.cfm

Tufts University Health & Nutrition Letter
> http://healthletter.tufts.edu

Tufts University Health & Nutrition Letter: Subscribe Form
> www.palmcoastd.com/pcd/document?imag_id=02410

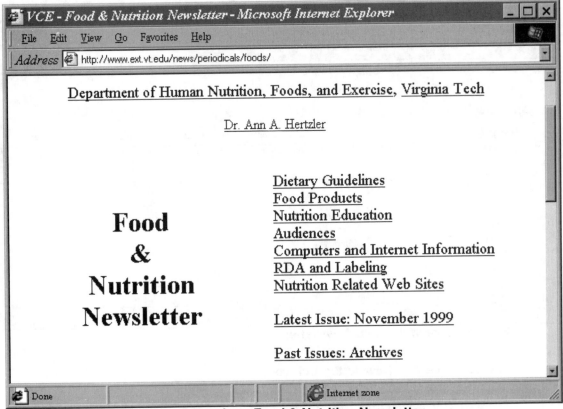

Virginia Cooperative Extension: Food & Nutrition Newsletter
> www.ext.vt.edu/news/periodicals/foods

Look It Up!

Are you curious about the nutritional content of that burger you just ate? Do you want to know more about how to read a food label? How much sodium is in a serving of black olives? Answers to these questions and more can be found at the sites below.

Circulation: Summary of a Scientific Conference on Preventive Nutrition
> http://circ.ahajournals.org/cgi/content/full/100/4/450

CSPI: A Diner's Guide to Health & Nutrition Claims on Restaurant Menus
> www.cspinet.org/reports/dinersgu.html

Dietsite.com: Food Label Terms
> www.dietsite.com/nutritionfacts/FoodLabels/Food%20label%20Descript
> ors

Fast Food Facts - Interactive Food Finder
> www.olen.com/food

FDA/CFSAN Dietary Supplement Health & Education Actof 1994
http://vm.cfsan.fda.gov/~dms/dietsupp.html

Mayo Clinic Health Oasis: Health Quiz
www.mayohealth.org/cgi-bin/apps/quiz.cgi/mayo/expert/htm/9603
quiz.txt?/mayo/common/htm/top.txt,/mayo/common/htm/bottom.txt

MotherNature.com: Library
www.mothernature.com/library/default.asp

PHYS
www.phys.com

Sante 7000 Search Form
http://209.98.30.12/sante7000/sante7000_search.cfm

Search the USDA Nutrient Database
www.nal.usda.gov/fnic/cgi-bin/nut_search.pl

Marketplace

Going shopping? Here's a few online stops selling everything from books to vitamins. Many offer information and links about their wares, but make yourself an informed consumer by first by verifying each site's credibility and security.

American Dietetic Association Marketplace
www.eatright.org/catalog/index.html

eNutrition
www.enutrition.com

Fitness Connection
www.fitness-connection.com

Food & Health Communications, Inc.
www.foodandhealth.com

Healthy Weight Network--Books & Resources
www.healthyweightnetwork.com/books.htm

IFIC: Ordering Information
http://ificinfo.health.org/order.htm

More.com
www.more.com

MotherNature.com
www.mothernature.com

Nature Mart
http://www2.naturemart.com/naturemart

Nature's Nutrition
www.naturesnutrition.com

Stayhealthy.com
www.stayhealthy.com/centers/nutrition.cfm

Symmetry International
www.go-symmetry.com

WholeFoods.com
www.wholefoods.com

Nutrition & Fun For Kids

Getting nutritious food and snacks into our children is often one of a parent's greatest challenges in our "fast food world." There are many sites with interactive nutrition games for kids and their folks. Some are actually a lot of fun. Give some a try.

24 Carrot Press: Nutrition for Kids
www.nutritionforkids.com

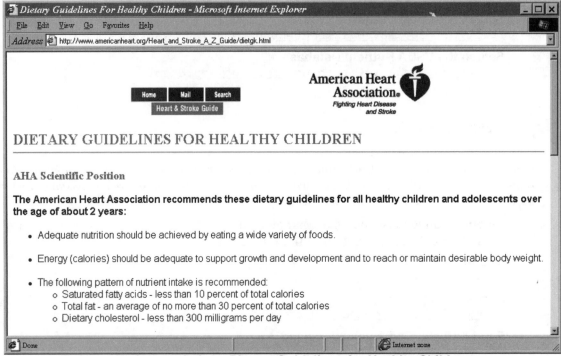

American Heart Association: Dietary Guidelines for Healthy Children
www.americanheart.org/Heart_and_Stroke_A_Z_Guide/dietgk.html

Children's Nutrition Research Center
www.bcm.tmc.edu/cnrc/newsletter/spr99let.html

CSPI: Suggestions for Better School Food
www.cspinet.org/kids/foodtips.htm

drkoop.com: Teen Nutrition
www.drkoop.com/wellness/nutrition/healthyliving/index.asp?id=35

drkoop.com: Toddler & Preschooler Nutrition
www.drkoop.com/wellness/nutrition/healthyliving/index.asp?id=34

Family Food Zone
www.familyfoodzone.com/fridge.html

Family Food Zone: Kids Cooking For Healthy Eating
www.familyfoodzone.com/cooking/index.html

Family Food Zone: Nutrition Café
www.familyfoodzone.com/game/index.html

FDA Kids Home Page
www.fda.gov/oc/opacom/kids

Feeding Kids Newsletter
www.nutritionforkids.com/Feeding_Kids.htm

Feeding Kids Newsletter: Subscribe
www.nutritionforkids.com/Subscribe2.htm

Florida Citrus Land For Kids
www.floridajuice.com/floridacitrus/kids/index.htm

FOOD Files: Amazing Records
http://library.advanced.org/11960/fun/records.htm

Food Fun For Kids
www.nppc.org/foodfun.html

Grab A Grape
http://exhibits.pacsci.org/nutrition/grape/grape.html

IFIC Insight: Extreme Eating - Are Teens Compromising Their Health?
http://ificinfo.health.org/insight/NovDec98/extremeeat.htm

Kids Food CyberClub
www.kidsfood.org

Kids Food CyberClub: Cyber Food Shopper
www.kidsfood.org/choices/shopper.html

Kids Food CyberClub: Food Guide Pyramid
www.kidsfood.org/f_pyramid/pyramid.html

Kids Food CyberClub: Nutrition Sleuths
www.kidsfood.org/sleuths/sleuths.html

Kids Food CyberClub: Rate Your Plate
www.kidsfood.org/rate_plate/rate.html

Kids Food CyberClub: Winning Choices
www.kidsfood.org/choices/winning/winning.html

Kidshealth.org: Food Guide Pyramid
http://kidshealth.org/kid/food/pyramid.html

Milk - It's On Everybody's Lips
www.whymilk.com

Nutrition for Kids: Recommended Links
www.nutritionforkids.com/Links.htm

Nutrition Sleuth
http://exhibits.pacsci.org/nutrition/sleuth/sleuth.html

Past Carrots - Nutrition for Kids
www.nutritionforkids.com/Carrots/All_Carrots.htm

Take the Food Pyramid Challenge
www.bennygoodsport.com/food.htm

This Week's Carrot - Nutrition for Kids
www.nutritionforkids.com/Carrots/Weekly_Carrot.htm

USA Pears - PearBear Healthy Kids
www.usapears.com/pbnw-kids.html

Washington State Dairy Council: Take Aim
www.eatsmart.org/html/game.html

Nutrition Concerns for Older Americans

Senior citizens have some dietary concerns that vary somewhat from those of other age groups. Although the food pyramid continues to be the basis of their nutritional health, as well as variety, balance, and moderation, these sites address the situations that arise as we mature.

American Dietetic Association: Nutrition & Health Campaign For Older Americans
www.eatright.org/olderamericans

American Dietetic Association:
Nutrition & Health for Older Americans: Antioxidants
www.eatright.org/olderamericans/antioxidants.html

American Dietetic Association: Nutrition & Health for Older Americans: Calcium
www.eatright.org/olderamericans/calcium.html

American Dietetic Association: Nutrition & Health for Older Americans: Fiber
www.eatright.org/olderamericans/fiber.html

American Dietetic Association: Nutrition & Health for Older Americans: Grains
www.eatright.org/olderamericans/grains.html

American Dietetic Association: Nutrition & Health for Older Americans: Protein
www.eatright.org/olderamericans/protein.html

American Dietetic Association: Nutrition & Health for Older Americans: Water
www.eatright.org/olderamericans/waterhydration.html

American Dietetic Association: Seniors - Eat Well for Good Health
www.eatright.org/nfs/nfs62.html

Colorado State University Cooperative Extension: Nutrition & Aging
www.colostate.edu/depts/CoopExt/PUBS/FOODNUT/09322.html

InteliHealth: Home to John Hopkins Health Information: The Aging Adult
www.intelihealth.com/IH/ihtIH?c=34061&t=8923&p=~br,IHW|~st,7165|~r,WSIHW000|~b,*|&d=dmtJHE

Nutrition During Pregnancy

Variety, balance, and moderation are still the mainstay of a pregnant woman's diet, but what about folic acid, calcium, iron, and protein? These sites offer insight to the nutritional needs of the pregnant woman.

A Good Start: Nutrition During Pregnancy
www.beef.org/nut_libr/preg_index.htm

FANSA: Folic Acid: A Reminder For Women Before & During Pregnancy
http://ift.micronexx.com/sc/sc_h04.html

Parent's Place: Calcium Supplements During Pregnancy
http://www4.parentsplace.com/pregnancy/nutrition

Parent's Place: Do I need Protein Supplements?
http://www4.parentsplace.com/pregnancy/nutrition/qa/0,3105,5690,00.html

Parent's Place: Foods That Interfere With Iron Absorption
http://www4.parentsplace.com/pregnancy/nutrition/qa/0,3105,12955,00.html

Parent's Place: Iron Supplementation in Pregnancy
http://www4.parentsplace.com/pregnancy/nutrition/qa/0,3105,715,00.html

Parent's Place: Non-Dairy Calcium Sources
http://www4.parentsplace.com/pregnancy/nutrition/qa/0,3105,5726,00.html

Parent's Place: Preparing For Pregnancy: A Nutritional Guide
http://www4.parentsplace.com/pregnancy/nutrition/qa/0,3105,11763,00.html

Parent's Place: Veganism & Pregnancy
http://www4.parentsplace.com/pregnancy/nutrition/qa/0,3105,5161,00.html

Parent's Place: Vitamin A in Pregnancy
http://www4.parentsplace.com/pregnancy/nutrition/qa/0,3105,5425,00.html

Parents Place: Pregnancy: Nutrition
http://www4.parentsplace.com/pregnancy/nutrition

Nutrition Issues for Women

Is it true that women need more calcium than men? What changes in diet must a pregnant woman undertake? These are web sites for women's nutrtition and the topics that are unique to their gender.

American Dietetic Association: Nutrition & Health Campaign for Women
www.eatright.org/womenshealth

American Dietetic Association: Nutrition & Health Campaign for Women: Breast Cancer & Nutrition
www.eatright.org/womenshealth/breastcancer.html

American Dietetic Association: Nutrition & Health Campaign for Women: Diabetes & Nutrition
www.eatright.org/womenshealth/diabetes.html

American Dietetic Association: Nutrition & Health Campaign for Women: Good News Guide For Healthy Women
www.eatright.org/womenshealth/guide.html

American Dietetic Association: Nutrition & Health Campaign for Women: Heart Disease & Nutrition
www.eatright.org/womenshealth/heartdisease.html

American Dietetic Association: Nutrition & Health Campaign for Women: Osteoporosis & Nutrition
www.eatright.org/womenshealth/osteoporosis.html

American Dietetic Association: Nutrition & Health Campaign for Women: Weight Management & Nutrition
www.eatright.org/womenshealth/weightmanagement.html

Colorado State University Cooperative Extension: Osteoporosis
www.colostate.edu/depts/CoopExt/PUBS/FOODNUT/09359.html

Colorado State University Cooperative Extension: Women's Health Issues
www.colostate.edu/depts/CoopExt/PUBS/FOODNUT/09360.html

drkoop.com: Nutrition During Pregnancy
www.drkoop.com/wellness/nutrition/healthyliving/index.asp?id=38

drkoop.com: Women's Nutrition
www.drkoop.com/wellness/nutrition/healthyliving/index.asp?id=36

InteliHealth: Home to John Hopkins Health Information: Nutrition for Mom
www.intelihealth.com/IH/ihtIH?t=4461&p=~br,IHW|~st,3324|~r,WSIH
W000|~b,*|&

Mayo Clinic Health Oasis: Pregnancy & Nutrition Update
www.mayohealth.org/mayo/9601/htm/pregvit.htm

New York Times on the Web: Women's Health: Diet & Exercise
www.nytimes.com/specials/women/whome/diet_exercise.html

Nutrition With Men in Mind

Chips and salsa, pretzels and beer, chili and beans. Is a man's food pyramid supposed to be any different from everyone else's? Try these sites for the facts.

American Dietetic Association: Questions Men Ask About Nutrition & Fitness
www.eatright.org/nfs/nfs51.html

American Heart Association: Dietary Guidelines for Healthy American Adults
www.americanheart.org/Heart_and_Stroke_A_Z_Guide/dietg.html

Ask the Dietician: Sports Nutrition
www.dietitian.com/sportnut.html

Men's Health
www.menshealth.com

Men's Health: Caloric Calculator
www.menshealth.com/features/eat_this/sports/index.html

Men's Health: Eat This
www.menshealth.com/features/eat_this/quick/index.html

Men's Health: Food, Nutrition, & Recipes
www.menshealth.com/food_nutrition/index.html

Men's Nutrition: Quiz
http://primusweb.com/fitnesspartner/library/nutrition/mensquiz.
htm

Professional Organization Sites

These are the some of the sites that may be considered as authorities; they wrote the book, so to speak, on nutrition. These are the places to visit when you want to verify the truth.

American Cancer Society
www.cancer.org

American Diabetes Association
www.diabetes.org

American Dietetic Association
www.eatright.org

American Dietetic Association Marketplace
www.eatright.org/catalog/index.html

American Dietetic Association: Search Daily Tips
www.eatright.org/cgi/searchtemp.cgi?dir=erm&template=searcherm.htm

American Dietetic Association: Tip of the Day
www.eatright.org/erm.html

American Heart Association
www.americanheart.org

American Society for Clinical Nutrition
www.faseb.org/ascn

California Dietetic Association
www.dietitian.org

Ready for a Quiz?

Test your nutritional knowledge with these fun quizzes. You didn't know learning could be so fun, did you?

American Diabetes Association: Feed Your Brain: Nutrition Quiz
www.diabetes.org/nutrition/i_quiz.asp

American Medical Association Health Insight: Interactive Health: Personal Nutritionist
www.ama-assn.org/insight/yourhlth/pernutri/pernutri.htm

CSPI: Fat or Fiction Quiz
www.cspinet.org/cgi-bin/quiz.cgi

CSPI: Rate Your Diet Quiz
www.cspinet.org/quiz/quiz_diet1.html

Diet & Nutrition Resource Center - Quizzes
www.mayohealth.org/mayo/common/htm/dietquiz.htm

Eat Well, Live Well Newsletter Archive
www.healthyeating.org/newsletters

Family Food Zone: Nutrition Café
www.familyfoodzone.com/game/index.html

FDA Kids Home Page
www.fda.gov/oc/opacom/kids

Grab A Grape
http://exhibits.pacsci.org/nutrition/grape/grape.html

Kids Food CyberClub: Cyber Food Shopper
www.kidsfood.org/choices/shopper.html

Kids Food CyberClub: Food Guide Pyramid
www.kidsfood.org/f_pyramid/pyramid.html

Kids Food CyberClub: Nutrition Sleuths
www.kidsfood.org/sleuths/sleuths.html

Kids Food CyberClub: Rate Your Plate
www.kidsfood.org/rate_plate/rate.html

Kids Food CyberClub: Winning Choices
www.kidsfood.org/choices/winning/winning.html

Mayo Clinic Health Oasis: Health Quiz
www.mayohealth.org/cgi-bin/apps/quiz.cgi/mayo/expert/htm/9603quiz.txt?/mayo/common/htm/top.txt,/mayo/common/htm/bottom.txt

Mayo Clinic Health Oasis: Quizzes From the Nutrition Center
www.mayohealth.org/mayo/common/htm/dietquiz.htm

Men's Nutrition: Quiz
http://primusweb.com/fitnesspartner/library/nutrition/mensquiz.htm

MotherNature.com: Quiz Central
www.mothernature.com/quiz/default.asp

NCI/CDC 5 A Day Online Tracking Chart
http://5aday.nci.nih.gov

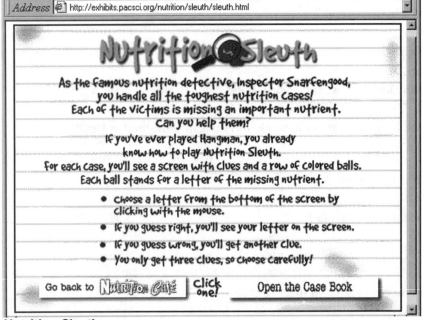

Nutrition Sleuth
http://exhibits.pacsci.org/nutrition/sleuth/sleuth.html

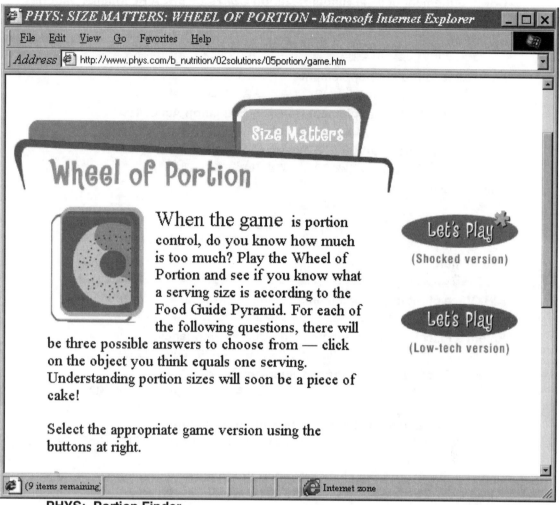

PHYS: Portion Finder
www.phys.com/b_nutrition/02solutions/05portion/game.htm

Take the Food Pyramid Challenge
www.bennygoodsport.com/food.htm

Washington State Dairy Council: Take Aim
www.eatsmart.org/html/game.html

Supplements: Are They Necessary?

Do we rreally need supplements? If we do, how much is enough? Can we take too much? Is it worth the money? It's a big industry, and there's a lot of money changing hands. These sites help to answer these questions, but the final decision is the buyer's alone.

American Dietetic Association: Straight Answers About Vitamin & Mineral Supplements
www.eatright.org/nfs/nfs66.html

Ask the Dietician: Vitamin Supplements
www.dietitian.com/vitamins.html

CSPI: Statement of Ilene Ringel Heller on CSPI's DESHEA Recommendations
www.cspinet.org/reports/diet_supplement.html

eNutrition
www.enutrition.com

FDA Guide to Dietary Supplements
http://vm.cfsan.fda.gov/~dms/fdsupp.html

FDA/CFSAN Dietary Supplement Health & Education Act of 1994
http://vm.cfsan.fda.gov/~dms/dietsupp.html

FDA/CFSAN: Food, Nutrition, & Cosmetics Q&As
http://vm.cfsan.fda.gov/~dms/qa-top.html

Fitness Connection
www.fitness-connection.com

Mayo Clinic Health Oasis: Buyer Beware
www.mayohealth.org/mayo/9707/htm/me_5sb.htm

Nature Mart
http://www2.naturemart.com/naturemart

NIH Office of Dietary Supplements
http://odp.od.nih.gov/ods/databases/ibids.html

Parent's Place: Calcium Supplements During Pregnancy
http://www4.parentsplace.com/pregnancy/nutrition

Parent's Place: Do I need Protein Supplements?
http://www4.parentsplace.com/pregnancy/nutrition/qa/0,3105,5690,00.html

Parent's Place: Foods That Interfere With Iron Absorption
http://www4.parentsplace.com/pregnancy/nutrition/qa/0,3105,12955,00.html

Parent's Place: Iron Supplementation in Pregnancy
http://www4.parentsplace.com/pregnancy/nutrition/qa/0,3105,715,00.html

Shape Up America! Fitness Center - Nutrition
www.shapeup.org/fitness/nutrition/fset3.htm

US Pharmacopeia: Just Ask
www.usp.org/pubs/just_ask/vitamin.htm

The Sweet Truth about Sugar & Sweeteners

Sugar gets blamed for causing hyperactivity in our children, and the artififcial sweeteners have been subject to carcinogenic accusations. These sites help us separate fact from fiction, and give us the sweet truth.

American Dietetic Association: Facts About Acesulfame Potassium
www.eatright.org/nfs/nfs69.html

American Dietetic Association: Facts About Aspartame
www.eatright.org/nfs/nfs32.html

Ask the Dietician: Sugar & Sweeteners
www.dietitian.com/sugar.html

Calorie Control Council: Low Calorie Sweeteners
www.caloriecontrol.org/lowcal.html

Colorado State University Cooperative Extension: Sugar & Sweeteners
www.colostate.edu/depts/CoopExt/PUBS/FOODNUT/09301.html

IFIC Review: Intense Sweeteners: Effect on Appetite & Weight Management
http://ificinfo.health.org/review/ir-intsw.htm

IFIC: Backgrounder on Sugars & Sweeteners
http://ificinfo.health.org/backgrnd/bkgr8.htm

IFIC: Everything You Need to Know About Acesulfame Potassium
http://ificinfo.health.org/brochure/aceK.htm

IFIC: Everything You Need to Know About Aspartame
http://ificinfo.health.org/brochure/aspartam.htm

IFIC: Everything You Need to Know About Sucralose
http://ificinfo.health.org/brochure/sucralose.htm

IFIC: Sweet Facts About Sugars & Health
http://ificinfo.health.org/review/swtfact.htm

IFIC: What You Should Know About Sugars
http://ificinfo.health.org/brochure/sugar.htm

Vitamins & Minerals

How much Vitamin C do we need? We know we need calcium, but how much? How much Vitamin B do we need? Use these sites to get the latest lowdown on vitamins and minerals.

American Dietetic Association: Catch the Calcium Craze
www.eatright.org/nfs/nfs72.html

American Dietetic Association: Nutrition & Health for Older Americans: Calcium
www.eatright.org/olderamericans/calcium.html

American Dietetic Association: Straight Answers About Vitamin & Mineral Supplements
www.eatright.org/nfs/nfs66.html

C For Yourself
www.cforyourself.com

Colorado State University Cooperative Extension: Fat-Soluble Vitamins
www.colostate.edu/depts/CoopExt/PUBS/FOODNUT/09315.html

Colorado State University Cooperative Extension: Water-Soluble Vitamins
www.colostate.edu/depts/CoopExt/PUBS/FOODNUT/09312.html

Delicious Decisions from the American Heart Association: Supplement Your Knowledge
www.deliciousdecisions.org/ff/tsd_supp_main.html

Dietsite.com: Fat Soluble Vitamins
www.dietsite.com/nutritionfacts/VitaminsMinerals/FatSolVit.html

Dietsite.com: Minerals
www.dietsite.com/nutritionfacts/VitaminsMinerals/minerals.html

Dietsite.com: Water Soluble Vitamins
www.dietsite.com/nutritionfacts/VitaminsMinerals/WatersolVitamins.html

drkoop.com: Vitamins & Minerals
www.drkoop.com/wellness/nutrition/vitamins_minerals

eNutrition
www.enutrition.com

FANSA: Folic Acid: A Reminder For Women Before & During Pregnancy
http://ift.micronexx.com/sc/sc_h04.html

IFIC Food Insight: Calcium for All Ages & Genders
http://ificinfo.health.org/insight/janfeb99/calcium.htm

IFIC Insight: Recommended Dietary Allowances
http://ificinfo.health.org/insight/septoct98/rdas.htm

IFIC: Brittle Bones: Osteoporosis Education for Asian Americans
http://ificinfo.health.org/insight/brittlebones.htm

InteliHealth: Home to John Hopkins Health Information:
Vitamin & Nutrition Resource Center
www.intelihealth.com/IH/ihtIH?t=325&p=~br,IHW|~st,325|~r,WSIHW000|~b,*|

Mayo Clinic Health Oasis: Vitamin & Nutritional Supplements
www.mayohealth.org/mayo/9707/htm/me_jun97.htm

On Safari Through the Vitamin Jungle
http://primusweb.com/fitnesspartner/library/nutrition/vitamins.htm

Parent's Place: Vitamin A in Pregnancy
http://www4.parentsplace.com/pregnancy/nutrition/qa/0,3105,5425,00.html

Physicians Committee for Responsible Medicine: Calcium & Strong Bones
www.strongbones.org

Vita-Web
www.vita-web.com

Vitamin Update
http://bookman.com.au/vitamins

What's Cooking? Healthy Recipe Sites

Visit these sites for cooking tips and recipe ideas that will make your meals more nutritious.

Cyberdiet's Low Fat Recipes
www.cyberdiet.com/recipe_index/recipe_index.html

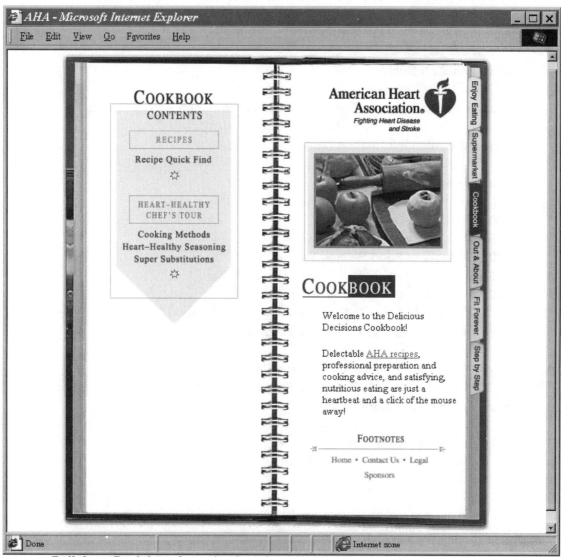

Delicious Decisions from the American Heart Association: Cookbook
www.deliciousdecisions.org/cb/index.html

Diet Depot Recipes
www.dietdepot.com/recipes.html

Official Recipes for the Carbohydrate Addict
www.carbohydrateaddicts.com/carecipe.html

Sugar Busters: Kitchen Form
www.sugarbusters.com/sbfiles/communicate/kitchen.html

Finding More on Nutrition - Directories

These directories will give you access to an ubelievable array of web sites about nutrition; they are excellent sources to satisfy your curiosity and they will satiate any hunger for knowledge. They are especially excellent for students who need to research any aspect of nutrition.

American Dietetic Association: Nutrition Resources for Consumers
www.eatright.org/nuresources.html

American Heart Association
www.americanheart.org

Arbor Nutrition Guide
www.arborcom.com

Arizona Health Sciences Center: Nutrition Information & Your Health
www.ahsc.arizona.edu/~lei/nutrition

Food & Nutrition Information Center
www.nal.usda.gov/fnic

HealthWeb: Nutrition
www.libraries.psu.edu/crsweb/hw/nutr

IFIC Foundation: Search
http://ificinfo.health.org/search.htm

IFIC: Glossary of Food-Related Terms
http://ificinfo.health.org/glossary.htm

IFIC: Organizations, Agencies, & Associations
http://ificinfo.health.org/resource/orgs.htm

Index of Food & Nutrition Internet Resources
www.nal.usda.gov/fnic/etext/fnic.html

Mayo Clinic: Diet & Nutrition Resource Center - Library References
www.mayohealth.org/mayo/common/htm/dietpg2.htm

Nutrient Data Laboratory
www.nal.usda.gov/fnic/foodcomp

Tufts University Health & Nutrition Letter
http://healthletter.tufts.edu

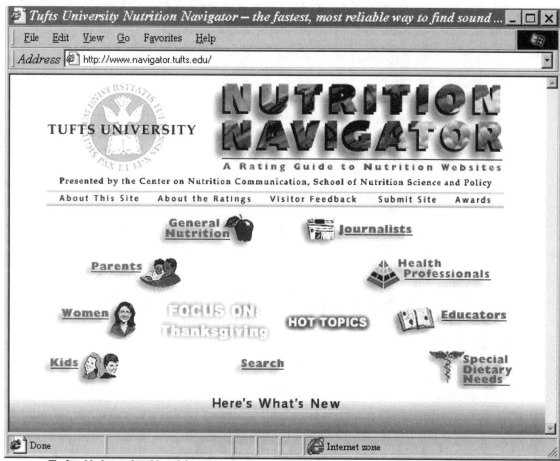

Tufts University Nutrition Navigator
www.navigator.tufts.edu

UDSA: Glossary of the Nutrient Data Laboratory
www.nal.usda.gov/fnic/foodcomp/Bulletins/glossary.html

University Nutrition Sites in the United States
www.sfu.ca/~jfremont/university.html

Virginia Cooperative Extension: Food & Nutrition Newsletter
www.ext.vt.edu/news/periodicals/foods

Finding More on Nutrition - Links

Visit these link-loaded web sites to help you research any nutrition subject which may be of interest to you.

American Dietetic Association: Links to Nutrition Web Sites
www.eatright.org/healthorg.html

American Dietetic Association: Nutrition Resources for Consumers
www.eatright.org/nuresources.html

Arbor Nutrition Guide
www.arborcom.com

Arizona Health Sciences Center: Nutrition Information & Your Health
www.ahsc.arizona.edu/~lei/nutrition

Food & Nutrition Information Center
www.nal.usda.gov/fnic

HealthWeb: Nutrition
www.libraries.psu.edu/crsweb/hw/nutr

Index of Food & Nutrition Internet Resources
www.nal.usda.gov/fnic/etext/fnic.html

Jean Frermont's Food & Nutrition on the Web
www.sfu.ca/~jfremont

La Leche League International: Useful Links
www.lalecheleague.org/links.html

New York Times on the Web: Women's Health: Diet & Exercise
www.nytimes.com/specials/women/whome/diet_exercise.html

Nutrient Data Laboratory
www.nal.usda.gov/fnic/foodcomp

Nutrition for Kids: Recommended Links
www.nutritionforkids.com/Links.htm

Oregon Dairy Council
www.oregondairycouncil.org

Stayhealthy.com
www.stayhealthy.com/centers/nutrition.cfm

Tufts University Nutrition Navigator
www.navigator.tufts.edu

University Nutrition Sites in the United States
www.sfu.ca/~jfremont/university.html

Virginia Cooperative Extension: Food & Nutrition Newsletter
www.ext.vt.edu/news/periodicals/foods

Adopting a Healthy Weight

300,000 people will die this year from causes directly related to obesity. Heart disease, cancer, and diabetes often stem from being overweight. This is an epidemic. Unfortunately there is no vaccine to intervene. How many times have we said that we've "got to drop a few pounds," and how many times have we been successful? How often do we regain those lost pounds - and maybe even more? These sites help us realize that a "diet" is not a temporary denial of the foods we love to eat, but rather the adoption of a healthy lifestyle.

Chat About Weight

These web sites are a great place to pose questions, find a weight loss partner for mutual support or share ideas, frustrations, and weight loss success.

American Association of Lifestyle Counselors: Forum
www.AALC.org/experts.htm

Cyberdiet's Forums
www.cyberdiet.com/messages

Dietsite.com: Discussion Forum
www.dietsite.com/weightloss

eDiets: Bulletin Boards
www.ediets.com/myediets/guest/webboard.cfm

PHYS: Chat
www.phys.com/c_tools/chat/chat.htm

Vegsource: The MacDougall Discussion Board
www.vegsource.com/mcdougall

Childhood Obesity

It is estimated that 20% of America's children are overweight, and there is a strong possibility that they will remain that way into adulthood. These sites provide guidelines and useful ideas to help our children adopt a healthy lifestyle.

Childhood Obesity
www.healthyeating.org/general/childhood_obesity.htm

Committed to Kids Pediatric Weight Management Program
www.committed-to-kids.com

Mayo Clinic Health Oasis: Childhood Obesity
www.mayohealth.org/mayo/9705/htm/overweig.htm

Mayo Clinic Health Oasis: Diet & Exercise Guidelines For Overweight Children
www.mayohealth.org/mayo/9705/htm/over_2sb.htm

Mayo Clinic Health Oasis: Managing Childhood Obesity
www.mayohealth.org/mayo/9705/htm/over_1sb.htm

Obesity Meds & Research News: Childhood Obesity Links
www.obesity-news.com/obchild.htm

University-Based Child/Adolescent Weight-Control Programs
www.niddk.nih.gov/health/nutrit/unversit/childho.htm

Drug & Herbal Therapies

There are countless purported "magic bullets" on the market. Some are available by prescription only, some have been withdrawn from the market entirely, yet others are of limited or no value. Get the facts.

American Dietetic Association: News: Using Diet Drugs
www.eatright.org/news

Dexfenfluramine
www.rxlist.com/cgi/generic/dexfen.htm

Dexfenfluuramine - Miracle Drug or Pandora's box?
www.weight.com/Dexfenfluramine.html

InteliHealth: Home to John Hopkins Health Information:
Index of Medication for Weight Control
www.intelihealth.com/IH/ihtIH?t=20705&c=225105&p=~br,IHW|~st,14
220|~r,WSIHW000|~b,*|&d=dmtContent

Meridia
www.4meridia.com

My Experience with Phen-fen
www.syspac.com/~hahn/phenfen.html

Redux & "Phen/fen" Medical Problems from Michael Myers M.D. Inc.
www.weight.com/medprob.html

Sibutramine from Michael Myers. M.D. Inc.
www.weight.com/sibutramine.html

WeightLoss2000.com: Drug Therapies
http://weightloss2000.com/drug

WeightLoss2000.com: Herbal Therapies
http://weightloss2000.com/herbs

Withdrawal of Dexfenfluramine/fenfluramine by Michael Myers M.D. Inc.
www.weight.com/withdrawal.html

Xenical
www.xenical.com/consumers/index.htm

E-Zines for Easy Reading

E-zines are colorful and often interactive web sites that feed us information in a concise and entertaining presentation. They are upbeat and motivational. They often contain compendiums of the latest research findings and statisitics regarding living a healthy lifestyle. Frequently, there are links in the articles if you wish to delve further into a particular subject.

InteliHealth: Home to John Hopkins Health Information: Weight Management Zone
www.intelihealth.com/IH/ihtIH?t=14220&p=~br,IHW|~st,14220|~r,WS IHW000|~b,*|

Obesity.com
www.obesity.com

PHYS: Weight Loss
www.phys.com/weightloss/01home/weightloss.html

Women.com: Weight Loss
www.healthyideas.com/weight/getstart.html

FAQs

Many times we think that we have a really original question, but often it has been asked before. Check these sites for the answer. Some sites will even let you send in your question if it hasn't been asked before.

Clinical FAQ of Michael Myers. M.D. Inc.
www.weight.com/faqclin.html

Healthy Weight--Healthy Eating
www.4meridia.com/consumer/archive/ask.cfm

Oxford University Libraries Automation Service
www.lib.ox.ac.uk/internet/news/faq/archive/dieting-faq.part1.html

Keeping Up-to-Date with the News in Weight Loss

It seems that every week there are news articles filled with statistics, survey results, and research findings on weight loss and obesity. These sites gather the latest weight loss and obesity news from around the world.

Barbara's Obesity Meds & Research News
www.obesity-news.com

Calorie Control Newsnet
www.caloriecontrol.org/ccnews.html

Cyberdiet's E-mail Newsletter
www.cyberdiet.com/subscribe

Cyberdiet's Food Facts
www.cyberdiet.com/foodfact/f_food.html

Diet & Weight Loss News Wire Summaries
http://www1.mhv.net/~donn/wire.html

Healthy Weight Network--Articles & News Releases
www.healthyweightnetwork.com/releases.htm

InteliHealth: Home to John Hopkins Health Information: Weight Management News Headlines
www.intelihealth.com/IH/ihtIH?t=20833&p=~br,IHW|~st,9103|~r,WSIHW000|~b,*|

Mayo Clinic Diet Center: Weight Loss
www.mayohealth.org/mayo/common/htm/dietpage.htm

Obesity.com
www.obesity.com

WeightLoss2000.com
http://weightloss2000.com

WeightLoss2000.com: Latest News
http://weightloss2000.com/news

Quizzes & Surveys

Some of these sites test your knowledge, some are surveys that invite your participation, and others are just for fun.

American Diabetes Association: Feed Your Brain: Nutrition Quiz
www.diabetes.org/nutrition/i_quiz.asp

American Health Association Health Insight: Interactive Health: Personal Nutritionist
www.ama-assn.org/insight/yourhlth/pernutri/pernutri.htm

CSPI: Fat or Fiction Quiz
www.cspinet.org/cgi-bin/quiz.cgi

CSPI: Rate Your Diet Quiz
www.cspinet.org/quiz/quiz_diet1.html

Diet & Nutrition Resource Center - Quizzes
www.mayohealth.org/mayo/common/htm/dietquiz.htm

Eat Well, Live Well Newsletter Archive
www.healthyeating.org/newsletters

Family Food Zone: Nutrition Café
www.familyfoodzone.com/game/index.html

FDA Kids Home Page
www.fda.gov/oc/opacom/kids

Grab A Grape
http://exhibits.pacsci.org/nutrition/grape/grape.html

Kids Food CyberClub: Cyber Food Shopper
www.kidsfood.org/choices/shopper.html

Kids Food CyberClub: Food Guide Pyramid
www.kidsfood.org/f_pyramid/pyramid.html

Kids Food CyberClub: Nutrition Sleuths
www.kidsfood.org/sleuths/sleuths.html

Kids Food CyberClub: Rate Your Plate
www.kidsfood.org/rate_plate/rate.html

Kids Food CyberClub: Winning Choices
www.kidsfood.org/choices/winning/winning.html

Mayo Clinic Health Oasis: Health Quiz
www.mayohealth.org/cgi-
bin/apps/quiz.cgi/mayo/expert/htm/9603quiz.txt?/mayo/common/htm
/top.txt,/mayo/common/htm/bottom.txt

Mayo Clinic Health Oasis: Quizzes From the Nutrition Center
www.mayohealth.org/mayo/common/htm/dietquiz.htm

Men's Nutrition: Quiz
http://primusweb.com/fitnesspartner/library/nutrition/mensquiz.htm

MotherNature.com: Quiz Central
www.mothernature.com/quiz/default.asp

NCI/CDC 5 A Day Online Tracking Chart
http://5aday.nci.nih.gov/

Nutrition Sleuth
http://exhibits.pacsci.org/nutrition/sleuth/sleuth.html

PHYS: Portion Finder
www.phys.com/b_nutrition/02solutions/05portion/game.htm

Take The Food Pyramid Challenge
www.bennygoodsport.com/food.htm

Washington State Dairy Council: Take Aim
www.eatsmart.org/html/game.html

Recipes for Weight Loss

View these web sites for some low-fat and low calorie cooking ideas.

Cyberdiet's Low Fat Recipes
www.cyberdiet.com/recipe_index/recipe_index.html

Delicious Decisions from the American Heart Association
www.deliciousdecisions.org

Delicious Decisions from the American Heart Association: Cookbook
www.deliciousdecisions.org/cb/index.html

Diet Depot Recipes
www.dietdepot.com/recipes.html

Low Fat Recipes
www.webvalue.net/recipes/lowfat/index.html

Shape Up America!: Cyberkitchen
www.shapeup.org/kitchen/frameset1.htm

Reference

These sites are good sources of information on weight loss. Many have searchable databases.

ALT.FOOD.FATFREE FAQs
www.fatfree.com/FAQ/alt-food-fat-free-faq

Barbara's Obesity Meds & Research News
www.obesity-news.com

Diet & Weight Loss News Wire Summaries
http://www1.mhv.net/~donn/wire.html

Dietsite.com: Food Diary
www.dietsite.com/Diets/WeightManagement/Food%20Diary.htm

Dietsite.com: Grades of Obesity
www.dietsite.com/Diets/WeightManagement/Grades%20Of%20Obesity.htm

Minnesota Obesity Center
http://www1.umn.edu/mnoc

Sites for Getting Some Advice & Motivation

These sites will help you motivate yourself and set goals to achieve a healthy lifestyle.

American Heart Association: Managing Your Weight
www.americanheart.org/Heart_and_Stroke_A_Z_Guide/obesity.html

Colorado State University Cooperative Extension:
Weight Loss Programs & Products
www.colostate.edu/depts/CoopExt/PUBS/FOODNUT/09363.html

Delicious Decisions from the American Heart Association
www.deliciousdecisions.org

Delicious Decisions from the American Heart Association: The Skinny on Dieting
www.deliciousdecisions.org/ff/tsd.html

Dietsite.com
www.dietsite.com

Dietsite.com: How to Write a Food Diary
www.dietsite.com/Diets/WeightManagement/Writing%20a%20Food%20Diary%20.htm

Getting Started on Your Diet
http://www1.mhv.net/~donn/start.html

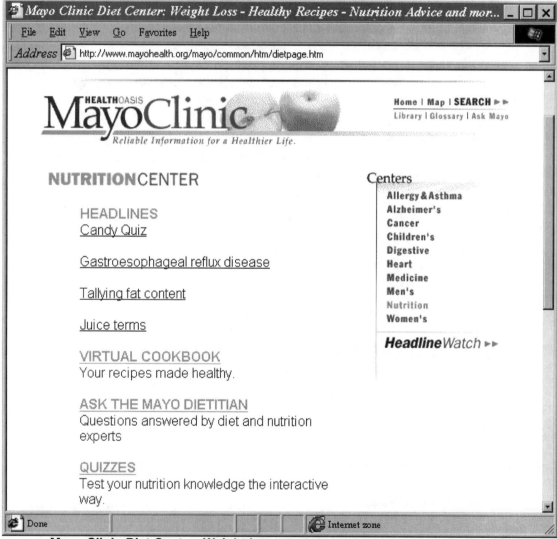

Mayo Clinic Diet Center: Weight Loss
www.mayohealth.org/mayo/common/htm/dietpage.htm

Mayo Clinic Health Oasis: Weight Control
www.mayohealth.org/mayo/9903/htm/weig_sb4.htm

Mayo Clinic Health Oasis: Weight Control: What Works & Why
www.mayohealth.org/mayo/9406/htm/main.htm

Obesity & Weight Control from Michael D. Myers. M.D. Inc.
www.weight.com

Why Do I Eat When I'm Not Hungry?
http://www1.mhv.net/~donn/hgr.html

Sites to Help Assess the Situation

Get out the measuring tape and bathroom scale. Many of these sites will calculate such things as your body mass index, calorie consumption, and calorie expenditure.

American Health Association Health Insight: Interactive Health
www.ama-assn.org/consumer/interact.htm

American Heart Association: Body Composition Tests
www.americanheart.org/Heart_and_Stroke_A_Z_Guide/body.html

Body Mass Index Calculator
www.kcnet.com/~marc/bmi.html

Burning Holiday Calories
http://primusweb.com/fitnesspartner/library/activity/holicals.htm

Calculating Your Body Mass Index
http://www1.mhv.net/~donn/bmi.htm

Calorie Control Council: Calorie Calculator
www.caloriecontrol.org/caloriecontrol/cgi-bin/calorie_calculator.cgi

Calorie Control Council: Enhanced Calorie Calculator
www.caloriecontrol.org/cgi-bin/Enhanced_calcalc/enhanced_calcalc.cgi

Calorie Control Council: Exercise Calculator
www.caloriecontrol.org/exercalc.html

Cyberdiet's Assessment Tools
www.cyberdiet.com/tools/assess.html

Cyberdiet's Daily Food Planner
www.cyberdiet.com/dfl

Cyberdiet's Eating Right
www.cyberdiet.com/ni/htdocs

Cyberdiet's Nutritional Profile
www.cyberdiet.com/profile/profile.cgi

Diet Analysis Web Page
http://dawp.anet.com

Dietsite.com: Diet & Recipe Analysis
www.dietsite.com/nutr/index.htm

Mayo Clinic Health Oasis: Weight Self-Assessment: Should You Shed Pounds?
www.mayohealth.org/mayo/9707/htm/weight.htm

MSNBC Calorie Calculator
www.msnbc.com/modules/quizzes/caloriecalc.asp

PHYS: Are You Fit or Fat?
www.phys.com/b_nutrition/01self_analysis/04fitorfat/fitorfat.cgi

PHYS: Snack Bandit
www.phys.com/c_tools/gadgets/snackbandit/snackbandit.html

PHYS: Self Analysis
www.phys.com/b_nutrition/01self_analysis/01home/self.htm

Shape Up America!: Body Mass Index
www.shapeup.org/bmi/index.html

The Learn Education Center
www.learneducation.com/weight.htm

Weight Table Comparison Study
http://www1.mhv.net/~donn/wtabl.html

Software

For those who count calories and like to be organized in the new millenium, these software sites can be helpful.

Heart Smart
www.siestasoftware.com/hsmart.htm

Hopkins Technology Health CD-ROMs
www.hoptechno.com/healthp.htm

Life Form
www.fitnesoft.com

Sante (For Good Health)
www.hoptechno.com/santeall.htm

Weight Commander Diet Program
www.interaccess.com/weightcmdr/dt.html

The Ups & Downs of Losing Weight

Imagine a talk show discussing weightloss and diets with participating experts from the American Dietetic Association, American Heart Association, and a few specialists from university medical centers. These sites are the virtual equivalent -- they help us understand weight loss and how to keep the weight off.

allHealth.com: Never Say Diet
www.allhealth.com/neversaydiet

American Dietetic Association: Weight Management
www.eatright.org/adap0197.html

American Health Association Health Insight: Interactive Health
www.ama-assn.org/consumer/interact.htm

American Heart Association: Commercial Weight Reduction Programs
www.americanheart.org/Heart_and_Stroke_A_Z_Guide/commw.html

American Heart Association:
Guidelines for Weight Management Programs for Healthy Adults
www.americanheart.org/Heart_and_Stroke_A_Z_Guide/commw.html

Calorie Control Council
www.caloriecontrol.org

Calorie Control Council: Winning Weights
www.caloriecontrol.org/winweigh.html

Causes of Obesity from Michael D. Myers M.D. Inc.
www.weight.com/causes.html

Childhood Obesity
www.healthyeating.org/general/childhood_obesity.htm

Colorado State University Cooperative Extension: Weight Loss Diets & Books
www.colostate.edu/depts/CoopExt/PUBS/FOODNUT/09364.html

Comprehensive Obesity Treatment by Michael Myers M.D.Inc.
www.weight.com/comprehensive.html

Cyberdiet's Food Facts
www.cyberdiet.com/foodfact/f_food.html

Cyberdiet's Health Club
www.cyberdiet.com/new_healthclub_site/health_club

Definition of Obesity from Michael D. Myers M.D.Inc.
www.weight.com/definition.html

Delicious Decisions from the American Heart Association: The Skinny on Dieting
www.deliciousdecisions.org/ff/tsd.html

Dietary Treatment of Obesity
www.weight.com/diets.html

Dietsite.com
www.dietsite.com

Dietsite.com: How to Write a Food Diary
www.dietsite.com/Diets/WeightManagement/Writing%20a%20Food%20Diary%20.htm

Eating Behaviors & Moods from Michael D. Myers M.D. Inc.
www.weight.com/eating.html

eDiets: Bulletin Boards
www.ediets.com/myediets/guest/webboard.cfm

Health Implications of Obesity
http://text.nlm.nih.gov/nih/cdc/www/49txt.html

Healthy Weight Network
www.healthyweightnetwork.com

Identifying Weight Loss Fraud & Quackery
www.healthyweightnetwork.com/fraud.htm

InteliHealth: Home to John Hopkins Health Information:
Weight Management Timeline
www.intelihealth.com/IH/ihtIH?t=14285&p=~br,IHW|~st,14220|~r,WSIHW000|~b,*|

Mayo Clinic Health Oasis: Weight Control: What Works & Why
www.mayohealth.org/mayo/9406/htm/main.htm

My Experience with Phen-fen
www.syspac.com/~hahn/phenfen.html

Newest Weight Loss Gimmicks from Michael D. Myers M.D. Inc.
www.weight.com/gimmick.html

NIH Technology Assessment-Voluntary Weight Loss
http://text.nlm.nih.gov/nih/ta/www/10.html

Obesity & Weight Control from Michael D. Myers. M.D. Inc.
www.weight.com

Obesity Complications from Michael D. Myers M.D. Inc.
www.weight.com/complications.html

Obesity: The World's Oldest Metabolic Disease
www.quantumhcp.com/obesity.htm

Shape Up America!: Cyberkitchen
www.shapeup.org/kitchen/frameset1.htm

The Hacker's Diet
www.fourmilab.ch/hackdiet/www/hackdiet.html

Understanding Adult Obesity
www.niddk.nih.gov/health/nutrit/pubs/unders.htm

University of Minnesota - Research Project Updates
http://www1.umn.edu/mnoc/topics/Updates.html

WeightLoss2000.com
http://weightloss2000.com

WeightLoss2000.com: Satisfying Eating
http://weightloss2000.com/satis

More Info - Directories

Use these online directories to find more sites about adopting a healthy weight..

About.com: Weight Loss
http://weightloss.about.com/health/fitness/weightloss/msubcalculators.htm?PM=68_708_T

Diet & Weight Loss/ Fitness Home Page
http://www1.mhv.net/~donn/diet.html

Healthy Weight Network
www.healthyweightnetwork.com

iVillage: Weight Loss Coach
www.ivillage.com/fitness/experts/wlcoach/archive

Mayo Clinic: Diet & Nutrition Resource Center - Library References
www.mayohealth.org/mayo/common/htm/dietpg2.htm

PHYS: Sitewide Search
www.phys.com/e_search/search.htm

University-Based Adult Weight-Control Programs
www.niddk.nih.gov/health/nutrit/unversit/univpro.htm

University-Based Child/Adolescent Weight-Control Programs
www.niddk.nih.gov/health/nutrit/unversit/childho.htm

Weight Control Information Network
www.niddk.nih.gov/health/nutrit/win.htm

More Info - Links

These links can take you deep into cyberspace and give you more than you're looking for. Rarely will you end up at a dead end.

About.com: Weight Loss
http://weightloss.about.com/health/fitness/weightloss/msubcalculators.htm?PM=68_708_T

Diet & Weight Loss/ Fitness Home Page
http://www1.mhv.net/~donn/diet.html

Diettalk
www.diettalk.com/index.shtml

iVillage: Weight Loss Coach
www.ivillage.com/fitness/experts/wlcoach/archive

Obesity Meds & Research News: Diet, Fitness, & Nutrition Links
www.obesity-news.com/dietweb.htm

Obesity Meds & Research News: Links to Diet Plans & Support Groups
www.obesity-news.com/dietlink.htm

Obesity Meds & Research News: Childhood Obesity Links
www.obesity-news.com/obchild.htm

Oxford University Libraries Automation Service
www.lib.ox.ac.uk/internet/news/faq/archive/dieting-faq.part1.html

Redux & "Phen/fen" Medical Problems from Michael Myers M.D. Inc.
www.weight.com/medprob.html

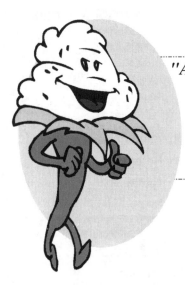

"Adequate food is the cradle of normal resistance, the playground of normal immunity, the workshop of good health, and the laboratory of long life."
*-- **Dr. Charles Mayo,**
celebrated American physician*

Weight Loss Programs
The Good, the Bad & the Ugly

Achieving a healthy weight is the goal of approximately 50 million Americans each year, and only 5% of these dieters succeed at keeping the weight off. In fact, it is estimated that we spend over $30 billion annually on weight loss products and programs. Unfortunately there is always someone who surfaces to exploit our weaknesses and our desperation. Trying to achieve a healthy weight can be compared to the difficulties faced by a smoker who is struggling through a smoking cessation program or an alcoholic who is trying to stop drinking. These sites represent a broad spectrum of programs, products, and strategies. Everyone's body is different -- so visit these sites and judge for yourself, or better yet, find one that looks interesting and then ask your doctor about it.

Adopting a Strategy to Achieve a Healthy Weight

These sites represent a myriad of approaches all aimed at achieving the same goal. Some are highly reputed, while others are highly controversial. See what works for you.

allHealth.com: Never Say Diet
www.allhealth.com/neversaydiet

American Heart Association: Commercial Weight Reduction Programs
www.americanheart.org/Heart_and_Stroke_A_Z_Guide/commw.html

American Heart Association: Dietary/Weight Loss Supplements
www.americanheart.org/Heart_and_Stroke_A_Z_Guide/dietw.html

American Heart Association:
Guidelines for Weight Management Programs for Healthy Adults
www.americanheart.org/Heart_and_Stroke_A_Z_Guide/commw.html

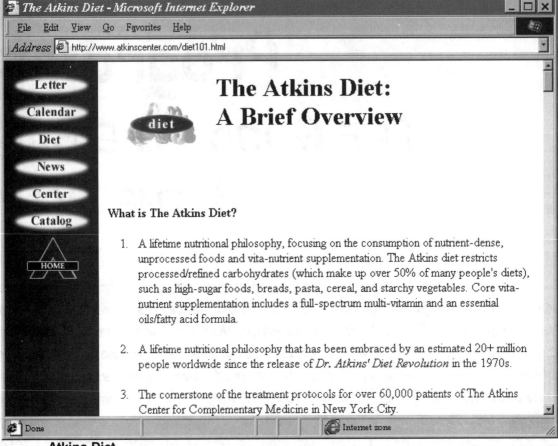

Atkins Diet
www.atkinscenter.com/diet101.html

Cambridge Diet
www.cambridgediet.com

Carbohydrate Addict's Official FAQ Page
www.carbohydrateaddicts.com/cafaq.html

Carbohydrate Addict's Official Home Page
www.carbohydrateaddicts.com

Carbohydrate Addict's Official Quick Quiz
www.carbohydrateaddicts.com/caquiz.html

Carbohydrate Addiction Defined
www.carbohydrateaddicts.com/cadfnd.html

Carbohydrate-Addicted Kids
www.carbohydrateaddicts.com/cakidsindex.html

Carbohydrate-Addicted Kids: A Definition
www.carbohydrateaddicts.com/cakidsdef.html

Catabolic Diet
www.catabolic.com/index2.htm

Choose to Lose Weight Loss/Healthy Eating Program
www.choicediets.com

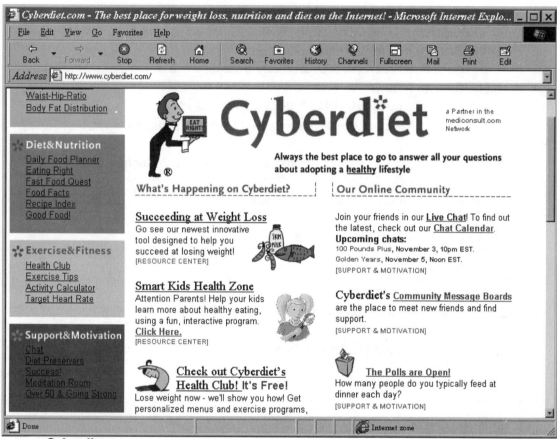

Cyberdiet
www.cyberdiet.com

Cyberdiet's Health Club
www.cyberdiet.com/new_healthclub_site/health_club

Cyberdiet's Over 50 & Going Strong
www.cyberdiet.com/seniors/over50.html

Cyberdiet: Succeeding at Weight Loss - A Program
www.cyberdiet.com/modules/wl/outline.html

Delicious Decisions from the American Heart Association: Approved Diets
www.deliciousdecisions.org/ff/tsd_diets_main.html

Delicious Decisions from the American Heart Association: Enjoy Eating
www.deliciousdecisions.org/ee/index.html

Delicious Decisions from the American Heart Association: Non AHA Approved Diets
www.deliciousdecisions.org/ff/tsd_nondiets_main.html

Diet Doctor
http://thedietdoctor.itool.com

Dietsite.com: Calorie Controlled Diet
www.dietsite.com/Diets/WeightManagement/Calorie%20Controlled%20
Diet.htm

Duke University: The Rice Diet Program
www.ricediet.com/us/index1.html

Duke University: The Rice Diet Program: What Will I Eat?
www.ricediet.com/us/program/eat.html

Eat Yourself Slim: The Montignac Method
http://global-m.com/montignac/montignac.htm

eDiets: Bulletin Boards
www.ediets.com/myediets/guest/webboard.cfm

eDiets: Custom Weight Loss Management & Dieting Programs
www.ediets.com

Help for Carbohydrate Addicts - Books by Drs. Richard & Rachael Heller
www.carbohydrateaddicts.com/cabooks.html

Identifying Weight Loss Fraud & Quackery
www.healthyweightnetwork.com/fraud.htm

IFIC Insight: The High Protein Myth
http://ificinfo.health.org/insight/septoct98/proteinmyth.htm

Liposuction Discussion Area
www.liposite.com/cgi-local/index.cgi

Liposuction Interactive Information Resource-Liposite
www.liposite.com

Nutri/System Program Features & Benefits
www.nutrisystem.com/fandb.html

Overeaters Anonymous
www.overeatersanonymous.org

Slim-Fast Online
www.slimfast.com

Sugar Busters
www.sugarbusters.com/sbfiles/home.html

Sugar Busters Comments & Experiences
www.sugarbusters.com/sbfiles/questions/comments.html

Sugar Busters Glossary
www.sugarbusters.com/sbfiles/questions/glossary.html

Sugar Busters Interview Form
www.sugarbusters.com/sbfiles/communicate/interview.html

Sugar Busters Q&A From The Book
www.sugarbusters.com/sbfiles/questions/questfirst.html

Sugar Busters: Questions Answered
www.sugarbusters.com/sbfiles/questions.html

Susan Powter
www.susanpowter.com

The Hacker's Diet
www.fourmilab.ch/hackdiet/www/hackdiet.html

Toppfast Diet Plan
www.toppfast.com/toppfast/default.htm

TOPS
www.tops.org

Zone Home
www.zonehome.com/index.htm

ZonePerfect.Com - The Official Home of the Zone Diet
www.enterthezone.com

ZonePerfect.Com: Discussion & Technical Support Center
http://conference.zoneperfect.com:8080/%7EZonePErfect

ZonePerfect.Com: Inside the Zone
www.enterthezone.com/Inside_The_Zone.html

ZonePerfect.Com: Overview of the ZonePerfect Nutrition Program
www.enterthezone.com/Outline.html

FAQs

Look for the answers here in these web sites to your questions.

Carbohydrate Addict's Official FAQ Page
www.carbohydrateaddicts.com/cafaq.html

Fen/Phen Crisis Center: FAQs
www.fenphen.com/faq.html

LipoSite: Frequently Asked Questions
www.liposite.com/faq

Oxford University Libraries Automation Service
www.lib.ox.ac.uk/internet/news/faq/archive/dieting-faq.part1.html

Plastic Surgery FAQs-Liposuction
www.plasticsurgery.org/faq/lipo.htm

Sugar Busters Q&A From The Book
www.sugarbusters.com/sbfiles/questions/questfirst.html

Sugar Busters: Questions Answered
www.sugarbusters.com/sbfiles/questions.html

ZonePerfect.Com: Overview of the ZonePerfect Nutrition Program
www.enterthezone.com/Outline.html

Online Shopping

Enjoy online shopping for everything from books to magic bullets. Just be sure the site is secure, and that you've checked out the sites on fraud for your own protection. If need to contact an ecommerce company offline, use iNet's WhoIs Gateway (`www.inet.net/cgi-bin/whoisqw`) to find name, phone and address information by typing in the short URL, such as "betrimtoo.com".

Allco Group - Independent Metabolife Distributors
> `www.allcogroup.com/metabolife/index.html`

AM-300 Natural Herbal Energizer
> `www.angelfire.com/biz2/am300herbal/index.html`

Amazing Micro Diet
> `www.microdiet.com`

Aoqili Fat Loss Soap
> `www.dfwbiznet.com/Soap.htm`

Attain Diet & Health Products
> `www.alldiets.com`

BeTrim Too
> `www.betrimtoo.com`

Cambridge Diet
> `www.cambridgediet.com`

Catabolic Diet
> `www.catabolic.com/index2.htm`

Cellasene: The One That Works
> `www.cellesene.com`

Chitosol
> `www.chitosol.com/product.htm`

Dermalife
> `www.furnspec.com/dermalife`

Diet Center Worldwide, Inc.
> `www.dietcenterworldwide.com`

Diet Depot: Digital Market
> `https://secure.gcci.com/cgi-bin_001/web_store.cgi`

Diet Magic Now!
> `www.dietmagicnow.com/4frame.htm`

Diet Results: Dr. Nagler's Safe Effective Way to Crash Off 5/10 lbs./wk
> `www.dietresults.com`

DietMate
> `www.dietmate.com`

Dr. Brad's Calorad
> `www.caloradnet.com/drbrad/index.htm`

Fast Trim
> `www.fast-trim.com/index.html`

Fat Absorb
> `www.fatabsorb.com`

Fat Magnets - Chitosan Food Supplements
www.fatmagnets.com/index.html

Fat Trapper System
www.fattrapper.com

For Weight Loss & More
http://fatabsorbers.com

Form YOU 3 International
www.formyou3.com/products.htm

Healthy Weight Network--Books & Resources
www.healthyweightnetwork.com/books.htm

Help for Carbohydrate Addicts - Books by Drs. Richard & Rachael Heller
www.carbohydrateaddicts.com/cabooks.html

Herbalife
www.herbalifediet.com

Home Enterprises - Beer Blok
www.homent.demon.co.uk/beerblok.htm

Home Enterprises - Diet & Health
www.homent.demon.co.uk/main.htm

Hunger Busters
www.hungerbusters.com

Jenny Craig Store
www.jennycraig.com/store/index.html

LEARN Education Center
www.learneducation.com

LosePounds.com
www.losepounds.com

Low Carb Connoisseur
www.low-carb.com/low-carb/index.html

Metabolife International
www.metabolife.com

My Personal Weight Loss Story
http://www1.mhv.net/~donn/prime.html

Natural Leaf Brand
www.naturalleaf.com

Nova Pharmaceutical, Inc.
www.novanx.com

Optifast
www.optifast.com

Overeaters Anonymous: Online Catalog
https://www.overeatersanonymous.org/catalog.htm

Physicians WEIGHT LOSS Centers
www.pwlc.com

Protein Power Plan
http://209.192.129.65

Seaweed Defat Soap
http://www5.icat.com/store/seaweedsoap/index.icl?ReferringURL=&colo=icat&affiliate=

Slim Form Patch
www.slimform.com

Star Power's Herbal 5000 Weight Loss Formula
www.starcom2.com/starpower

Sugar Busters Order Form
www.sugarbusters.com/sbfiles/preorder.html

Susan Powter: Bookstore
www.susanpowter.com/bookstore.htm

Thermobolics Weight Loss Center on the Web
www.t-24.com

Toppfast Diet Plan
www.toppfast.com/toppfast/default.htm

Weight Loss Patch
www.weight-loss-patch.com/jump.html

Weight Management Centers - Healthy Living Product Directory
http://commerce1.webboy.com/acbnew/Directory.cfm?&DID=16&User_ID=483&st=7949&st2=-684967812&st3=58625106

Weight Perfect - Diet & Weight Loss Plan
www.weightperfect.com

ZonePerfect Store
http://store.zoneperfect.com

Sites About the Zone

Perhaps no other diet program has generated so much controversy in recent years. Although other high protein diets exist, Barry Sears' best selling books have brought his "Zone" under the microscopes of both critics and supporters. Here are some sites that range all the way from sanctification to damnation of the Zone.

IFIC Insight: The High Protein Myth
http://ificinfo.health.org/insight/septoct98/proteinmyth.htm

McDougall Newsletter: The Great Debate: High vs. Low Protein Diets
www.drmcdougall.com/debate.html

Nutrition Action: Carbo-Phobia-Zoning Out on the New Diet Books
www.cspinet.org/nah/zone.html

Vegsource: Debunking the Zone Diet
www.vegsource.org/attwood/zone.htm

Zone Amigos List
www.zonehome.com/amiglist.htm

Zone Home
www.zonehome.com/index.htm

ZonePerfect Store
http://store.zoneperfect.com

ZonePerfect.Com - The Official Home of the Zone Diet
www.enterthezone.com

ZonePerfect.Com: Discussion & Technical Support Center
http://conference.zoneperfect.com:8080/%7EZonePErfect

ZonePerfect.Com: Inside the Zone
www.enterthezone.com/Inside_The_Zone.html

ZonePerfect.Com: Overview of the ZonePerfect Nutrition Program
www.enterthezone.com/Outline.html

Sites Promoting Fad Diets

Fad diets have always been around and they have always been controversial. Dieticians will argue that they fall short of achieving variety, balance, and moderation, and that they can be dangerous for your health. Nevertheless, we come home from work carrying a photocopy of a "great diet that really works." These sites harbor a few of the many "fad diets."

3 Day Diet
www.dietnutrition.com/3daydiet.html

4 Day Diet
www.dietnutrition.com/4daydiet.html

5 Day Miracle Diet
www.dietnutrition.com/5daydiet.html

7 Day Diet
www.dietnutrition.com/7daydiet.html

American Heart Association: Fad Diets
www.americanheart.org/Heart_and_Stroke_A_Z_Guide/fad.html

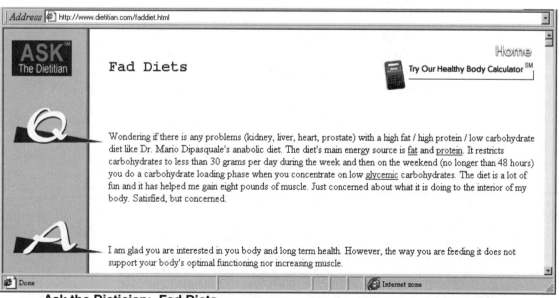

Ask the Dietician: Fad Diets
www.dietitian.com/faddiet.html

Cabbage Soup Diet: Mayo Clinic
www.mayohealth.org/mayo/9704/htm/wabout1.htm

**Delicious Decisions from the American Heart Association:
Non AHA Approved Diets**
www.deliciousdecisions.org/ff/tsd_nondiets_main.html

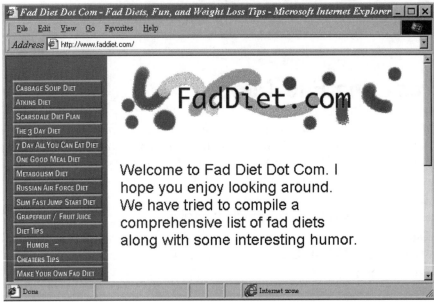

Fad Diet.com
www.faddiet.com

Fad Diet.com: 7 Day All You Can Eat Diet
www.faddiet.com/faddiet/7dayallyouca.html

Fad Diet.com: Cheater's Tips
www.faddiet.com/faddiet/cheaterstips.html

Fad Diet.com: Grapefruit/Juice Diet
www.faddiet.com/faddiet/grapfruitjui.html

Fad Diet.com: Make Your Own Fad Diet
www.faddiet.com/faddiet/makyourownfa.html

Fad Diet.com: Russian Air Force Diet
www.faddiet.com/faddiet/rusairfordie.html

Mayo Clinic Health Oasis: There Is No "Mayo Clinic Diet"
www.mayohealth.org/mayo/9806/htm/mayodiet.htm

Metabolism Diet
www.dietnutrition.com/metabolism.html

Scarsdale Diet
www.dietnutrition.com/scarsdale.html

Top 10 Fad Diet Plans in the USA
www.dietnutrition.com/faddiets.html

Wellness MD - Cabbage/Chicken Soup Fat Burning Diet
www.wellnessmd.com/fatburn.html

Sites With Recipes

Some of these sites have searchable databases, allowing you to find many good low cal and low fat recipes.

Cyberdiet's Low Fat Recipes
www.cyberdiet.com/recipe_index/recipe_index.html

Delicious Decisions from the American Heart Association: Cookbook
www.deliciousdecisions.org/cb/index.html

Diet Depot Recipes
www.dietdepot.com/recipes.html

Official Recipes for the Carbohydrate Addict
www.carbohydrateaddicts.com/carecipe.html

Sugar Busters: Kitchen Form
www.sugarbusters.com/sbfiles/communicate/kitchen.html

Surgical Options for Obesity

Morbid obesity is a scary sounding term, and surgery as treatment is also a frightening thought. But the potential mortality of continued obesity may be outweighed by the potential benefits of bariatric surgery. Liposuction is considered to be more in the realm of body sculpting rather than a strategy for weightloss. It's for those love handles that won't go away after diet and exercise have succeeded. Investigate the options here.

Academy of Bariatric Surgeons
www.obesityhelp.com/abs

Academy of Bariatric Surgeons: FAQs
www.obesityhelp.com/abs/faq.htm

Academy of Bariatric Surgeons: Meet Patients
www.obesityhelp.com/abs/patients.htm

Academy of Bariatric Surgeons: Types of Surgery
www.obesityhelp.com/abs/surgerytypes.htm

Association for Morbid Obesity Support
www.obesityhelp.com/morbidobesity

Atlantic Surgery Associates: Gastric Surgery Information
www.stomachstapling.com/surgery.html

Atlantic Surgery Associates: Resources
www.stomachstapling.com/resources.html

Atlantic Surgical Associates
www.stomachstapling.com

International Laparoscipic Obesity Surgery Team
www.obesitylapbandsurgery.com/teammain.htm

Lipoinfo.com
www.lipoinfo.com

Lipoplasty Society
www.lipoplasty.com

LipoSite-Liposuction Online Chat
www.liposite.com/chat

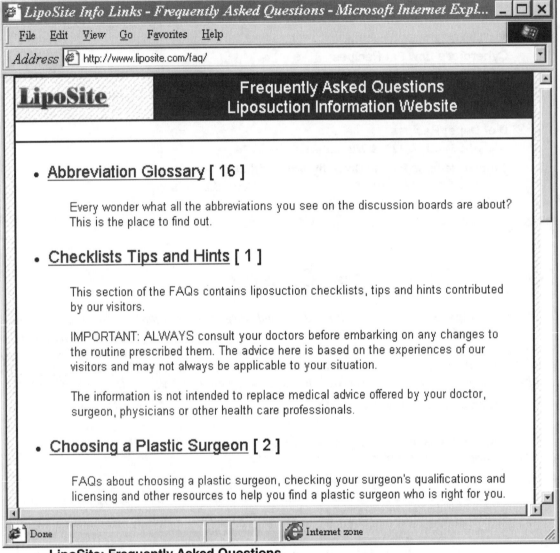

LipoSite: Frequently Asked Questions
www.liposite.com/faq

Liposuction
www.geocities.com/HotSprings/5142/liposuction/liposuctions.html

Liposuction Before & After Photos
www.liposite.com/photos

Liposuction Discussion Area
www.liposite.com/cgi-local/index.cgi

Liposuction Interactive Information Resource-Liposite
www.liposite.com

Liposuction True Life Journals
www.liposite.com/journals

LipoSymposium
www.liposymposium.com

LipoSymposium Forum
www.liposymposium.com/forum

MSO Surgery Information
www.drrossfox.com/surgery.html

MSO-Weight Loss Surgery for the Treatment of Obesity
www.drrossfox.com/home.html

Olwen's Links on Obesity Surgery
http://homepages.ihug.co.nz/~olwen/ocwlnkws.htm

Pacific Bariatric Surgical Medical Group
www.pbsmg.com

Plastic Surgery FAQs-Liposuction
www.plasticsurgery.org/faq/lipo.htm

Surgical Treatment of Obesity
www.weight.com/obesitysurgery.html

Surgilite
http://surgilite.hypermart.net

University Institute for the Surgery of Morbid Obesity
www.shedweight.com

We're All In This Together: Sites for Support

The journey to a healthy weight is a road fraught with temptations, distractions, and frustrations. Try these web sites for some support and inspiration.

At Home With Richard Simmons
www.richardsimmons.com

Better Health: Never Say Diet
www.betterhealth.com/neversaydiet

Beyond Dieting
www.beyonddieting.com

CADIS Information
www.toon.org/~cadis/info/cadis.html

CADIS: Carohydrate Addict's Diet Information & Support
www.toon.org/~cadis/info/subscribe.html

Carbohydrate Addiction Support Online
www.carbohydrateaddicts.com/caonline.html

Circle of Hope: Free Weight Loss Support Group
www.swlink.net/~colonel/coh.html

Cyberdiet's Success Stories
www.cyberdiet.com/success/s197.html

Diet & Weight Loss Tips Collection
http://www1.mhv.net/~donn/tips.html

Good Housekeeping: Fitness Connection: Starting Your Weight Loss Journal
   http://homearts.com/gh/health/1196opb3.htm

HotJ: Heavyweights on the Journey
   http://recovery.hiwaay.net/hotj/index.html

InteliHealth: Home to John Hopkins Health Information:
Five Tips For Planning & Losing Weight
   www.intelihealth.com/IH/ihtIH?t=20704&c=224700&p=~br,IHW|~st,14
   220|~r,WSIHW000|~b,*|&d=dmtContent

Jenny Craig: Guide to Feeling Fit
   www.jennycraig.com/guide/index.html

Magic of Believing-A Weight Loss Support Group
   www.swlink.net/~colonel

Obesity.com: Community Board & Support
   http://weightloss2000.com/support/support_00_intro.htm

Overeaters Anonymous
   www.overeatersanonymous.org

TOPS
   www.tops.org

Zone Amigos List
   www.zonehome.com/amiglist.htm

ZonePerfect.Com: Discussion & Technical Support Center
   http://conference.zoneperfect.com:8080/%7EZonePErfect

Links to More Weight Loss Sites

The links on these pages can be very useful for someone who wants to know more. They're also useful for students who may need to research this subject.

Atlantic Surgery Associates: Resources
   www.stomachstapling.com/resources.html

LipoSymposium
   www.liposymposium.com

Olwen's Links on Obesity Surgery
   http://homepages.ihug.co.nz/~olwen/ocwlnkws.htm

Oxford University Libraries Automation Service
   www.lib.ox.ac.uk/internet/news/faq/archive/dieting-
   faq.part1.html

Redux & "Phen/fen" Medical Problems from Michael Myers M.D. Inc.
   www.weight.com/medprob.html

ZonePerfect.Com: Inside the Zone
   www.enterthezone.com/Inside_The_Zone.html

Vegetarian, Vegan & Other Lifestyle Diets

If you knew that vegetarians have lower incidences of heart disease, cancer, and diabetes than people who eat meat, would you consider taking on that lifestyle? If you knew that their life expectancy is longer than those who eat meat, would you give that diet some thought? These sites contain information for everyone, from the avowed vegetarian to the curious cattleman.

A Fruitful Lifestyle?

What does the fruitarian food pyramid look like? Perhaps it is easier to say what a fruitarian eats rather than what he or she doesn't eat. But just imagine the time you could save by throwing out most of your pots and pans, and "eating it raw." These sites tell us all about it.

All Raw Times: Juicers
www.rawtimes.com/index.html

Bionomic Nutrition Forum
http://venus.nildram.co.uk/veganmc/forum.htm

Drinking Your Veggies
www.salton-maxim.com

Encyclopedia of Fruitarianism & Rational Living
www.student.nada.kth.se/~f95-mwi/fun/encyclopedia.html

Fresh Network
http://easyweb.easynet.co.uk/karenk/top.html

Fruitarian Club - Join
www.fruitarian.com/ar/TheFruitarianClub.htm

Fruitarian Foundation
www.fruitarian.com/ar/AboutFruitarianFoundation.htm

Fruitarian Network
http://spot.acorn.net/fruitarian

Fruitarian Site
www.fruitarian.com

Fruitarian Universal Network
www.student.nada.kth.se/~f95-mwi/fun

Fruitarian Universal Network: FAQs
www.student.nada.kth.se/~f95-mwi/fun/faq.html

Fruitarian Universal Network: Nutrition Calculator
www.student.nada.kth.se/~f95-mwi/fun/calc.html

Fruitarian Universal Network: What Do Fruitarians Eat?
www.student.nada.kth.se/~f95-mwi/fun/whatEat.html

Fruitarian Universal Network: What is a Fruitarian?
www.student.nada.kth.se/~f95-mwi/fun/whatIs.html

Fruitarian Universal Network: Why Become a Fruitarian?
www.student.nada.kth.se/~f95-mwi/fun/why.html

Fruitarian Universal Network: How to Become a Fruitarian
www.student.nada.kth.se/~f95-mwi/fun/howTo.html

Fruitarian, Vegetarian, & Raw Food Links
http://www1.islandnet.com/~arton/fruitlink.html

Fruitarian Network Around the World
http://www3.islandnet.com/~arton/fruitnet.html

Living & Raw Food: Recipes
www.living-foods.com/recipes

Living & Raw Foods
www.rawfoods.com/index.shtml

Living & Raw Foods: Articles & Information
www.living-foods.com/articles

Living & Raw Foods: Chat
www.living-foods.com/chat

Living & Raw Foods: City Guide
www.living-foods.com/cityguide/index.cgi?db=default&uid=

Living & Raw Foods: Discussion Board
www.living-foods.com/board/new/list.cgi

Living & Raw Foods: FAQ
www.living-foods.com/faq.html

Living & Raw Foods: How to Become a Fruitarian
www.living-foods.com/articles/fruitarian.html

Living & Raw Foods: Marketplace
http://wwww.living-foods.com/marketplace

Living & Raw Foods: Register for Membership
www.living-foods.com/register.html

Living & Raw Foods: The Personals
www.living-foods.com/personals

Living & Raw Foods: In the News
www.living-foods.com/news

Original Fruitarian Guidebook: How to Become a Fruitarian
www.islandnet.com/~arton/fruitext.html

Salton - The Industry Leader in Home Products
www.salton-maxim.com

A Little Help From My Friends

Are you looking for some help, maybe a bit of support with your diet? These sites are useful for both the veteran vegetarian and the neophyte.

All Raw Times: E-mail Resources
www.rawtimes.com/email.html

Better Health: Never Say Diet
www.betterhealth.com/neversaydiet

Living & Raw Foods: Register for Membership
www.living-foods.com/register.html

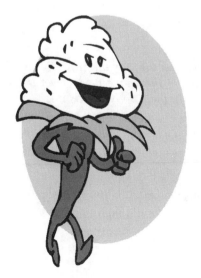

"You ask people why they have deer heads on the wall. They always say, 'Because it's such a beautiful animal.' There you go. I think my mother's attractive, but I have photographs of her."
--Ellen DeGeneres
("Famous Vegeterians" on ChickPages.Com)

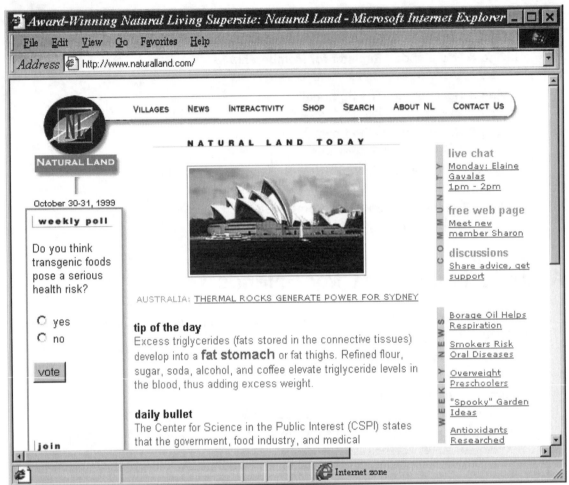

Natural Land: Support Platform Discussion
www.naturalland.com/disc/support.htm

Accepting Yourself the Way You Are

These sites are for those who have decided to accept themselves just the way they are. Perhaps they've tried every diet in the book and on the Internet, or maybe they have never even tried one. The bottom line is they are, or want to be, comfortable within their body just as it is.

Body Positive
www.bodypositive.com

National Association to Advance Fat Acceptance
http://naafa.org

Obesity Meds & Research News: Fat Acceptance Links
www.obesity-news.com/fataccep.htm

Directories

Try these directories to look further into lifestyle diets.

EatVeg Menu
www.newveg.av.org/menu.htm

Living & Raw Foods: City Guide
www.living-foods.com/cityguide/index.cgi?db=default&uid=

Sufi Center Bookstore
www.rosanna.com/books/cookbooks.htm

Vegetarian & Health Food Restaurants
www.ecomall.com/eat.htm

Vegetarian Central
http://vegetariancentral.org/siteindex

Vegetarian Central: Nutrition & Health
http://vegetariancentral.org/siteindex/Nutrition_and_Health

Vegetarian Cuisine
http://vegetarian.miningco.com

Vegetarian Pages
www.veg.org/veg

Vegetarian Resource Center
www.tiac.net/users/vrc/index.htm

Vegetarian Times' Virtual Vegetarian
www.vegetariantimes.com

Vegetarianism: Glossary of Terms
www.macalester.edu/~kwiik/Veggie/terms.htm

Vegetarianism: Vegetarian Organizations
www.macalester.edu/~kwiik/Veggie/orgs.htm

Vegsource: Your Friendly Vegetarian Resource
www.vegsource.com

World Guide to Vegetarianism
www.veg.org/veg/Guide

E-Zines

E-zines are handy for obtaining quick information. They have concise articles and very often will provide links if you desire further study on a topic. Many are loaded with colorful graphics and interactive pages. The only downside is that you can't take this magazine to the bathroom with you.

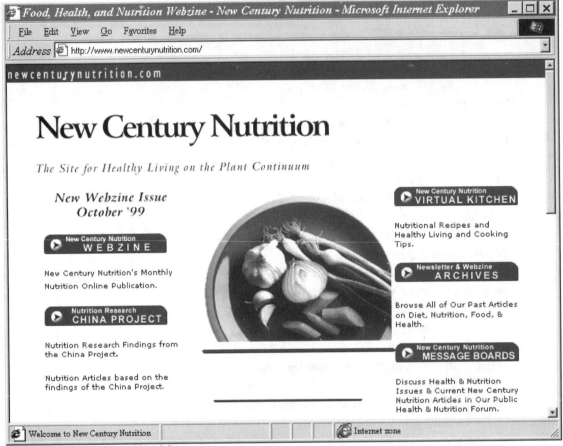

New Century Nutrition
www.newcenturynutrition.com

Vegetarian Journal
www.vrg.org/journal

Vegetarian Voice Online
www.cyberveg.org/navs/voice/voice.html

Veggie Life Magazine
www.veggielife.com

WholeFoods.com: Whole Living Magazine
www.wholefoods.com/magazine/index.html

FAQs

Just the thought of adopting an alternative diet can raise a myriad of questions. Chances are they've been asked before, and you can find the answers on these sites.

Living & Raw Foods: FAQ
www.living-foods.com/faq.html

Macrobiotic Questions & Answers
www.macrobiotic.org/letters1.html

Veganet: The Centurion's Choice
http://library.advanced.org/20922/index.shtml

Vegetarian Nutrition - FAQ
http://members.aol.com/sauromalus/vegnutr.htm

Vegetarian Pages
www.veg.org/veg

Veggies Unite!
http://vegweb.com

Fasting

This isn't exactly a lifestyle diet, nor is it a recommended weight loss strategy. What's important is what you don't eat. Check out the benefits of an occasional fast on these web pages.

Benefits of Fasting
www.healthpromoting.com/articles/benefit.doc

Fasting - Health Promoting Online
www.healthpromoting.com/fast.html

Health Promoting Online
www.healthpromoting.com/indexframe.htm

Just For Fun

Check out these sites for some vegetarian fun online.

101 Reasons Why I'm A Vegetarian
www.geocities.com/RainForest/2062/101.HTML

Famous Vegetarians
www.chickpages.com/veggiefarm/famousveg

Last Sane Cow in England
www.sanecow.tasmanians.com

Stupid Things Vegetarians Hear
www.boutell.com/vegetarian/stupid.html

Links

These sites may well take you deep into cyberspace. Just leave a popcorn trail so you can return safely.

About.com: Vegetarian Cuisine
http://vegetarian.about.com

All Raw Times: E-mail Resources
www.rawtimes.com/email.html

Club Veg: Links of Vegetarian Interest
www.clubveg.org/links.htm

Cybermacro Links
www.cybermacro.com/addlink/storage/macro.html

Cybermacro Natural Health Links
www.cybermacro.com/addlink/storage/health.html

Fruitarian, Vegetarian, & Raw Food Links
http://www1.islandnet.com/~arton/fruitlink.html

Good Karma Café - Our Karma, Our Bodies
www.goodkarmacafe.com/body/karma.shtml

Living & Raw Foods
www.rawfoods.com/index.shtml

Marcus' Vegetarian Page
http://marcussharpe.com/veg1.htm

Natural Home & Travel Guide
www.naturalusa.com/index.html

Obesity Meds & Research News: Fat Acceptance Links
www.obesity-news.com/fataccep.htm

Vegetarian Resource Center
www.tiac.net/users/vrc/index.htm

Vegetarian Times' Virtual Vegetarian
www.vegetariantimes.com

Veggies Anonymous: Resources for Vegetarians, Vegans, & Other Non-Carnivores
www.geocities.com/HotSprings/4664

Veggies Unite!
http://vegweb.com

Macrobiotic Web Sites

Macrobiotics is not just a diet, but an approach to living. It encompasses the physical, emotional, and spiritual aspects of the whole being. Chew your rice at least 100 times while surfing these sites.

Alchemy Pages: An Introduction
www.creative.net/~kaareb/index.html/intro.html

Alchemycal Pages: General Dietary Recommendations
www.creative.net/~kaareb/index.html/dietrec.html

Alchemycal Pages: What is Macrobiotics?
www.creative.net/~kaareb/index.html/qa.html

Australian School of Macrobiotics
www.comcen.com.au/~safe77/index.html

Carbondale Center for Macrobiotic Studies
www.macrobiotic.org/

Carbondale Center: Macrobiotic Center
www.macrobiotic.org/CCMS_Classes.htm

Carbondale Center: The Importance of Chewing
www.macrobiotic.org/health16.html

Cybermacro Home Page
www.cybermacro.com

Cybermacro Links
www.cybermacro.com/addlink/storage/macro.html

Cybermacro Natural Health Links
www.cybermacro.com/addlink/storage/health.html

Cybermacro: Articles
www.cybermacro.com/articles11.html

Cybermacro: Chat
www.cybermacro.com/chat.html

Cybermacro: Discussion Forums
www.cybermacro.com/forum1/forums.html

Cybermacro: Recipes
www.cybermacro.com/recipes.html

Foundation for the Macrobiotic Way
www.enjoy-life.com/health

Foundation for the Macrobiotic Way: A Macrobiotic Diet
www.enjoy-life.com/health/corepages/macrodiet.html

Kushi Institute
www.macrobiotics.org/ki.html

Macrobiotic Questions & Answers
www.macrobiotic.org/letters1.html

Macrobiotics Online
www.macrobiotics.org

Macrobiotics Today
www.natural-connection.com/resource/macro.html

MacroNews: Cooklets
www.macronews.com/cooklet.htm

Natural Home & Travel Guide
www.naturalusa.com/index.html

One Peaceful World
www.macrobiotics.org/OPW.html

Rosanna's Macrobiotic Kitchen
www.rosanna.com

Sufi Center Bookstore
www.rosanna.com/books/cookbooks.htm

Vega Study Center
www.vega.macrobiotic.net

Message Boards

You can post messages, share thoughts, or discuss hot topics here. Also, you can share recipes on the recipe exchange.

Food & Recipe Message Board
www.webvalue.net/recipes/bbsp/index.html

Good Karma Café - Vegetarian Recipe Exchange
http://freshpages.com/Vegetarian_Recipes/Vegetarian_Recipes.html

Good Karma Café - Welcome to Recipe Central
www.goodkarmacafe.com/recipes/recipes.shtml

Vegan Outreach: Forums
www.veganoutreach.org/forum/cgi-bin/Ultimate.cgi?action=intro

Vegetarian Times' Virtual Vegetarian
www.vegetariantimes.com

Vegsource: Veganism
www.vegsource.com/wwwboard/veganism/wwwboard.html

VegWeb - Recipe Exchange
www.vegweb.com/exchange

Newsletters

If you subscribe, some of these newsletters come to you weekly via your e-mail for free. Try one.

Natural Land: Free E-mail Newsletter & Free Magazine Trial Subscription
www.naturalland.com/sub.htm

Vegan Street
www.veganstreet.com

Vegetarian Epicure
www.vegetarianepicure.com

VegWeb - Newsletter
http://vegweb.com/newsletter

Online Shops

Find books, food, and even appliances using these web stores.

All Raw Times: Juicers
www.rawtimes.com/index.html

BizDistrict Bookseller - Vegetarian Books
www.bizdistrict.com/bookstore/vegbooks.html

Earthy Delights
http://earthy.com

Farm Catalog: Vegetarian Cookbooks
www.farmcatalog.com/cgi-bin/Web_store/web_store.cgi?page=cookbooks.html&cart_id=3673722.19484

Living & Raw Foods: Marketplace
http://www.living-foods.com/marketplace

MacroNews: Cooklets
www.macronews.com/cooklet.htm

Miracle Exclusives Online
www.miracleexclusives.com

Salton - The Industry Leader in Home Products
www.salton-maxim.com

Vegan.com Bookstore
www.vegan.com/bookstore/index.htm

WholeFoods.com
www.wholefoods.com

WholeFoods.com: Marketplace
www.wholefoods.com/market/index.html

Recipes

There are thousands of recipes to be found on these sites. Some are searchable. Try one out for your next potluck dinner.

Cybermacro: Recipes
www.cybermacro.com/recipes.html

Fatfree: The Low Fat Vegetarian Recipe Archive
www.fatfree.com/

Food & Recipe Message Board
www.webvalue.net/recipes/bbsp/index.html

Fruitarian Universal Network: What Do Fruitarians Eat?
www.student.nada.kth.se/~f95-mwi/fun/whatEat.html

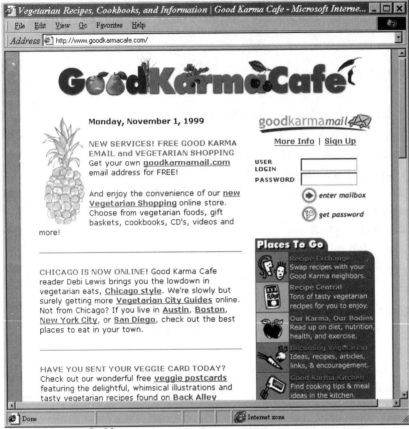

Good Karma Café
www.goodkarmacafe.com

Good Karma Café - Vegetarian Recipe Exchange
http://freshpages.com/Vegetarian_Recipes/Vegetarian_Recipes.html

Good Karma Café - Welcome to Recipe Central
www.goodkarmacafe.com/recipes/recipes.shtml

Good Stuff Recipes Online
www.goodstuffonline.com/index.html

Great Vegetarian Recipes
www.webvalue.net/recipes

Healthy Gourmet Vegetarian Food Page
www.bizdistrict.com/food.html

International Vegetarian Union: Recipes Around the World
www.ivu.org/recipes

Joanne Stepaniak - Recipes
www.vegsource.org/joanne/recipes.htm

Light Living
www.lightliving.com

Living & Raw Food: Recipes
www.living-foods.com/recipes

Living & Raw Foods
www.rawfoods.com/index.shtml

Natural Land: Cooking Village
www.naturalland.com/cv.htm

Natural Land: eNaturalMall
www.naturalland.com/shop.htm

Porridge People
www.geocities.com/HotSprings/Sauna/7015

Recipes from the Vegging Out Kitchen
www.execpc.com/~veggie/recipes.html

Small Household Vegetarian Recipes
www.boutell.com/vegetarian/index.html

Tarla Dalal
www.tarladalal.com

Taste of Heaven & Earth
www.amacord.com/taste

Vegan Recipe Index
www.hut.fi/~jstalvio/cookbook1/Vegan-index.html

Vegan Recipes
http://cooties.punkrock.net/veg/recipes

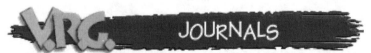

Vegetarian Epicure
www.vegetarianepicure.com

THE
VEGETARIAN
RESOURCE
GROUP   **VRG.**   JOURNALS

Vegetarian Journal: Recipes from the Archives
www.vrg.org/journal/index.htm

Vegetarian Resource Group: Recipes
www.vrg.org/recipes

Vegetarianism: Recipes
www.macalester.edu/~kwiik/Veggie/recipes.htm

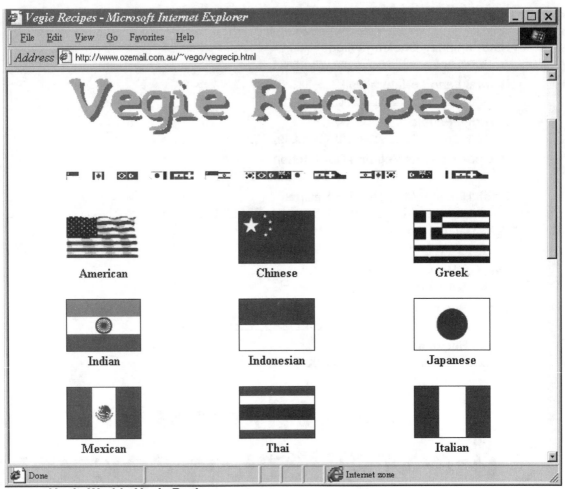

Vegie World: Vegie Recipes
www.ozemail.com.au/~vego/vegrecip.html

Vegsource: Best of the Net Recipes
www.vegsource.com/recipe

VegWeb - Recipe Exchange
www.vegweb.com/exchange

VegWeb - Recipe Directory
www.vegweb.com/food

WWW Cookbook
www.hut.fi/~jstalvio/cookbook1

Seeking A Balanced Vegetarian Diet

"Where do you get your protein?" and "If you don't do dairy, where do you get your calcium?" The vegetarian food pyramid demonstrates how variety, balance, and moderation can be achieved. Details about the pyramid and other ways to maintain a balanced diet can be found at these sites.

Four Food Groups
www.vegsource.com/food_groups.htm

Good Vegan Calcium Sources
www.interlog.com/~john13/recipes/calcium.htm

Vegetarian Diet Pyramid
www.oldwayspt.org/html/p_veg.htm

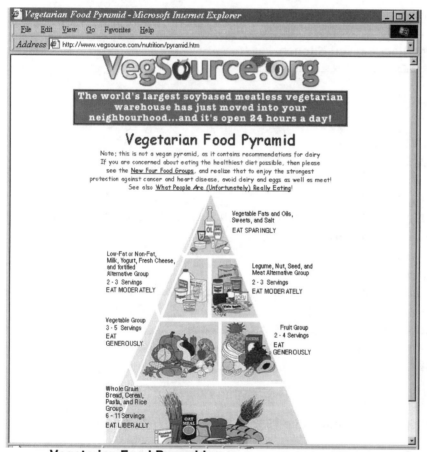

Vegetarian Food Pyramid
www.vegsource.com/nutrition/pyramid.htm

Vegie World: The Calcium Myth
www.ozemail.com.au/~vego/calcium.html

VegWeb - Vitamins & Minerals
www.vegweb.com/veginfo/vitamins.shtml

Sites for Vegan Diets

Vegans usually exclude animal flesh, animal products such as eggs and dairy, and they may exclude honey as well. Some even exclude yeast products. They also do not wear or use animal products. So the question begs to be asked: "So where do they get their calcium?" These sites answer not only that question, but help us to understand the vegan diet.

Eatveg.com
www.newveg.av.org

Good Vegan Calcium Sources
www.interlog.com/~john13/recipes/calcium.htm

Grass Roots Veganism with Joanne Stepaniak
www.vegsource.org/joanne

Porridge People
www.geocities.com/HotSprings/Sauna/7015/

Recipes from the Vegging Out Kitchen
www.execpc.com/~veggie/recipes.html

Vegan Bikers
http://venus.nildram.co.uk/veganmc

Vegan News
www.bury-rd.demon.co.uk

Vegan Outreach
www.veganoutreach.org

Vegan Outreach: Forums
www.veganoutreach.org/forum/cgi-bin/Ultimate.cgi?action=intro

Vegan Outreach: Why Vegan?
www.veganoutreach.org/wv

Vegan Recipe Index
www.hut.fi/~jstalvio/cookbook1/Vegan-index.html

Vegan Recipes
http://cooties.punkrock.net/veg/recipes

Vegan Society: Teen Vegans
www.vegansociety.com/info/info07.html

Vegan Street
www.veganstreet.com

Vegan.com - Disparaging Meat Since 1997
www.vegan.com

Vegan.com Bookstore
www.vegan.com/bookstore/index.htm

Veganet: The Centurion's Choice
http://library.advanced.org/20922/index.shtml

Veganism for the Over 60
www.vegansociety.com/info/info05.html

Vegetarian Recipes Around the World
www.ivu.org/recipes

Vegetarian Resource Group: Vegan Diet During Pregnancy & Lactation
www.vrg.org/nutrition/veganpregnancy.htm

Vegsource: Veganism
www.vegsource.com/wwwboard/veganism/wwwboard.html

Someone To Talk To

These are sites for chatting. Some may require registration, but log on, ask questions, share recipes, get advice, or make some veggie-cyber friends.

Cybermacro: Chat
www.cybermacro.com/chat.html

Living & Raw Foods: Chat
www.living-foods.com/chat

Living & Raw Foods: Discussion Board
www.living-foods.com/board/new/list.cgi

Natural Land: Chat Room
www.naturalland.com/chat.htm

Natural Land: Support Platform Discussion
www.naturalland.com/disc/support.htm

Natural Land: Community Platform Discussion
www.naturalland.com/disc/community.htm

VegWeb - Chat
www.vegweb.com/chat

Trying Out a Different Kind of Diet

Eating meatless meals does not require religious convictions or conversion to Hinduism. Nor is it necessary to harbor a strong pro-environmental stance. It could merely stem from a desire to serve a different kind of meal to your family. These sites contribute some thoughts and discussion about various lifestyle diets.

Bionomic Nutrition Forum
http://venus.nildram.co.uk/veganmc/forum.htm

Cybermacro: Articles
www.cybermacro.com/articles11.html

Cybermacro: Discussion Forums
www.cybermacro.com/forum1/forums.html

EarthSave: Healthy People, Healthy Planet
www.earthsave.org

Encyclopedia of Fruitarianism & Rational Living
www.student.nada.kth.se/~f95-mwi/fun/encyclopedia.html

Good Karma Café - Our Karma, Our Bodies
www.goodkarmacafe.com/body/karma.shtml

Hinduism Online: Discussing Vegetarianism With a Meateater
www.hinduismtoday.kauai.hi.us/ashram/Resources/Ahimsa/WinMeatEaterArgument.html

Living & Raw Foods: How to Become a Fruitarian
www.living-foods.com/articles/fruitarian.html

Natural Land: Nutrition Village
www.naturalland.com/nv.htm

Natural Land: Community Platform Discussion
www.naturalland.com/disc/community.htm

Vegie World: Tips for Making the Change
www.ozemail.com.au/~vego/tips.html

Vegetarian Sites

There are several different kinds of vegetarians. Lacto-ovo vegetarians use egg and dairy products, lacto vegetarians use dairy, and ovo vegetarians consume eggs. A semi-vegetarian may choose to eat some fish or chicken, but does not eat beef. Vegetarian sites abound on the WWW. Some sites offer tremendous resources while others may be personal web pages that bring us just a smile to go with our food. Grab a veggie burger and log on.

101 Reasons Why I'm A Vegetarian
www.geocities.com/RainForest/2062/101.HTML

About.com: Vegetarian Cuisine
http://vegetarian.about.com

American Dietetic Association: Position on Vegetarian Diets
www.eatright.org/adap1197.html

American Heart Association: Vegetarian Diets
www.americanheart.org/Heart_and_Stroke_A_Z_Guide/vegdiet.html

Carrot & Stick News Articles
www.goldfever.com/fatbrat/Page2.htm

Challenges to Vegetarianism
http://vegetarian.about.com/library/weekly/aa080299.htm?pid=2757&cob=home

Chickertarian Information Page
www.newveg.av.org/animals/chicketarian.htm

Club Veg
www.clubveg.org

Club Veg: Links of Vegetarian Interest
www.clubveg.org/links.htm

Dilip's Vegetarian Resource Page
www.cs.unc.edu/~barman/vegetarian.html

EarthSave: Healthy People, Healthy Planet
www.earthsave.org

Earthy Delights
http://earthy.com

EatVeg Menu
  www.newveg.av.org/menu.htm

European Vegetarian Union
  www.ivu.org/evu

Famous Vegetarians
  www.chickpages.com/veggiefarm/famousveg

Farm Catalog: Vegetarian Cookbooks
  www.farmcatalog.com/cgi-
  bin/Web_store/web_store.cgi?page=cookbooks.html&cart_id=3673722
  .19484

Fatfree: The Low Fat Vegetarian Recipe Archive
  www.fatfree.com

Food & Recipe Message Board
  www.webvalue.net/recipes/bbsp/index.html

Four Food Groups
  www.vegsource.com/food_groups.htm

Frequently Asked Questions About Vegetarianism
  www.veg.org/veg/FAQ/rec.food.veg.html

Fruitarian, Vegetarian, & Raw Food Links
  http://www1.islandnet.com/~arton/fruitlink.html

Going Vegetarian: Part II
  http://vegetarian.about.com/library/weekly/aa030298.htm?pid=275
  7&cob=home

Going Vegetarian: Part I
  http://vegetarian.about.com/library/weekly/aa022398.htm?pid=275
  7&cob=home

Good Karma Café
  www.goodkarmacafe.com/

Good Karma Café - Vegetarian Recipe Exchange
  http://freshpages.com/Vegetarian_Recipes/Vegetarian_Recipes.html

Good Karma Café - Welcome to Recipe Central
  www.goodkarmacafe.com/recipes/recipes.shtml

Good Nutrition - A Look at Vegetarian Basics
  http://mars.superlink.com/user/dupre/navs/nutri.html

Good Stuff Recipes Online
  www.goodstuffonline.com/index.html

Great Vegetarian Recipes
  www.webvalue.net/recipes/

Healthy Gourmet Vegetarian Food Page
  www.bizdistrict.com/food.html

Hinduism Online: Discussing Vegetarianism With a Meateater
  www.hinduismtoday.kauai.hi.us/ashram/Resources/Ahimsa/WinMeatEa
  terArgument.html

International Vegetarian Union
  www.ivu.org/evu

International Vegetarian Union: Recipes Around the World
  www.ivu.org/recipes

Jennie's Vegetarian Info Page
www.frognet.net/~jsq22/VEGINFO.html

Jewish Holiday Fare
http://vegetarian.about.com/msubholjewish.htm?pid=2757&cob=home

Jewish Vegetarians of North America
www.orbyss.com/jvna.htm

Joanne Stepaniak - Recipes
www.vegsource.org/joanne/recipes.htm

Jupiter Rising: Online Vegetarian Resource
http://members.aol.com/khlisson/vegetarian.html

Last Sane Cow in England
www.sanecow.tasmanians.com

Living & Raw Foods: Marketplace
http://www.living-foods.com/marketplace

MacroNews: Cooklets
www.macronews.com/cooklet.htm

Marcus' Vegetarian Page
http://marcussharpe.com/veg1.htm

McDougall - Online Wellness Center
www.drmcdougall.com

Meat.org
www.meat.org

Miracle Exclusives Online
www.miracleexclusives.com

Natural Home & Travel Guide
www.naturalusa.com/index.html

Natural Kitchen
www.natural-connection.com/kitchen/default.html

Natural Land: Chat Room
www.naturalland.com/chat.htm

Natural Land: Cooking Village
www.naturalland.com/cv.htm

Natural Land: eNaturalMall
www.naturalland.com/shop.htm

Natural Land: Free E-mail Newsletter & Free Magazine Trial Subscription
www.naturalland.com/sub.htm

Natural Land: Nutrition Village
www.naturalland.com/nv.htm

Natural Land: Support Platform Discussion
www.naturalland.com/disc/support.htm

Natural Land: Award Winning Natural Living Supersite
www.naturalland.com

Natural Land: Community Platform Discussion
www.naturalland.com/disc/community.htm

New Century Nutrition
www.newcenturynutrition.com

North American Vegetarian Society
www.cyberveg.org/navs

Physicians Committee for Responsible Medicine: Vegetarian Starter Kit
www.pcrm.org/health/VSK/starterkit.html

Small Household Vegetarian Recipes
www.boutell.com/vegetarian/index.html

Stupid Things Vegetarians Hear
www.boutell.com/vegetarian/stupid.html

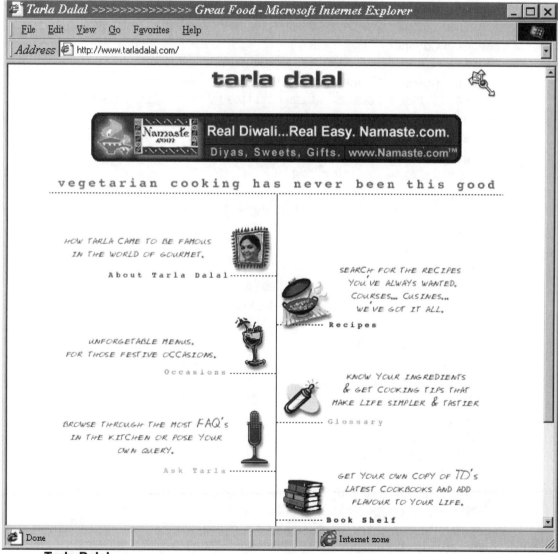

Tarla Dalal
www.tarladalal.com

Taste of Heaven & Earth
www.amacord.com/taste

Transition Tips to Vegetarianism
www.newveg.av.org/transition/transition.htm

US Soy Foods Directory
http://soyfoods.com

VegDining.Com
www.vegdining.com

Vegetarian & Health Food Restaurants
www.ecomall.com/eat.htm

Vegetarian Central
http://vegetariancentral.org/siteindex

Vegetarian Central: Nutrition & Health
http://vegetariancentral.org/siteindex/Nutrition_and_Health

Vegetarian Cuisine
http://vegetarian.miningco.com

Vegetarian Cuisine: Definitive Collection of NetLinks
http://vegetarian.about.com/mlibrary.htm?COB=home&PID=2757

Vegetarian Diet Pyramid
www.oldwayspt.org/html/p_veg.htm

Vegetarian Epicure
www.vegetarianepicure.com

Vegetarian Food Pyramid
www.vegsource.com/nutrition/pyramid.htm

Vegetarian Journal
www.vrg.org/journal

Vegetarian Journal: Subscribe
www.vrg.org/journal/subscribe.htm

Vegetarian Journal: Recipes from the Archives
www.vrg.org/journal/index.htm

Vegetarian Nutrition - FAQ
http://members.aol.com/sauromalus/vegnutr.htm

Vegetarian Nutrition for Teenagers
www.vrg.org/nutrition/teennutrition.htm

Vegetarian Pages
www.veg.org/veg

Vegetarian Resource Group
www.vrg.org

Vegetarian Resource Group: Choosing & Using a Dietician
www.vrg.org/journal/dietitian.htm

Vegetarian Resource Group: Recipes
www.vrg.org/recipes

Vegetarian Resource Group: The Vegetarian Game
www.vrg.org/game

Vegetarian Resource Group: Vegetarianism in a Nutshell
www.vrg.org/nutshell/nutshell.htm

Vegetarian Ring
www.geocities.com/RainForest/4083/vegring2.html

Vegetarianism: Eat to Your Health
www.macalester.edu/~kwiik/Veggie/health.htm

Vegetarianism: Recipes
www.macalester.edu/~kwiik/Veggie/recipes.htm

Vegetarianism: Vegetarian Fun Facts
www.macalester.edu/~kwiik/Veggie/funfact.htm

Vegetarianism: Vegetarian Organizations
www.macalester.edu/~kwiik/Veggie/orgs.htm

Veggie Kids
www.execpc.com/~veggie/tips.html

Veggie Life Magazine
www.veggielife.com

Veggies Anonymous: Resources for Vegetarians, Vegans, & Other Non-Carnivores
www.geocities.com/HotSprings/4664

Veggies Unite!
http://vegweb.com

Vegging Out
www.execpc.com/~veggie/index.html

Vegging Out: Salt Talk - The Debate About Sodium & Your Health
www.execpc.com/~veggie/salt.html

Vegie Info: Why Vegetarian?
www.ozemail.com.au/~vego/whyveg.html

Vegie World: The Calcium Myth
www.ozemail.com.au/~vego/calcium.html

Vegie World: Three Simple Steps to Go Vegetarian
www.ozemail.com.au/~vego/3steps.html

Vegie World: Tips for Making the Change
www.ozemail.com.au/~vego/tips.html

Vegie World: Vegie Recipes
www.ozemail.com.au/~vego/vegrecip.html

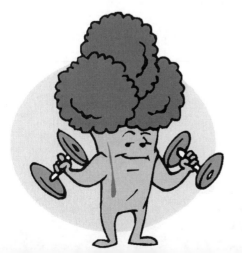

"Nothing will benefit health and increase chances for survival of life on Earth as the evolution to a vegetarian diet"
- Albert Einstein

Vegsource: Your Friendly Vegetarian Resource
www.vegsource.com

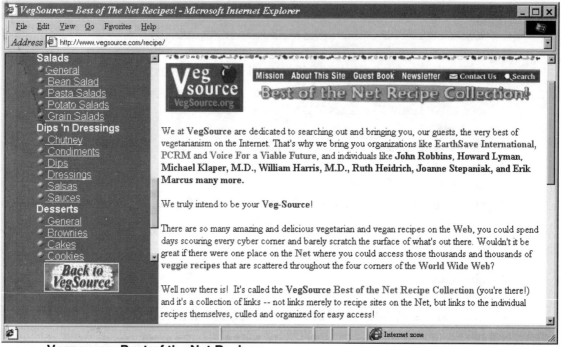

Vegsource: Best of the Net Recipes
www.vegsource.com/recipe

VegWeb - Recipe Exchange
www.vegweb.com/exchange

VegWeb - Chat
www.vegweb.com/chat

VegWeb - Newsletter
http://vegweb.com/newsletter

VegWeb - Recipe Directory
www.vegweb.com/food

VegWeb - Vitamins & Minerals
www.vegweb.com/veginfo/vitamins.shtml

Very Vegetarian Sites
www.cyber-kitchen.com/index/html/gp35.html

VitaPro
www.vitapro.com

Vita-Soy International
www.vitasoy-usa.com

Virtual Vegetarian
www.vegetariantimes.com

Viva Vegie Society
www.earthbase.org/vivavegie/home.html

WholeFoods.com
www.wholefoods.com

WholeFoods.com: Marketplace
www.wholefoods.com/market/index.html

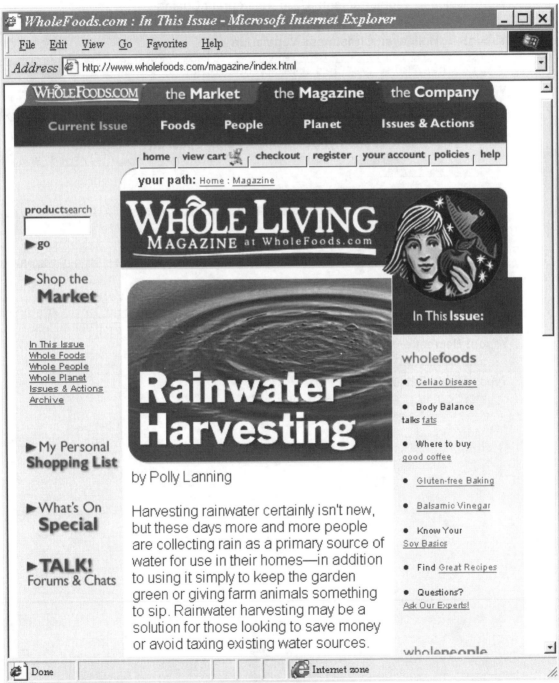

WholeFoods.com: Whole Living Magazine
www.wholefoods.com/magazine/index.html

Wildwood Natural Foods
www.wildwoodnaturalfoods.com/frame.html

World Guide to Vegetarianism
www.veg.org/veg/Guide

World Guide to Vegetarianism: USA: National Organizations
www.veg.org/veg/Guide/USA/National_Vegetarian_Organizations.html

World Guide to Vegetarianism: USA: Restaurant Chains
www.veg.org/veg/Guide/USA/Restaurant_Chains.html

Yahoo! . . . Holidays: Christmas: Vegetarian
http://dir.yahoo.com/Society_and_Culture/Food_and_Drink/Cooking
/Recipes/Holidays/Christmas/Vegetarian

Yahoo! . . . Holidays: Thanksgiving: Vegetarian
http://dir.yahoo.com/Society_and_Culture/Food_and_Drink/Cooking
/Recipes/Holidays/Thanksgiving/Vegetarian

Yahoo! Business & Economy: Companies: Food: Specialty: Vegetarian
http://dir.yahoo.com/Business_and_Economy/Companies/Food/Specia
lty/Vegetarian

Yahoo! Net Events: Vegetarians
http://events.yahoo.com/Net_Events/Society_and_Culture/Cultures
_and_Groups/Vegetarians

Yahoo! Society & Culture: Cultures & Groups: Vegetarians
http://dir.yahoo.com/Society_and_Culture/Cultures_and_Groups/Ve
getarians

Yahoo! Society & Culture: Food & Drink: Cooking: Recipes: Vegetarian
http://dir.yahoo.com/Society_and_Culture/Food_and_Drink/Cooking
/Recipes/Vegetarian

Yahoo! Recreation: Travel: Vegetarian
www.yahoo.co.uk/Recreation/Travel/Vegetarian

Yves' Veggie Cuisine
www.yvesveggie.com/main.html

Preventative Nutrition & Control of Disease

Our genetic makeup is not the only factor that determines whether or not we will be led down the path toward illnesses such as cancer of heart disease. The sites in this chapter help us to understand the immense control we can have in determining our own longevity. Other sites show us diet strategies to help us keep symptoms of some illnesses we already bear under control, such as diabetes. Visiting some of these sites could save your life.

Diabetes-Related Sites

There are many good sites to help the diabetic with meal planning and to understand nutrition. Learn more about the exchange system or about carbohydrate counting. Most importantly, always consult your healthcare provider and your registered dietician before you attempt any change in your diet.

American Diabetes Association: FAQs About Nutrition & Diabetes
www.diabetes.org/nutrition/faqs.asp

American Diabetes Association: Feed Your Brain: Nutrition Quiz
www.diabetes.org/nutrition/i_quiz.asp

American Diabetes Association: Healthy Restaurant Eating: Is It Possible?
www.diabetes.org/nutrition/restauranteating.asp

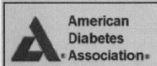 American
Diabetes
Association

Nutrition

Click Here
to
Customize

Home

Learn About ADA
About ADA
Career Opportunities
Annual Report
Disclaimer

Donate Now
How and Why to Donate
Memorial Contributions
Establish a Planned Gift
The Elizabeth Knight
Fund

Diabetes Info
General Information
In the News
Newly Diagnosed
Nutrition
Exercise
Take the Risk Test
Tip of the Day
Recipe of the Day
Clinical Practice
Recommendations
African American Program

**Become a Member
/ Subscribe**
Professional Membership
General Membership

The Nutrition Area is sponsored in part
by a grant from Archway Cookies.
www.archwaycookies.com

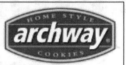

NEW! Discover the ins and outs of
Healthy Restaurant Eating.

NEW! Learn how to Eat Healthy with
the Food Pyramid as Your Guide.

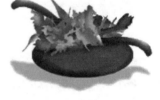

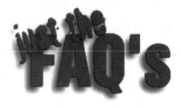

" *THE **WEBB** COOKS* "
Robyn Webb, Author
A twice monthly article on
cooking and nutrition.

**Read the Interview
with Hope Warshaw.**

**Frequently Asked Questions
About Nutrition**

American Diabetes Association: Nutrition
www.diabetes.org/nutrition

American Diabetes Association: Recipe of the Day
www.diabetes.org/recipes/072099.asp

American Diabetes Association: Wordplay
www.diabetes.org/nutrition/herbs_puzzle.asp

American Dietetic Association: Diabetes Meal Planning
www.eatright.org/nfs/nfs37.html

**American Dietetic Association: Nutrition & Health Campaign for Women:
Diabetes & Nutrition**
www.eatright.org/womenshealth/diabetes.html

Ask the Dietician: Diabetes
www.dietitian.com/diabetes.html

Ask the Dietician: Diabetic Exchange & Carbo Counting
www.dietitian.com/diabexch.html

Children With Diabetes: Ask The Diabetes Team: Meal Planning, Food & Diet
www.childrenwithdiabetes.com/dteam/d_0d_01b.htm

Children With Diabetes: Carbohydrate Counting
www.childrenwithdiabetes.com/d_08_d00.htm

Children With Diabetes: Computerized Meal Planning
www.childrenwithdiabetes.com/d_08_400.htm

Children With Diabetes: Cookbooks
www.childrenwithdiabetes.com/d_08_300.htm

Children With Diabetes: Fast Food Facts
www.childrenwithdiabetes.com/d_08_700.htm

Children With Diabetes: Food Guide Pyramid
www.childrenwithdiabetes.com/d_08_800.htm

Children With Diabetes: Meal Planning Aids
www.childrenwithdiabetes.com/d_08_430.htm

Children With Diabetes: Readers' Favorite Recipes
www.childrenwithdiabetes.com/d_08_200.htm

Children With Diabetes: Sugar Substitutes
www.childrenwithdiabetes.com/d_08_b00.htm

Circulation: Summary of a Scientific Conference on Preventive Nutrition
http://circ.ahajournals.org/cgi/content/full/100/4/450

Diabetes.com: Healthy Diet & Exercise
www.diabetes.com/health_library/diet_and_exercise.html

Diabetes.com: Simple Secrets of Low-Fat, Controlled Carbohydrate Eating
www.diabetes.com/health_library/articles/13t103205.html

Diabetes.com: What You Need to Know About Exchange Lists
www.diabetes.com/health_library/features/fst10338.html

Diabetes.Store
http://merchant.diabetes.org/adabooks/Default.asp

Dietsite.com: Diabetes
www.dietsite.com/Diets/Diabetes/diabetesfs.htm

Dietsite.com: Emergency Food Exchanges
www.dietsite.com/Diets/Diabetes/SickDayManagement/Emergency%20Food%20Exchange%20Groups.htm

Dietsite.com: Hyperglycemia
www.dietsite.com/Diets/Diabetes/SickDayManagement/HYPERglycemia.htm

Dietsite.com: Hypoglycemia or Insulin Reaction
www.dietsite.com/Diets/Diabetes/SickDayManagement/HYPOglycemia.htm

Dietsite.com: No Concentrated Sweet Food List
www.dietsite.com/Diets/Diabetes/DiabeticDiets/No%20Concentrated%20Sweet%20Food%20List.htm

Dietsite.com: No Concentrated Sweets, Low Fat Diet
www.dietsite.com/Diets/Diabetes/DiabeticDiets/No%20Concentrated%20Sweets%20Low%20Fat%20Diet.htm

Dietsite.com: Sick Day Guidelines For the Insulin Dependent Diabetic
www.dietsite.com/Diets/Diabetes/SickDayManagement/Sick%20Day%20Therapy%20for%20Type%201%20Diabetes.htm

Dietsite.com: Sick Day Management For the Non-insulin Dependent Diabetid
www.dietsite.com/Diets/Diabetes/SickDayManagement/Sick%20Day%20Therapy%20for%20Type%20II%20Diabetes.htm

Dietsite.com: The Diabetic Diet
www.dietsite.com/Diets/Diabetes/DiabeticDiets/diabetic_diet.htm

Dietsite.com: The Exchange System
www.dietsite.com/Diets/Diabetes/exchange_system.htm

drkoop.com: A Growing Problem
www.drkoop.com/wellness/nutrition/healthyliving/index.asp?id=192

Eating Healthy With The Diabetes Food Pyramid As Your Guide
www.diabetes.org/nutrition/article031799.asp

Feeding the Child With Diabetes - Grade School Through Middle School
www.uchsc.edu/misc/diabetes/nwsntrn1.html

Joslin Diabetes Center
www.joslin.org

Joslin Diabetes Center: Carbohydrate Counting
www.joslin.org/education/library/wcarbsug.html

Joslin Diabetes Center: Diet Strategies For Women With Diabetes: Why Some Work & Some Don't
www.joslin.org/education/library/wmagdiet.html

Joslin Diabetes Center: Eating For Life: Discussion
www.joslin.org/managing/eating.html

Joslin Diabetes Center: Facts About Fiber
www.joslin.org/education/library/wiber.html

Joslin Diabetes Center: Fitting Alcohol Into Your Meal Plan
www.joslin.org/education/library/walohol.html

Joslin Diabetes Center: Fitting Sugar Into Your Meal Plan
www.joslin.org/education/library/wcarbsug.html

Joslin Diabetes Center: Portion Control
www.joslin.org/education/library/wcarbsug.html

Joslin Diabetes Center: There's No Such Thing As A Diabetic Diet
www.joslin.org/education/library/nodiet2.html

Joslin Diabletes Center: Recommended Cookbooks & Resource Books
www.joslin.org/education/library/wcbook.html

NutriGenie Diabetes Meal Planner
http://users.aol.com/nutrigenie/ngdmp44.html

NutriGenie: Managing Diabetes Version 3.6 For Windows
http://users.aol.com/nutrigenie/nsmd36.html

Parent's Place: Blood Sugar Control During Pregnancy
http://www4.parentsplace.com/pregnancy/nutrition/qa/0,3105,1119
5,00.html

Treating Diabetes With Good Nutrition
www.cyberdiet.com/modules/diabetes/outline.html

Diet & Alzheimer's

The relationship between diet and Alzheimer's is a subject of continuing investigation. There may be a link between thiamine deficiencies and Alzheimer's, and maybe between magnesium and Alzheimer's as well. Of great importance is the need for optimizing nutrition in the Alzheimer's patient.

American Dietetic Association:
Nutrition Care of Your Loved One With Alzheimer's Disease
www.eatright.org/nfs/nfs61.html

Better Health: Malnutrition Ups Death Risk in Alzheimer's Patients
www.betterhealth.com/seniors/caregiving/news/0,4800,1959_127311
,00.html

Combating Alzheimer's Disease With Diet
www.awesomelibrary.org/alzheimer.html

Prevention of Major Medical Problems With Diet
www.neat-schoolhouse.org/diet-prev.html

Diet & Hypertension

High blood pressure can be susceptible to changes in diet. Check out the DASH diet, and other sites here.

DASH Diet Navigation Page
http://dash.bwh.harvard.edu./dashdiet.html

DASH Diet: Hints for Success
http://dash.bwh.harvard.edu./dashdiettips.html

DASH Diet: Salt & Losing Weight
http://dash.bwh.harvard.edu./dashdietsalt.html

DASH Diet: Sample Menus
http://dash.bwh.harvard.edu./dashdietsamplemenus.html

Dietary Approaches to Stop Hypertension
http://dash.bwh.harvard.edu./

drkoop.com: DASH Away High Blood Pressure
www.drkoop.com/wellness/nutrition/healthyliving/index.asp?id=216

Following the DASH Diet
http://dash.bwh.harvard.edu./dashdietservings.html

Heart Information Network: DASH Diet Lowers Blood Pressure
www.heartinfo.com/news97/dash61797.htm

Mayo Clinic Health Oasis: The DASH Diet - It May Benefit Your Blood Pressure
www.mayohealth.org/mayo/9805/htm/dash.htm

Mayo Clinic Health Oasis: The DASH Diet
www.mayohealth.org/mayo/9805/htm/dash_sb.htm

National Institutes of Health: The DASH Diet
www.nih.gov/news/pr/apr97/Dash.htm

Diets that May Decrease Risk of Cancer

Of the 500,000 deaths that occur annually as a result of cancer, one third of them can be attributed to dietary factors. It's a no-brainer that we should check out some of these sites and reduce our risk of getting cancer by a third!

American Cancer Society: Alternative & Complementary Methods
www.cancer.org/alt_therapy/index.html

American Cancer Society: Commitment to Nutrition & Cancer Prevention
http://www2.cancer.org/prevention/index.cfm?prevention=commitment

American Cancer Society: Common Questions About Diet & Cancer
http://www2.cancer.org/prevention/index.cfm?prevention=questions

American Cancer Society: Dietary & Herbal Remedies
www.cancer.org/alt_therapy/index.html

American Cancer Society: Fat Consumption & Breast Cancer Risk
http://www2.cancer.org/zine/dsp_SecondaryStories.cfm?sc=001&archiveLink=001_04261999_0

American Cancer Society: Healthy Eating Cookbook
www.cancer.org/bookstore/cook_exc.html

American Cancer Society: Importance of Nutrition in Cancer Prevention
http://www2.cancer.org/prevention/index.cfm?prevention=1

American Cancer Society: Prevention
http://www2.cancer.org/prevention/index.cfm?prevention=factors

American Cancer Society: Recommendations
http://www2.cancer.org/prevention/index.cfm?prevention=recommendations

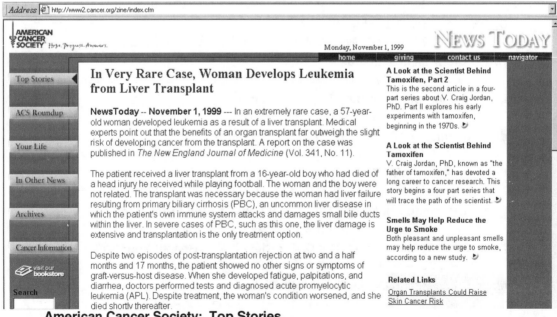

American Cancer Society: Top Stories
http://www2.cancer.org/zine/index

American Dietetic Association: Nutrition & Health Campaign for Women: Breast Cancer & Nutrition
www.eatright.org/womenshealth/breastcancer.html

Ask the Dietician: Cancer
www.dietitian.com/cancer.html

CancerGuide: Bovine Cartilage
http://cancerguide.org/btc.html

CancerGuide: PSK
http://cancerguide.org/psk.html

CancerGuide: Simone Shark Cartilage Protocol
http://cancerguide.org/simone_prot.html

CancerNet
http://cancernet.nci.nih.gov

CancerNet: Eating Hints For Cancer Patients
http://cancernet.nci.nih.gov/eating_hints/eatintro.html

CancerNet: Eating Hints Glossary
http://cancernet.nci.nih.gov/eating_hints/eatglossary.html

CancerNet: Eating Well During Cancer Treatment
http://cancernet.nci.nih.gov/eating_hints/eatwell.html

CancerNet: Managing Eating Problems During Treatment
http://cancernet.nci.nih.gov/eating_hints/eatmanage.html

CancerNet: Special Diets For Special Needs
http://cancernet.nci.nih.gov/eating_hints/eatdiets.html

Colorado State University Cooperative Extension: Nutrition & Cancer
www.colostate.edu/depts/CoopExt/PUBS/FOODNUT/09313.html

IFIC: Diet & Environment in Cancer Risk
http://ificinfo.health.org/insight/dietenv.htm

IFIC: Experts Agree on Key Advice to Reduce Cancer Risk
http://ificinfo.health.org/insight/novdec97/cancerrisk.htm

IFIC: Questions & Answers About Cancer, Diet, & Fats
http://ificinfo.health.org/qanda/diet_cancer.htm

JHS Natural Products: Coriolus
www.jhsnp.com/about_coriolus.html

JHS Natural Products: PSK Mushrooms
www.jhsnp.com/index2.html

Mayo Clinic Health Oasis: Cancer - What You Eat Can Affect Your Risk
www.mayohealth.org/mayo/9509/htm/cancer.htm

National Cancer Institute: Information For People With Cancer
http://rex.nci.nih.gov/PATIENTS/INFO_PEOPL_DOC.html

OncoLink FAQ: Nutrition During Bone Marrow Transplant
www.oncolink.upenn.edu/support/faq/faq_bmt_diet.html

OncoLink: Nutrition During Cancer Treatment: FAQs
www.oncolink.upenn.edu/support/nutrition/faq

OncoLink: Onco Tip: Macrobiotic Diet
www.oncolink.upenn.edu/support/tips/tip24.html

OncoLink: Onco Tip: Megadose Vitamin C
www.oncolink.upenn.edu/support/tips/tip25.html

OncoLink: Tips For Conquering Eating Problems
www.oncolink.upenn.edu/specialty/med_onc/bmt/newsletter/N34/eat_tips.html

OncoLink: NCI/PDQ Physician Statement: Nutrition
www.oncolink.upenn.edu/pdq_html/3/engl/304467.html

People Against Cancer Home Page
http://main.dodgenet.com/nocancer/index.html

Prevention of Major Medical Problems With Diet
www.neat-schoolhouse.org/diet-prev.html

Recipes For Better Nutrition During Cancer Treatment
http://cancernet.nci.nih.gov/eating_hints/eatrecipes.html

University of Texas Center for Alternative Medicine Research in Cancer
www.sph.uth.tmc.edu:8052/utcam

University of Texas Center for Alternative Medicine Research in Cancer: Gerson Program
www.sph.uth.tmc.edu:8052/utcam/summary/gerson.htm

University of Texas Center for Alternative Medicine Research in Cancer: Green Tea
www.sph.uth.tmc.edu:8052/utcam/summary/greentea.htm

University of Texas Center for Alternative Medicine Research in Cancer: Hoxsey
www.sph.uth.tmc.edu:8052/utcam/summary/hoxsey.htm

University of Texas Center for Alternative Medicine Research in Cancer: Macrobiotics
www.sph.uth.tmc.edu:8052/utcam/therapies/macrobiotic.htm

University of Texas Center for Alternative Medicine Research in Cancer: Mistletoe
www.sph.uth.tmc.edu:8052/utcam/summary/mistletoe.htm

University of Texas Center for Alternative Medicine Research in Cancer: Research in Progress
www.sph.uth.tmc.edu:8052/utcam/resact.htm

University of Texas Center for Alternative Medicine Research in Cancer: Corilous Versicolor
www.sph.uth.tmc.edu:8052/utcam/summary/coriolus.htm

University of Texas Center for Alternative Medicine Research in Cancer: Reviews of Therapies
www.sph.uth.tmc.edu:8052/utcam/therapy.htm

FAQs

FAQs are frequently asked questions. These are a few sites where your questions may already have been answered. If you don't see the answer, some sites allow you to submit your question.

American Cancer Society: Common Questions About Diet & Cancer
http://www2.cancer.org/prevention/index.cfm?prevention=questions

American Diabetes Association: FAQs About Nutrition & Diabetes
www.diabetes.org/nutrition/faqs.asp

Children With Diabetes: Ask The Diabetes Team: Meal Planning, Food & Diet
www.childrenwithdiabetes.com/dteam/d_0d_01b.htm

IFIC: Questions & Answers About Cancer, Diet, & Fats
http://ificinfo.health.org/qanda/diet_cancer.htm

Ketogenic Option: FAQs
http://members.aol.com/ketoption4/faq.htm

OncoLink: Nutrition During Cancer Treatment: FAQs
www.oncolink.upenn.edu/support/nutrition/faq

Stanford Medical Center: FAQs About the Ketogenic Diet
www.stanford.edu/group/ketodiet/FAQ.html

Food Allergies

According to the American Dietetic Association, one of three people believe they have a food allergy, but the fact is that only 1% of adults have a true food allergy. Learn more about food allergies and food intolerances with these sites.

American Dietetic Association: Food Allergies
www.eatright.org/nfs/nfs47.html

Ask the Dietician: Allergies
www.dietitian.com/allergie.html

Dietsite.com: Information on Flours & Thickening Agents
www.dietsite.com/Diets/FoodSensitivities/Gluten%20Free%20Flours
%20&%20Thickening%20Agents.htm

Eat Well, Live Well: Food Allergy
www.healthyeating.org/general/food-allergy.htm

Food Allergy Network
www.foodallergy.org

Food Allergy Network: Facts & Fiction
www.foodallergy.org/facts_fiction.html

Food Allergy Network: Food Allergy Research
www.foodallergy.org/research.html

Mayo Clinic Health Oasis: Food Allergies - Widely Misunderstood
www.mayohealth.org/mayo/9908/htm/foodal.htm?ref=nutrition

    National Food Safety Database: Beware the Unknown Brew: Herbal Teas & Toxicity
        www.foodsafety.org/sf/sf184.htm

    National Food Safety Database: Consumer's Guide to Natural Toxicants in Food
        www.foodsafety.org/fs/fs044.htm

Gluten-Free Diets

Celiac disease is marked by an intolerance of gluten and may affect as many as 1 in 300 people. The Web has some good sites for finding help for living with a gluten-free diet.

    American Dietetic Association: Food Allergies
        www.eatright.org/nfs/nfs47.html

    Ask the Dietician: Allergies
        www.dietitian.com/allergie.html

    Dietsite.com: Information on Flours & Thickening Agents
        www.dietsite.com/Diets/FoodSensitivities/Gluten%20Free%20Flours%20&%20Thickening%20Agents.htm

    Eat Well, Live Well: Food Allergy
        www.healthyeating.org/general/food-allergy.htm

    Food Allergy Network
        www.foodallergy.org

    Food Allergy Network: Facts & Fiction
        www.foodallergy.org/facts_fiction.html

    Food Allergy Network: Food Allergy Research
        www.foodallergy.org/research.html

    Mayo Clinic Health Oasis: Food Allergies - Widely Misunderstood
        www.mayohealth.org/mayo/9908/htm/foodal.htm?ref=nutrition

    National Food Safety Database: Beware the Unknown Brew: Herbal Teas & Toxicity
        www.foodsafety.org/sf/sf184.htm

    National Food Safety Database: Consumer's Guide to Natural Toxicants in Food
        www.foodsafety.org/fs/fs044.htm

Living With HIV/AIDS

Unfortunately, there is no diet to decrease the risk of contracting HIV. However, there are many nutrition sites to help maximize the body's defenses. Be sure to visit the food safety sites, which are of paramount importance.

    AIDS Project LA: Positive Living Newsletter: Good Nutrition & HIV
        www.thebody.com/apla/sep98/nutrition.html

    AIDS-Related Quackery & Fraud
        www.quackwatch.com/01QuackeryRelatedTopics/aids.html

American Dietetic Association:
Nutrition Intervention in the Care of Persons With HIV
  www.eatright.org/ahivinter.html

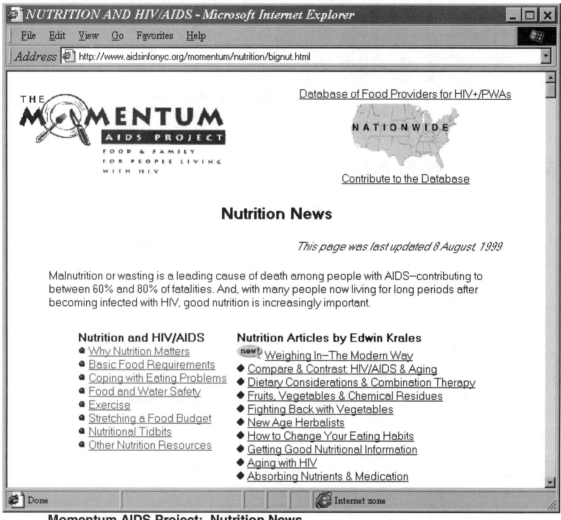

Momentum AIDS Project: Nutrition News
  www.aidsinfonyc.org/momentum/nutrition/bignut.html

POZ Magazine
  www.poz.com

POZ Partner: Grandma's Recipe
  www.thebody.com/poz/survival/7_99/diet.html

POZ: All You Can Eat
  www.thebody.com/poz/survival/4_99/diet.html

The Body:
Alternative & Complementary Treatments, Including Natural & Herbal Remedies
  www.thebody.com/treat/herbal.html

The Body: An AIDS & HIV Information Resource
  www.thebody.com/index.shtml

The Body: Diet & Nutrition
www.thebody.com/dietnut.html

The Body: Diet & Nutrition: Vitamins
www.thebody.com/dietnut/vitamins.html

The Body: Forum On Wasting, Diet, Nutrition & Exercise
www.thebody.com/cgi/wastingans.html

USDA/FSIS: Food Safety for Persons With AIDS
www.fsis.usda.gov/OA/pubs/aids.htm

Wellness Web: Nutrition Tips For People Living With AIDS
www.wellweb.com/nutri/living_with_aids.htm

Migraines & Food Triggers

Many things can trigger a migraine headache. These sites discuss food triggers. Click quietly and check out these web sites.

American Dietetic Association: Migraine Headaches & Food
www.eatright.org/nfs/nfs48.html

Ask the Dietician: Headaches & Migraines
www.dietitian.com/headaches.html

Migraine Awareness Group
www.migraines.org

Migraines and MSG
www.magicnet.net/~btnature

National Institutes of Health: Headache: Hope Through Research
www.ninds.nih.gov/patients/disorder/headache/head2.htm

Quizzes

Check your knowledge base by taking some quick tests.

American Diabetes Association: Feed Your Brain: Nutrition Quiz
www.diabetes.org/nutrition/i_quiz.asp

American Diabetes Association: Wordplay
www.diabetes.org/nutrition/herbs_puzzle.asp

Delicious Decisions from the AHA: Step by Step
www.deliciousdecisions.org/ss/index.html

Recipes

Sample some recipes from these sites if you're interested in lifestyle changes for your health.

American Diabetes Association: Recipe of the Day
www.diabetes.org/recipes/072099.asp

Children With Diabetes: Readers' Favorite Recipes
www.childrenwithdiabetes.com/d_08_200.htm

DASH Diet Navigation Page
http://dash.bwh.harvard.edu./dashdiet.html

Delicious Decisions from the American Heart Association
www.deliciousdecisions.org

Dietsite.com: Sample Menu For Gluten Free Diet
www.dietsite.com/Diets/FoodSensitivities/Menu%20For%20Gluten%20
Free%20Diet.htm

Gluten-Free Recipes & Cooking Tips
www.celiac.com/recipes.html

Ketogenic Diet
www.ketogenic.org

Recipes For Better Nutrition During Cancer Treatment
http://cancernet.nci.nih.gov/eating_hints/eatrecipes.html

Reducing Risk of Heart Disease & Stroke

Heart and blood vessel diseases remain America's number one killer. As our population ages, more people are at a higher risk. These sites help us to adopt lifestyle changes so that we may reduce risk factors that make us vulnerable to these diseases.

American Dietetic Association: Soluble Fiber & Heart Disease
www.eatright.org/nfs/nfs88.html

American Heart Association
www.americanheart.org

American Heart Association: An Eating Plan For Healthy Americans
www.americanheart.org/catalog/Health_catpage5.html

American Heart Association: Cholesterol
www.americanheart.org/Heart_and_Stroke_A_Z_Guide/choldi.html

American Heart Association: Diet & Nutrition
www.americanheart.org/catalog/Health_catpage4.html

American Heart Association: Dietary Recommendations
www.americanheart.org/catalog/Health_catpage5.html

American Heart Association: Dietary/Lifestyle Interventions & the AHA Diet
www.americanheart.org/Heart_and_Stroke_A_Z_Guide/dietlife.html

Better Health: Dean Ornish M.D.: Key Elements of His Program
www.betterhealth.com/ornish/articles/gen/0,4260,6754_125300,00.html

Better Health: Dean Ornish, M.D.
www.betterhealth.com/ornish/

Delicious Decisions from the AHA: Step by Step
www.deliciousdecisions.org/ss/index.html

Healthy Heart Handbook for Women
www.nih.gov/health/chip/nhlbi/heart

Healthy Heart Handbook for Women: Major Risk Factors
www.nih.gov/health/chip/nhlbi/heart/bheart.htm

Healthy Heart Handbook for Women: Prevention
www.nih.gov/health/chip/nhlbi/heart/cheart.htm

Healthy Heart Handbook for Women: The Healthy Heart
www.nih.gov/health/chip/nhlbi/heart/aheart.htm

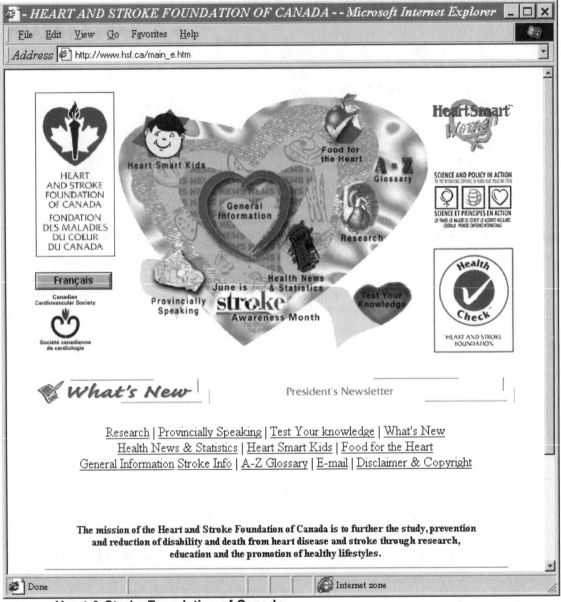

Heart & Stroke Foundation of Canada
www.hsf.ca/main_e.htm

Heart Watch Newsletter
www.betterhealth.com/heartwatch/jul99

Heart Watch Newsletter: Can Vitamin E Pills Protect the Heart?
www.betterhealth.com/seniors/alternative/nejm/0,4802,1958_124100,00.html

Heart Watch: Fiber Lowers Heart Disease Risk in Women
www.betterhealth.com/nejm/0,4802,7016_127321,00.html

HeartInfo Nutrition Guide
www.heartinfo.com/nutrition/nutrhrtdisease1297.htm

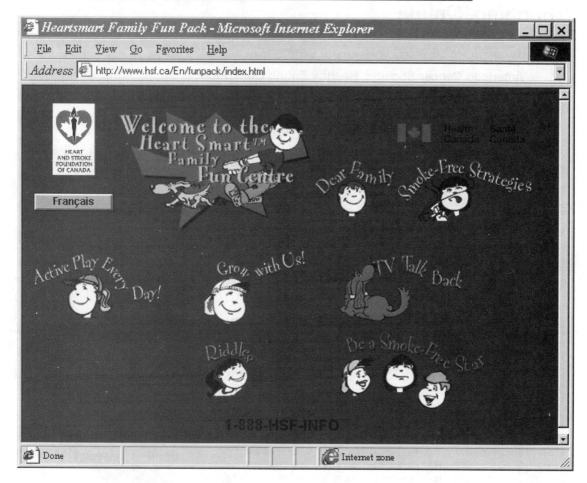

Heartsmart Family Fun Pack
www.hsf.ca/En/funpack/index.html

Nutrition Action Healthletter: Healing Broken Hearts
www.cspinet.org/nah/6_99/heart.htm

Prevention of Major Medical Problems With Diet
www.neat-schoolhouse.org/diet-prev.html

Women of the Baby Boom: Time to Get Heart Smart
http://primusweb.com/fitnesspartner/library/activity/femheart.htm

Shopping Online

Buy everything online from cookbooks to mushrooms.

American Cancer Society: Healthy Eating Cookbook
www.cancer.org/bookstore/cook_exc.html

Diabetes.Store
http://merchant.diabetes.org/adabooks/Default.asp

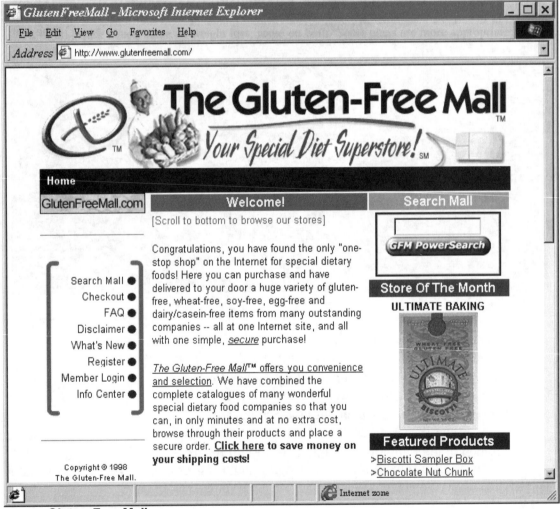

Gluten-Free Mall
www.glutenfreemall.com

JHS Natural Products: Coriolus
www.jhsnp.com/about_coriolus.html

JHS Natural Products: PSK Mushrooms
www.jhsnp.com/index2.html

Sites for Underweight People

Although being underweight is not necessarily a disease in itself, it can be a problem. Sudden, unexplained weight loss deserves the attention of your doctor. But if it's a chronic condition that you'd like to remedy, try these sites.

**American Dietetic Association: Gaining Weight -
A Healthy Plan for Adding Pounds**
www.eatright.org/nfs/nfs10.html

Ask the Dietician: Underweight
www.dietitian.com/underwei.html

Dietsite.com: High Calorie & Protein Diet
www.dietsite.com/SportsNutrition/high_calorie_and_protein_diet.htm

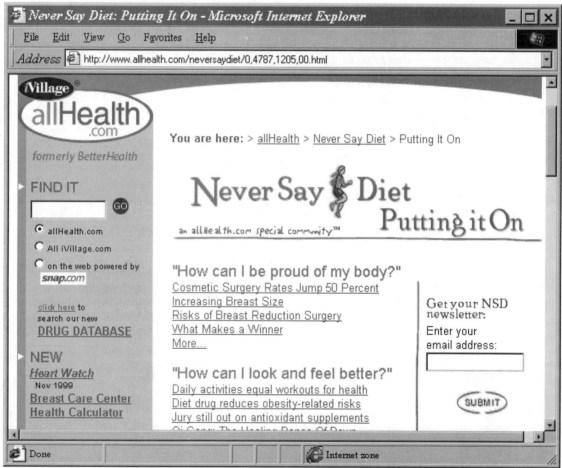

Never Say Diet: Putting It On
www.betterhealth.com/neversaydiet/0,4787,1205,00.html

Weight Gain Products
www.jumbomart.com/products/index.php/c/3

Software

You can download these software programs and give them a try.

Ketogenic Diet Software
www.infinet.com/~ophir/keto

NutriGenie Diabetes Meal Planner
http://users.aol.com/nutrigenie/ngdmp44.html

NutriGenie: Managing Diabetes Version 3.6 For Windows
http://users.aol.com/nutrigenie/nsmd36.html

Supplements for Alternative Medicine

The sites listed here can supply you with the supplements you may need if you're pursuing alternative treatment for your particular kind of cancer. Of course, your doctor or oncologist must be kept informed, and hopefully, in agreement.

CancerGuide: Bovine Cartilage
http://cancerguide.org/btc.html

CancerGuide: PSK
http://cancerguide.org/psk.html

CancerGuide: Simone Shark Cartilage Protocol
http://cancerguide.org/simone_prot.html

JHS Natural Products: Coriolus
www.jhsnp.com/about_coriolus.html

University of Texas Center for Alternative Medicine Research in Cancer: Green Tea
www.sph.uth.tmc.edu:8052/utcam/summary/greentea.htm

University of Texas Center for Alternative Medicine Research in Cancer: Corilous Versicolor
www.sph.uth.tmc.edu:8052/utcam/summary/coriolus.htm

Treating Epilepsy With Ketogenic Diets

The ketogenic diet is a special method of treating seizure disorders. If you are considering undertaking something like this, seek help from your healthcare provider first. Find out the details of what this diet is and how it works.

Keto Perfect
http://lonestar.texas.net/~jsaravia/epilepsy.html

Ketogenic Diet
www.ketogenic.org

Ketogenic Diet Programs
www.stanford.edu/group/ketodiet/ketocenters.html

Ketogenic Diet Software
www.infinet.com/~ophir/keto

Ketogenic Option, The
http://member.aol.com/ketooption

Ketogenic Option: FAQs
http://members.aol.com/ketoption4/faq.htm

Stanford Medical Center: FAQs About the Ketogenic Diet
www.stanford.edu/group/ketodiet/FAQ.html

Stanford Medical Center: Ketogenic Diet Program
www.stanford.edu/group/ketodiet

Stanford Medical Center: Ketogenic Diet Resources
www.stanford.edu/group/ketodiet/ketores.html

Women & Heart Disease

Coronary heart disease is also a woman's concern. Over ten million American women of all ages suffer from heart disease and over 245,000 women die each year. But by taking an active role in their own disease prevention they can dramatically cut their risks. To that end, check out these sites.

American Dietetic Association: Nutrition & Health Campaign for Women: Breast Cancer & Nutrition
www.eatright.org/womenshealth/breastcancer.html

American Heart Association: Women, Heart Disease and Stroke
www.americanheart.org/Heart_and_Stroke_A_Z_Guide/women.html

American Heart Association: Women, Heart Disease and Stroke Statistics
www.americanheart.org/Heart_and_Stroke_A_Z_Guide/womens.html

Healthy Heart Handbook for Women
www.nih.gov/health/chip/nhlbi/heart

Healthy Heart Handbook for Women: Major Risk Factors
www.nih.gov/health/chip/nhlbi/heart/bheart.htm

Healthy Heart Handbook for Women: Prevention
www.nih.gov/health/chip/nhlbi/heart/cheart.htm

Healthy Heart Handbook for Women: The Healthy Heart
www.nih.gov/health/chip/nhlbi/heart/aheart.htm

Heart Watch: Fiber Lowers Heart Disease Risk in Women
www.betterhealth.com/nejm/0,4802,7016_127321,00.html

Women of the Baby Boom: Time to Get Heart Smart
http://primusweb.com/fitnesspartner/library/activity/femheart.htm

More Sites - Directories & Links

For further in-depth study on any of these subjects, these directories will help you out.

American Heart Association
www.americanheart.org

American Heart Association: Heart and Stroke A to Z Guide
www.americanheart.org/Heart_and_Stroke_A_Z_Guide

HeartInfo Nutrition Guide
www.heartinfo.com/nutrition/nutrhrtdisease1297.htm

Joslin Diabetes Center: Recommended Cookbooks & Resource Books
www.joslin.org/education/library/wcbook.html

Ketogenic Diet
www.ketogenic.org

Stanford Medical Center: Ketogenic Diet Resources
www.stanford.edu/group/ketodiet/ketores.html

The Body:
Alternative & Complementary Treatments, Including Natural & Herbal Remedies
www.thebody.com/treat/herbal.html

The Body: An AIDS & HIV Information Resource
www.thebody.com/index.shtml

The Body: Diet & Nutrition
www.thebody.com/dietnut.html

Fitness & High Performance

A healthy weight and lifestyle must include some forms of exercise. Unfortunately, many Americans lead an overly sedate life. We are rendered inactive by automobiles, remote controls, online shopping, and cordless phones among the many other comforts of modern living. According to the AMA, we are the most physically inactive generation that has ever lived. The first law of thermodynamics when applied to nutrition would say that a change in weight is equal to caloric intake minus caloric output. Therefore, if we combine dieting with exercise, we stand a greater chance of losing weight and staying trim. In fact, to lose one pound of fat requires the loss of 3,500 calories. This chapter serves to motivate us and to raise our awareness of the need to exercise.

Calculators, Assessments & Quizzes

How do you measure up? Some of these sites will help you figure your body mass index, how many calories you burn when you do practically anything, and you can even calculate your fitness profile. Try out these interactive and easy to use sites.

American Medical Association Health Insight: Interactive Health
www.ama-assn.org/consumer/interact.htm

Burning Holiday Calories
http://primusweb.com/fitnesspartner/library/activity/holicals.htm

Calorie Control Council: Exercise Calculator
www.caloriecontrol.org/exercalc.html

Calories Burned During Physical Activity
http://www1.mhv.net/~donn/calorie.html

Fitness Zone: Fitness Profile
www.fitnesszone.com/profiles

Healthy Weight--Healthy Steps
www.4meridia.com/consumer/archive/steps/fitness.cfm

Healthy Weight--Healthy Steps Calorie Burning Guide
www.4meridia.com/consumer/archive/steps/cal.cfm

Healthy Weight--Healthy Steps--Walking Test
www.4meridia.com/consumer/archive/steps/walkingtest.cfm

InteliHealth: Home to John Hopkins Health Information: Fitness Quiz
www.intelihealth.com/IH/ihtIH?t=2415&c=81&p=~br,IHW|~st,334|~r,
WSIHW000|~b,*|&d=dmtQuiz

InteliHealth: Home to John Hopkins Health Information: Gadgets & Quizzes
www.intelihealth.com/IH/ihtIH?t=20705&c=225043&p=~br,IHW|~st,14
220|~r,WSIHW000|~b,*|&d=dmtContent

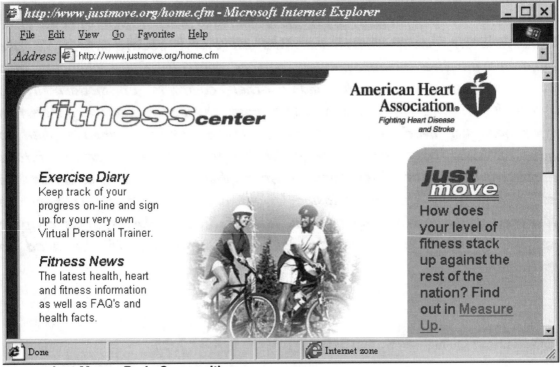

Just Move: Body Composition
www.justmove.org/myfitness/actarticles/acframes.cfm?Target=body
comp.html

Just Move: Healthy Heart Workout Quiz
www.justmove.org/myfitness/lowarticles/lowframes.cfm?Target=www
.justmove.org/myfitness/workoutquiz.cfm

Just Move: Measure Up
www.justmove.org/measureup

Just Move: My Fitness
www.justmove.org/myfitness

Just Move: Physical Activity Calorie Use Chart
www.justmove.org/myfitness/actarticles/acframes.cfm?Target=calo
riechart.html

Just Move: Target Heart Rates
www.justmove.org/myfitness/actarticles/acframes.cfm?Target=hart
rates.html

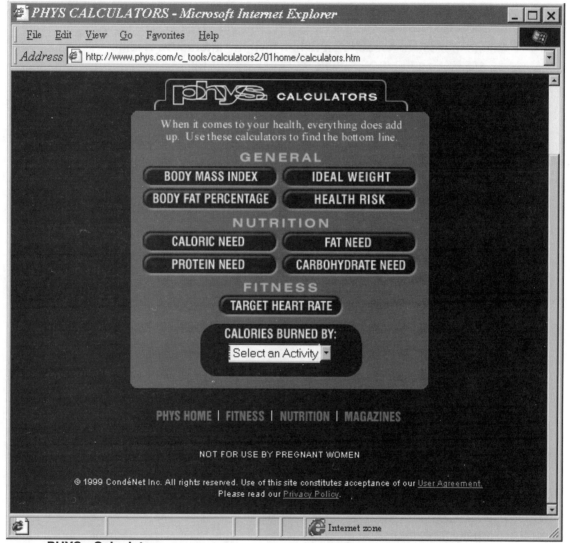

PHYS: Calculators
www.phys.com/c_tools/calculators2/01home/calculators.htm

Shape Up America! Fitness Center - Assessment
www.shapeup.org/fitness/assess/fset2.htm

Thriveonline.com: Are You Fit?
www.thriveonline.com/shape/wgames/gen/shape.fit.html

WeightLoss2000.com: Aerobics: Finding Your Target Heart Rate
http://weightloss2000.com/health_library/exercise/exer_11_aerob
ics.html

WeightLoss2000.com: How Fit Are You?
http://weightloss2000.com/health_library/exercise/exer_01_howfit.html

Getting Started on an Exercise Program

Developing your own fitness plan is not difficult. The hard part is merely getting started. After you've checked in with your healthcare provider, a program can be as simple as a short walk. These sites serve to motivate and inform us about getting started. Ready, set, point and click.

American Medical Association Health Insight: Developing Your Fitness Program
www.ama-assn.org/insight/gen_hlth/trainer/index.htm

American Medical Association Health Insight: Interactive Health
www.ama-assn.org/consumer/interact.htm

American Medical Association: Health Insight: Fitness Basics
www.ama-assn.org/insight/gen_hlth/fitness/fitness.htm

Cardiovascular Machine Workouts
http://primusweb.com/fitnesspartner/library/activity/cardiowork.htm

Colorado State University Cooperative Extension: Nutrition for the Athlete
www.colostate.edu/depts/CoopExt/PUBS/FOODNUT/09362.html

Delicious Decisions from the American Heart Association: Fit Forever
www.deliciousdecisions.org/ff/index.html

Dietsite.com
www.dietsite.com

Drink Up!
http://primusweb.com/fitnesspartner/library/nutrition/fluids.htm

drkoop.com: 10 Basic Stretches
http://drkoop.com/wellness/fitness/exercise/stretch.asp

drkoop.com: Exercise & Diabetes
http://drkoop.com/wellness/fitness/facts/exercise-diabetes.asp

drkoop.com: Exercise & Heart Disease
http://drkoop.com/wellness/fitness/facts/exercise-heart-disease.asp

drkoop.com: Exercise & Obesity
http://drkoop.com/wellness/fitness/facts/exercise-obesity.asp

drkoop.com: Stretching
http://drkoop.com/wellness/fitness/facts/stretching.asp

Fitness Forum
http://primusweb.com/fitnesspartner/forum/forum.htm

Fitness Online: Community
http://216.33.170.201/community.asp

InteliHealth: Home to John Hopkins Health Information: Fundamentals of Fitness
www.intelihealth.com/IH/ihtIH?t=8901&p=~br,IHW|~st,7165|~r,WSIHW000|~b,*|

Just Move: Cyberteams
www.justmove.org/cyberteams

Just Move: Physical Activity
www.justmove.org/myfitness/actarticles/acframes.cfm?Target=exercise.html

Motivation to Move
http://primusweb.com/fitnesspartner/library/activity/motomove.htm

Physical Activity & Health: A Report of the Surgeon General
www.cdc.gov/nccdphp/sgr/sgr.htm

WeightLoss2000.com: Easy Exercises
http://weightloss2000.com/exer

WeightLoss2000.com: What's Stopping You?
http://weightloss2000.com/health_library/exercise/exer_03_whats stop.html

Aerobic & Cardiovascular Exercise

The idea is to get moving, and to enjoy it. Try these sites for a "jump" start.

Aerobics & Fitness Association of America
www.afaa.com

Aerobics & Fitness Association of America: FitTown
www.afaa.com/10010.ASP?1=&1=12

Cardiovascular Exercise Principles & Guidelines: Part I
http://primusweb.com/fitnesspartner/library/activity/gf_guide1.htm

Cardiovascular Exercise Principles & Guidelines: Part II
http://primusweb.com/fitnesspartner/library/activity/gf_guide2.htm

Cyberdiet's Exercise & Fitness Tips
www.cyberdiet.com/exer/exercise.html

drkoop.com: Aerobics
http://drkoop.com/wellness/fitness/facts/aerobics.asp

drkoop.com: Spinning
www.drkoop.com/wellness/fitness/files/spinning.asp

drkoop.com: Swimming
http://drkoop.com/wellness/fitness/facts/swimming.asp

Fitness Find: Cross Training
www.fitnessfind.com/crosstrain.html

Just Move!
www.justmove.org/home.cfm

Just Move: AHA Events Calendar
www.justmove.org/events/August.html

Just Move: Exercise & Your Heart - A Guide to Physical Activity
www.justmove.org/myfitness/actarticles/acframes.cfm?Target=ex_y rhart.html

Just Move: Exercise Diary
www.justmove.org/diary/login.cfm?CFID=22458&CFTOKEN=30300

Just Move: My Fitness
www.justmove.org/myfitness

PHYS: Aerobics
www.phys.com/f_fitness/03encyclopedia/02database/aerobics.html

Understanding Your Training Heart Rate
http://primusweb.com/fitnesspartner/library/activity/thr.htm

WeightLoss2000.com: Aerobics: Finding Your Target Heart Rate
http://weightloss2000.com/health_library/exercise/exer_11_aerobics.html

Bicycling

Bicycling is a fairly stress-free way to exercise. It helps you condition your lower body and can be aerobic. There is no high impact or continuous pounding. The family can also enjoy biking together. Check these sites for a look into the world of bicycling.

drkoop.com: Bicycling
http://drkoop.com/wellness/fitness/facts/bicycling.asp

drkoop.com: Spinning
www.drkoop.com/wellness/fitness/files/spinning.asp

Fitness Find: Bicycling
www.fitnessfind.com/bicycling.html

GORP: Great Outdoor Recreation Pages: Biking
www.gorp.com/gorp/activity/biking.htm

PHYS: Bicycling
www.phys.com/f_fitness/03encyclopedia/02database/bicycling.html

PHYS: Spinning
www.phys.com/f_fitness/03encyclopedia/02database/spinning.html

Thriveonline.com: Biking Tips
www.thriveonline.com/outdoors/bike/biketips/toc.mtbiking.html

E-Zines

E-zines are online magazines. Most articles are concise and make for great, informative reading. Plus, e-zine web sites are colorful, and often have interactive quizzes, calculators, and surveys.

Fitness Zone
www.fitnesszone.com

Fitness Zone: Fitnesszine
www.fitnesszone.com/features

Fitness Zone: Fitnesszine: Archives
www.fitnesszone.com/features/archives

Fitness Zone: Fitnesszine: Sports Nutrition Myths
www.fitnesszone.com/features/archives/jul198/3070698.html

Fitness Zone: Fitnesszine: Staying With the Program
www.fitnesszone.com/features/archives/tips.html

GORP: Great Outdoors Recreation Pages
www.gorp.com/default.htm

Healthy Athlete
   http://bewell.com/healthy/athlete/index.asp

PHYS: Exercise Guide
   www.phys.com/f_fitness/03encyclopedia/01home/exercise.html

PHYS: Fitness Main Page
   www.phys.com/f_fitness/00home/home.htm

Thriveonline.com: Biking Tips
   www.thriveonline.com/outdoors/bike/biketips/toc.mtbiking.html

Thriveonline.com: Fitness
   www.thriveonline.com/fitness/index.html

Thriveonline.com: Hiking & Backpacking
   www.thriveonline.com/outdoors/hike/hikingindex.html

Thriveonline.com: Running
   www.thriveonline.com/outdoors/run/runindex.html

Thriveonline.com: The G.O. Guide
   www.thriveonline.com/outdoors/go-guide/goindex.html

Women.com: Fitness
   www.women.com/fitness

Exercise & Pregnancy

Should you stop exercising when you are pregnant? Should you change your routine? Visit these sites for ideas about structuring or restructuring your fitness plan.

drkoop.com: Exercise & Pregnancy
   http://drkoop.com/wellness/fitness/facts/exercise-pregnancy.asp

FitnessMatters: Running on Full
   http://lifematters.com/rofintro.html

Parent's Place: Exercise During Pregnancy
   http://www4.parentsplace.com/pregnancy/nutrition/gen/0,3375,111
   82,00.html

Pregnancy Today Online: ACOG Guidelines for Exercise in Pregnancy
   www.pregnancytoday.com

Exercise For Older Americans

Older Americans are not exempt from adopting a healthy lifestyle. Slow down the aging clock by logging onto these sites .

drkoop.com: Exercise & the Elderly
   http://drkoop.com/wellness/fitness/facts/exercise-elderly.asp

drkoop.com: Fitness Facts For Older Americans
   http://drkoop.com/wellness/fitness/facts/exercise-older.asp

Fitness News: Health Facts - Exercise Tips For Older Americans
   www.justmove.org/fitnessnews/healthf.cfm?Target=eldertips.html

InteliHealth: Home to John Hopkins Health Information: Fitness & the Elderly
www.intelihealth.com/IH/ihtIH?t=8923&p=~br,IHW|~st,7165|~r,WSIH
W000|~b,*|&

Slowing the Aging Clock
http://primusweb.com/fitnesspartner/library/activity/agingclock.htm

Exercise Sites For Kids & Teens

Our children are becoming increasingly sedate. Their time is filled with passive moments in front of computers, televisions, and video games. Usually their activity level is a reflection of their parents'. Here are some sites to help you find some methods to motivate them.

drkoop.com: Exercise & Your Child
http://drkoop.com/wellness/fitness/facts/exercise-child.asp

Fitness News: Health Facts - Children & the Need for Physical Activity Fact Sheet
www.justmove.org/fitnessnews/healthf.cfm?Target=kidsfacts.html

Fitness News: Health Facts - Exercise & Children
www.justmove.org/fitnessnews/healthf.cfm?Target=exerckids.html

Make Fitness Fun For Kids
http://primusweb.com/fitnesspartner/library/activity/funkids.htm

Mayo Clinic Health Oasis: Diet & Exercise Guidelines For Overweight Children
www.mayohealth.org/mayo/9705/htm/over_2sb.htm

Meet Benny Goodsport & the Goodsport Gang
www.bennygoodsport.com

Frequently Asked Questions

Got a question about fitness? There's a good chance that it's already been asked and the answer you're looking for is here in these sites.

Dietsite.com: Creatine & Sports Performance
www.dietsite.com/SportsNutrition/Creatine%20and%20Sports%20Perf
ormance.htm

Fitness Partner Connection: FAQs
http://primusweb.com/fitnesspartner/library/features/fpcfaq.htm

Fitness Zone: Library
www.fitnesszone.com/library

Fitnessmatters: Frequently Asked Fitness Questions
http://lifematters.com/jackfaq.html

Go Ask Alice: Fitness & Nutrition
www.goaskalice.columbia.edu/Cat3.html

Sports Nutrition Connection: Questions & Answers
http://rampages.onramp.net/~msam/qa.html

I Need Somebody! Chat & Message Boards

Whether you're looking for an online fitness buddy, or you just want to post a message, hang out in these chat rooms and message boards to satisfy your need for interaction.

American Association of Lifestyle Counselors: Forum
www.AALC.org/experts.htm

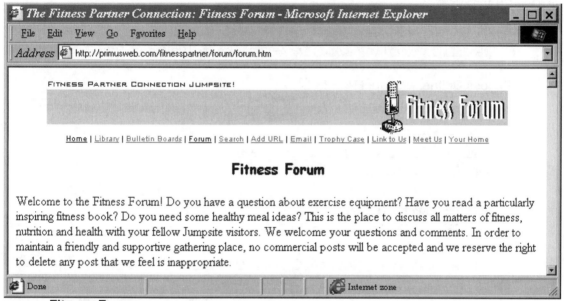

Fitness Forum
http://primusweb.com/fitnesspartner/forum/forum.htm

Fitness Online: Community
http://216.33.170.201/community.asp

Fitness Partner Connection
http://primusweb.com/fitnesspartner/boards/bb01.htm

Fitness Partner Connection: Bulletin Board: Fitness Equipment
http://primusweb.com/fitnesspartner/boards/bb03.htm

Fitness Zone: Forums
www.fitnesszone.com/forums

Just Move: Cyberteams
www.justmove.org/cyberteams

Men's Fitness: Chat
http://216.33.170.200:4080/chat/world/html/login.html?uri=/*index

Men's Fitness: Discussion
http://216.33.170.201/magcommunity/threads.asp?topicID={84F6F35B-281F-11D3-9691-0090277C0BFE}

PHYS: Forums
www.phys.com/d_forums/allforums.html

Thriveonline.com: Message Boards - Backpacking
www.thriveonline.com/cgi-bin/webx.cgi?14@^6762@.ee8ccee

Men & Exercise

Are you looking for that lean and ripped look? Abs of steel? Or are you just looking for some good routines for general fitness? Try these sites.

Bill Pearl Enterprises, Inc.
www.billpearl.com

Fitness Online
www.fitnessonline.com/index.asp

Fitness Online: Fitness Goals
www.fitnessonline.com/fitnessonline/folCategoryTemplates/category.asp?Catid=16

Fitness Online: Personal Profile
www.fitnessonline.com/fitnessonline/folPersonalization/membership.asp

Man's Life: Fitness
www.manslife.com/fitness/bigsweat

Man's Life: Fitness Forum
www.manslife.com/stickit/display/ml_fitness?TOPID=u9Myaxw3

Man's Life: Psycho Trainer
www.manslife.com/fitness/trainer

Men's Fitness
www.mensfitness.com/mensfitness/index.asp?catid=184

Men's Fitness: Chat
http://216.33.170.200:4080/chat/world/html/login.html?uri=/*index

Men's Fitness: Discussion
http://216.33.170.201/magcommunity/threads.asp?topicID={84F6F35B-281F-11D3-9691-0090277C0BFE}

Men's Fitness: Ten Gym Mistakes Beginners Make
www.mensfitness.com/magazines/magViewer/FitnMagArt.asp?Catid=234&Objid={49EC4C5A-2382-11D3-ACE5-00A0244A08DA}&curpage=1&curCatID=184

Men's Health: Personal Trainer
www.menshealth.com/personaltrainer/index.html

Men's Health: Personal Trainer - Scrawny to Brawny
www.menshealth.com/personaltrainer/t2_routines/original_index.html

Men's Health: Personal Trainer - Unbelievable Abs
www.menshealth.com/personaltrainer/t4_routines/original_index.html

Runner's World: Claim Check
www.runnersworld.com/nutrition/nu4supps.html

Runner's World: Energy To Go
www.runnersworld.com/nutrition/gels.html

Runner's World: Performance Pick-Me-Ups
www.runnersworld.com/nutrition/nuperform.html

Runner's World: Taking the Bar
www.runnersworld.com/nutrition/nuenergybar2.html

Runner's World: You Can Take It With You
www.runnersworld.com/nutrition/nuenergybar.html

Sports Nutrition Connection: Dietary Intake & Supplementation: Effects On Testosterone
http://rampages.onramp.net/~msam/misc/testoste.html

News in the World of Fitness

Stay abreast of the latest in fitness research and news with these web sites.

Fitness News from the American Heart Association
www.justmove.org/fitnessnews

Just Move: AHA Events Calendar
www.justmove.org/events/August.html

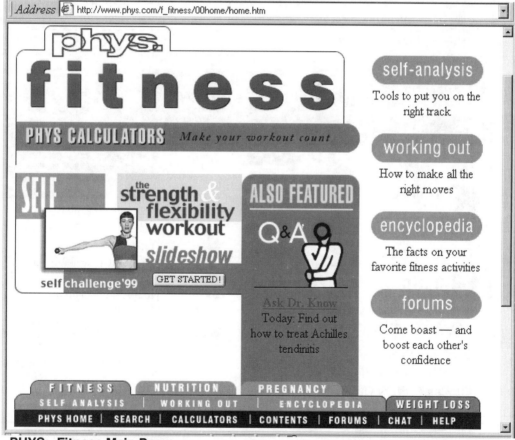

PHYS: Fitness Main Page
www.phys.com/f_fitness/00home/home.htm

Online Shopping

Are you looking for andro or DHEA? How about some fitness equipment? Just make sure the site you choose to use is secure.

American Sports Nutrition
www.fitness-connection.com/American_Sports_Nutrition.htm

AST Sports Science
www.ast-ss.com

BigFitness.com
www.bigfitness.com

Century Sports Nutrition
www.ginns.com/centurysportsnutrition/index.html

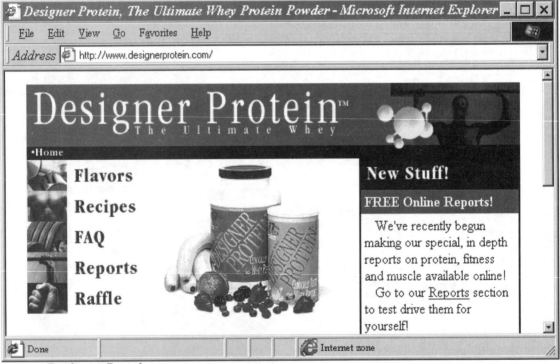

Designer Protein
www.designerprotein.com

Fitness Factory Outlet
www.fitnessfactory.com

Fitness Online: Marketplace
www.fitnessonline.com/marketplace/index.asp?magazine=fitnessonline

Fitness Partner Connection: Bulletin Board: Fitness Equipment
http://primusweb.com/fitnesspartner/boards/bb03.htm

Fitness Zone
www.fitnesszone.com

Fitness Zone: Classifieds
www.fitnesszone.com/classifieds

Fitness Zone: Shop
http://fitnesszone.viper.net/index.htm

MET-Rx Engineered Nutrition
www.met-rx.com

Nutripeak.com: Sports Nutrition For the Serious Athlete
www.nutripeak.com

PowerBar Online
www.powerbar.com

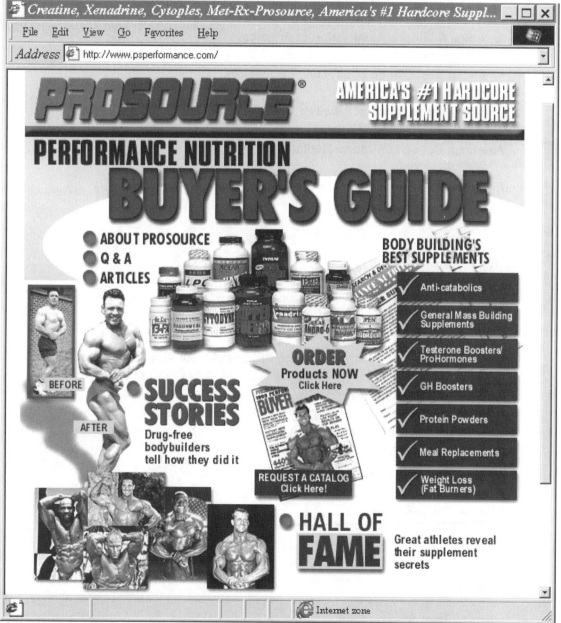

Prosource
www.psperformance.com

USA Sportslabs Inc.
www.usalabs.com/SNGrowth.htm

Valusport.com
http://valusport.com/lib/nutrionline/index.html

Professional Organizations

Some of these Professional Organizations host impressive web sites for the general public as well as for their members.

Aerobics & Fitness Association of America
www.afaa.com

American Association of Lifestyle Counselors
www.AALC.org

American Association of Lifestyle Counselors: Forum
www.AALC.org/experts.htm

American College of Sports Medicine
www.acsm.org

American Council on Exercise
www.acefitness.org

Running

These web sites are designed for both the newcomer and the marathon runner.

Cool Running
www.coolrunning.com

Cool Running: A Walking & Running Program for All Abilities
www.coolrunning.com/major/97/training/swit0214.htm

Cool Running: Basic Training Site
www.coolrunning.com/training/indexbegin.shtml

Cool Running: Sole Searching
www.coolrunning.com/training/shoes.shtml

Cyberdiet's Exercise & Fitness Tips
www.cyberdiet.com/exer/exercise.html

drkoop.com: Jogging
http://drkoop.com/wellness/fitness/facts/jogging.asp

Fitness Find: Running
www.fitnessfind.com/running.html

New Runner
www.newrunner.com

New Runner: Step by Step
www.newrunner.com/step

New Runner: Why Run?
www.newrunner.com/whyrun.html

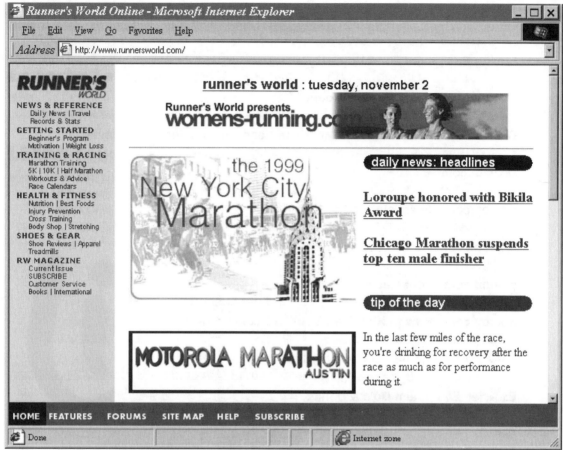

Runner's World Online
www.runnersworld.com

Runner's World: Fluid Fluency
www.runnersworld.com/nutrition/nufluids.html

Thriveonline.com: Running
www.thriveonline.com/outdoors/run/runindex.html

Motivation & Support

Even after we're exercising, there comes a time when we get bored with it, or we wonder if it is really worth the time and effort. These sites give us some ideas to turn it up a notch when we are faltering.

Active Living Canada
http://activeliving.ca/activeliving/alc.html

American Medical Association Health Insight: Developing Your Fitness Program
www.ama-assn.org/insight/gen_hlth/trainer/index.htm

American Medical Association: Health Insight: Fitness Basics
www.ama-assn.org/insight/gen_hlth/fitness/fitness.htm

Battling Boredom
http://primusweb.com/fitnesspartner/library/activity/battlebore dom.htm

Buying Equipment For a Home Gym
http://primusweb.com/fitnesspartner/library/features/0298hmgym.htm

Cardiovascular Machine Workouts
http://primusweb.com/fitnesspartner/library/activity/cardiowork.htm

Delicious Decisions from the American Heart Association: Fit Forever
www.deliciousdecisions.org/ff/index.html

Dietsite.com
www.dietsite.com

drkoop.com: Exercising to Lose Weight
www.drkoop.com/wellness/fitness/files/ex2-lose-wght.asp

drkoop.com: Fitness Center
www.drkoop.com/wellness/fitness

drkoop.com: Four Get Fit
http://drkoop.com/wellness/fitness/four_fit

drkoop.com: How to Kick Start Your Exercise Program
www.drkoop.com/wellness/fitness/files/exercise-program.asp

Easy Ways to Boost Your Activity Level
http://primusweb.com/fitnesspartner/library/activity/activity.htm

Exercise Equipment Do's & Don'ts
http://primusweb.com/fitnesspartner/library/equipment/equip01.htm

Exercise Errors
http://primusweb.com/fitnesspartner/library/activity/errors.htm

Fitness Jumpsite!
http://primusweb.com/fitnesspartner/index.html

Fitness Online: Fitness Goals
www.fitnessonline.com/fitnessonline/folCategoryTemplates/catego ry.asp?Catid=16

Fitness Partner Connection
http://primusweb.com/fitnesspartner/boards/bb01.htm

Fitness Zone: Fitnesszine: Archives
www.fitnesszone.com/features/archives/

Fitness Zone: Fitnesszine: Staying With the Program
www.fitnesszone.com/features/archives/tips.html

Fitness Zone: Join
www.fitnesszone.com/join

Fitting In Fitness
http://primusweb.com/fitnesspartner/library/activity/fittingfit nessin.htm

InteliHealth: Home to John Hopkins Health Information: Fitness & Sports Medicine
www.intelihealth.com/IH/ihtIH?t=7165&p=~br,IHW|~st,7165|~r,WSIH W000|~b,*|

InteliHealth: Home to John Hopkins Health Information: Fundamentals of Fitness
www.intelihealth.com/IH/ihtIH?t=8901&p=~br,IHW|~st,7165|~r,WSIH
W000|~b,*|

InteliHealth: Home to John Hopkins Health Information: Starting a Fitness Program
www.intelihealth.com/IH/ihtIH?t=8916&p=~br,IHW|~st,7165|~r,WSIH
W000|~b,*|

Just Move: My Fitness
www.justmove.org/myfitness

Just Move: Physical Activity
www.justmove.org/myfitness/actarticles/acframes.cfm?Target=exercise.html

Just Move: The Benefits of Daily Physical Activity
www.justmove.org/myfitness/actarticles/acframes.cfm?Target=dailybene.html

Making Time For Strength Training
http://primusweb.com/fitnesspartner/library/activity/traintime.htm

Mass Attack
www.geocities.com/HotSprings/Spa/9598/home.html

Motivation to Move
http://primusweb.com/fitnesspartner/library/activity/motomove.htm

PHYS: Exercise Guide
www.phys.com/f_fitness/03encyclopedia/01home/exercise.html

Shape Up America! Fitness Center
www.shapeup.org/fitness/index.htm

Shape Up America! Fitness Center - Improvement
www.shapeup.org/fitness/improve/fset4.htm

Starting An Exercise Program
http://primusweb.com/fitnesspartner/library/activity/startexercise.htm

Stretching & Flexibility
http://galway.informatik.uni-kl.de/staff/weidmann/pages/stretch/stretching_toc.html

Thriveonline.com: Fitness
www.thriveonline.com/fitness/index.html

WeightLoss2000.com: A Little Exercise:
Weight Loss Is Just One of Many Benefits
http://weightloss2000.com/health_library/exercise/exer_02_alittle.html

WeightLoss2000.com: What's Stopping You?
http://weightloss2000.com/health_library/exercise/exer_03_whatsstop.html

What's Your Excuse?
http://primusweb.com/fitnesspartner/library/activity/excuses.htm

Sports Nutrition

Sports drinks, energy bars, ergogenic aids, DHEA, creatine, whey: these are but a few of the supplements athletes are trying for enhanced performance. Do they work? These sites will guide you through the confusing maze of sports nutrition.

American Dietetic Association: Athletes Fuel Up For Fitness
www.eatright.org/nfs/nfs0.html

American Dietetic Association:
Nutrition for Physical Fitness & Athletic Performance
www.eatright.org/afitperform.html

American Dietetic Association: Tip: Sports Nutrition Game Plan
www.eatright.org/erm/erm012699.html

Colorado State University Cooperative Extension: Nutrition for the Athlete
www.colostate.edu/depts/CoopExt/PUBS/FOODNUT/09362.html

Dietsite.com: Creatine & Sports Performance
www.dietsite.com/SportsNutrition/Creatine%20and%20Sports%20Perf
ormance.htm

Dietsite.com: Diet to Improve Performance
www.dietsite.com/SportsNutrition/improved%20Performance%20Diet.htm

Dietsite.com: Dietary Goals for Improved Performance
www.dietsite.com/SportsNutrition/Performance%20Diet's%20Goals.htm

Dietsite.com: Ergogenic Aids
www.dietsite.com/SportsNutrition/Ergogenic%20Aids.html

Dietsite.com: Guidelines for Using Sports Food
www.dietsite.com/SportsNutrition/guidelines_for_using_sports_food.
htm

Dietsite.com: High Calorie & Protein Diet
www.dietsite.com/SportsNutrition/high_calorie_and_protein_diet.htm

Dietsite.com: High Calorie/High Protein Recipes
www.dietsite.com/Diets/AIDSCancer/CalorieProtein/High%20Calorie
%20&%20Protein%20Recipes.htm

Dietsite.com: Nutrients for Athletes
www.dietsite.com/SportsNutrition/NutrientsAthletes/nutrients_2.htm

Dietsite.com: Ranking the Sports Drinks
www.dietsite.com/SportsNutrition/Ranking%20the%20Sports%20Drinks.h
tml

Dietsite.com: Sports Drinks
www.dietsite.com/SportsNutrition/Sports%20Drinks.htm

Dietsite.com: Sports Nutrition
www.dietsite.com/SportsNutrition/index.htm

Dietsite.com: Sports Performance & Caffeine
www.dietsite.com/SportsNutrition/Caffeine%20and%20Sports%20Perf
ormance.htm

Fitness Zone: Fitnesszine: Sports Nutrition Myths
www.fitnesszone.com/features/archives/jul98/3070698.html

FitnessLink: Choosing Bodybuilding Supplements
www.fitnesslink.com/food/supps.htm

FitnessLink: Eating For Energy
www.fitnesslink.com/food/energy.htm

FitnessLink: Searching the Galaxy For the Ultimate Thirst Quencher
www.fitnesslink.com/food/water.htm

FitnessLink: Sports Nutrition Supplements Mislabeled & Misleading
www.fitnesslink.com/food/mislabel.htm

Healthy Athlete: Energy Bars & Gels
http://bewell.com/healthy/athlete/1999/barsgels/index.asp

InteliHealth: Home to John Hopkins Health Information: Sports Nutrition
www.intelihealth.com/IH/ihtIH?t=8933&p=~br,IHW|~st,7165|~r,WSIH
W000|~b,*|

Mayo Clinic Health Oasis: DHEA - Hype or Health
www.mayohealth.org/mayo/9612/htm/dhea.htm

Mayo Clinic Health Oasis: Energy Gels
www.mayohealth.org/mayo/9510/htm/energyge.htm

Mayo Clinic Health Oasis: Muscle-Building: Do Andro & Creatine Work?
www.mayohealth.org/mayo/9811/htm/muscle.htm

Men's Health: Sports Nutrition
www.menshealth.com/features/eat_this/sports/index.html

MET-Rx Engineered Nutrition
www.met-rx.com

Peakhealth.net: Pre & Post Workout Nutrition: Research Review
www.peakhealth.net/article.cfm?article_id=12435&action=article

PowerBar Online
www.powerbar.com

Sports Nutrition Connection
http://rampages.onramp.net/~msam/home.html

Sports Nutrition Connection: An Overview of Ketogenic Diets
http://rampages.onramp.net/~msam/index.html

Sports Nutrition Connection:
Basic Nutritional Considerations For the Endurance Athlete
http://rampages.onramp.net/~msam/enduranc/basicE.html

Sports Nutrition Connection:
Basic Nutritional Considerations for the Strength Athlete/Bodybuilder
http://rampages.onramp.net/~msam/strength/basicS.html

Sports Nutrition Connection:
Dietary Intake & Supplementation: Effects On Testosterone
http://rampages.onramp.net/~msam/misc/testoste.html

Sports Nutrition Connection: How to Get Lean & Ripped
http://rampages.onramp.net/~msam/strength/ripped.html

Sports Nutrition Connection: Nutrition For Gaining Muscle Mass
http://rampages.onramp.net/~msam/strength/weightga.html

Sports Nutrition Connection: Questions & Answers
http://rampages.onramp.net/~msam/qa.html

Sports Nutrition Connection: **The Beneficial Effects of Fat**
http://rampages.onramp.net/~msam/enduranc/fat.html

Sports Nutrition Connection: **Why Water Is The Most Important Nutrient**
http://rampages.onramp.net/~msam/enduranc/water.html

Wellness Web: **Chromium Picolinate**
www.wellweb.com/nutri/chromium_picolinate.htm

Strength Training

It isn't just for men anymore. Recent research is revealing the importance of strength training for the bone health of everyone. You really don't have to have mirrored walls, or grunt, and make funny faces either!

American Dietetic Association: Fitness & Bone Health
www.eatright.org/nfs/nfs38.html

Bill Pearl Enterprises, Inc.
www.billpearl.com

Cyberpump!
www.cyberpump.com

drkoop.com: Muscular Fitness Exercise
http://drkoop.com/wellness/fitness/facts/muscular-fitness.asp

FitnessLink: Pre-Contest Dieting Simplified
www.fitnesslink.com/food/contest.htm

Fitness Online: Strength Training
www.fitnessonline.com/fitnessonline/folCategoryTemplates/category.asp?Catid=12

Griffin's Weightlifting Page: Weighty Matters
http://weber.u.washington.edu/~griffin/weights.html

IFIC: A Fountain of Youth
http://ificinfo.health.org/insight/janfeb98/fountain.htm

JPFS Workouts
www.jeanpaul.com/workouts.html

Making Time For Strength Training
http://primusweb.com/fitnesspartner/library/activity/traintime.htm

Mayo Clinic Health Oasis: Weight Training
www.mayohealth.org/mayo/9905/htm/weight.htm

PHYS: Weight Training
www.phys.com/f_fitness/03encyclopedia/02database/weights.html

Sports Nutrition Connection:
Basic Nutritional Considerations for the Strength Athlete/Bodybuilder
http://rampages.onramp.net/~msam/strength/basicS.html

Strength Training Basics
http://primusweb.com/fitnesspartner/library/activity/trainbasics.htm

Walking

Here's an exercise for both the rich and poor. The equipment needed is minimal. Dress for the weather and go for a walk. Plus, these sites have many good ideas to help keep your walks interesting.

Cool Running: A Walking & Running Program for All Abilities
www.coolrunning.com/major/97/training/swit0214.htm

Cyberdiet's Exercise & Fitness Tips
www.cyberdiet.com/exer/exercise.html

drkoop.com: Walking
http://drkoop.com/wellness/fitness/facts/walking.asp

Fitness Find: Walking
www.fitnessfind.com/walking.html

Health Steps
www.ghc.org/health_info/self/fitness/hlthstep.html

Healthy Weight--Healthy Steps--Walking Test
www.4meridia.com/consumer/archive/steps/walkingtest.cfm

PHYS: Walking
www.phys.com/f_fitness/03encyclopedia/02database/walking.html

Physician & Sports Medicine: Exercising When You're Overweight
www.physsportsmed.com/issues/oct_96/weight.htm

Seven Simple Steps to Help You Walk Your Weight Off
www.4meridia.com/consumer/archive/steps/tips.cfm

Thriveonline.com: Hiking & Backpacking
www.thriveonline.com/outdoors/hike/hikingindex.html

Thriveonline.com: Message Boards - Backpacking
www.thriveonline.com/cgi-bin/webx.cgi?14@^6762@.ee8ccee

Walking Connection
www.walkingconnection.com/index.html

Walking Connection With Jo Ann Taylor
www.walkingconnection.com/Walking_Training.html

Walking Connection: FAQs, Concerns, & Potential Problems
www.walkingconnection.com/Walking_Tips.html

Walking For Exercise & Pleasure
www.hoptechno.com/book9.htm

WeightLoss2000.com: Walking: Getting Started
http://weightloss2000.com/health_library/exercise/exer_07_walkstart.html

WeightLoss2000.com: Walking: Humanity's Oldest Exercise Helps Control Weight
http://weightloss2000.com/health_library/exercise/exer_06_walkintro.html

Women's Fitness

These sites approach fitness and exercise from a woman's perspective, and address concerns unique to women.

Bill Pearl Enterprises, Inc.
www.billpearl.com

Fitness Online
www.fitnessonline.com/index.asp

Fitness Online: Fitness Goals
www.fitnessonline.com/fitnessonline/folCategoryTemplates/category.asp?Catid=16

Fitness Online: Personal Profile
www.fitnessonline.com/fitnessonline/folPersonalization/membership.asp

New York Times on the Web: Women's Health: Diet & Exercise
www.nytimes.com/specials/women/whome/diet_exercise.html

Women & Physical Activity: A Historical Journey
http://primusweb.com/fitnesspartner/library/activity/womenhistory.htm

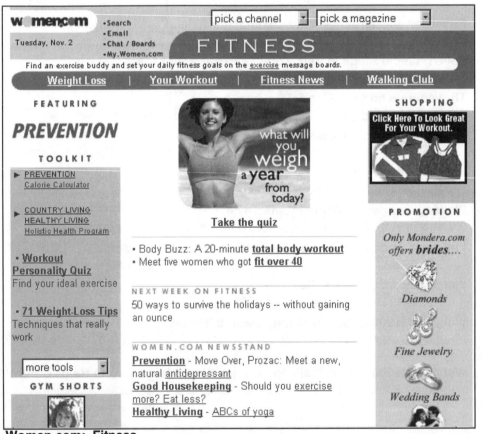

Women.com: Fitness
www.women.com/fitness

Yoga

Yoga exercises are designed to ease muscle tension and to improve the flexibility of the body's joints and ligaments. It is a complete fitness program and will releae endorphins in the brain as well as any other exercise. Yoga can also be very relaxing with its meditative qualities. Visit these sites for more information about Yoga.

Fitness Online: Mind & Body
www.fitnessonline.com/fitnessonline/folCategoryTemplates/SuperCategory.asp?CatID=6

World of Yoga
www.yogaworld.org

Yoga for Beginners
www.mv.com/ipusers/howell/ejh

Yoga for Busy People
www.indolink.com/Health/Yoga/yoga2.html

YogaClass.com
www.yogaclass.com

More Exercise Online - Directories & Links

If you are interested in investigating an aspect of exercise or fitness in greater depth, try these sites for further study.

Fitness Find: Bicycling
www.fitnessfind.com/bicycling.html

Fitness Find: Cross Training
www.fitnessfind.com/crosstrain.html

Fitness Find: Running
www.fitnessfind.com/running.html

Fitness Find: Walking
www.fitnessfind.com/walking.html

Fitness Jumpsite!
http://primusweb.com/fitnesspartner/index.html

GORP: Great Outdoors Recreation Pages
www.gorp.com/default.htm

Healthy Athlete
http://bewell.com/healthy/athlete/index.asp

Mayo Clinic Health Oasis: DHEA - Hype or Health
www.mayohealth.org/mayo/9612/htm/dhea.htm

NetSweat.com: The Internet's Fitness Resource
www.netsweat.com/

New York Times on the Web: Women's Health: Diet & Exercise
www.nytimes.com/specials/women/whome/diet_exercise.html

PHYS: Aerobics
www.phys.com/f_fitness/03encyclopedia/02database/aerobics.html

PHYS: Sports Activity Database
www.phys.com/f_fitness/03encyclopedia/01home/activity.html

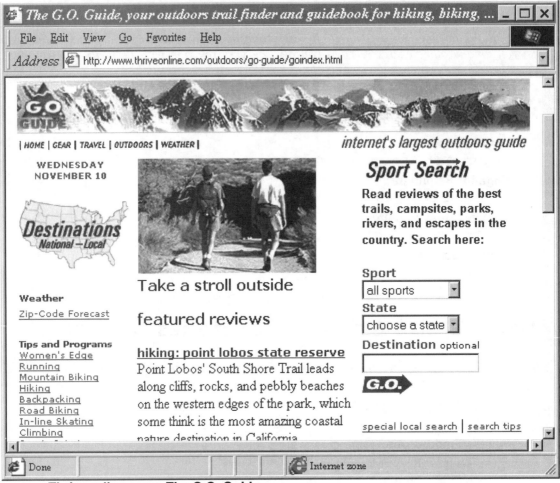

Thriveonline.com: The G.O. Guide
www.thriveonline.com/outdoors/go-guide/goindex.html

Worldguide: Health & Fitness Forum
www.worldguide.com/home/dmg/Fitness/hf.html

Issues in Food Safety

"What are you eating now?" Mothers have asked their children that question through the ages. Now, more than ever, we must ask ourselves this same question. The issues of food poisoning, irradiation and biotechnology affect us all; it is of the utmost importance for immunocompromised people who undergo cancer treatment and for those who have contracted HIV. It is our responsibility to understand these issues and to be informed about just what is happening to our food and water. Wash your hands and surf through these sites.

FAQs & Quizzes

Take a few food safety quizzes, then check out the answers. If you've got questions, you'll most likely find the answers in the frequently asked question (FAQ) sites.

FDA/CFSAN: Can Your Kitchen Pass the Food Safety Test?
http://vm.cfsan.fda.gov/~dms/fdkitchn.html

IFIC: Questions & Answers About Food Irradiation
http://ificinfo.health.org/qanda/qairradi.htm

National Food Safety Database: Test Your Food Safety IQ
www.foodsafety.org/register.htm

Pure-food.com: Facts About Herbicides & Pesticides
www.pure-food.com/pesticid.htm

USDA/FSIS: Panic Button Food Safety Questions
www.fsis.usda.gov/OA/pubs/panicbut.htm

Food Biotechnology

"Genetic engineering," "cloning," "biotechnology," and "biogenetics." These are words many of us were not taught in school. But now we have eco-guerrillas destroying field test crops around the world. Just what is going on with our food supply? Should we be concerned, or should we rest comfortably knowing that scientissts are tinkering with our food? Logon to the world of biotechnology and decide for yourself.

American Dietetic Association: Food Biotechnology
www.eatright.org/nfs/nfs9.html

Biotechnology in Agriculture: Challenges For The Future
www.nal.usda.gov/bic/Audio/BT-MD.html

Campaign For Food Safety: Dangers of Genetic Engineered Food
www.purefood.org/gelink.html

Campaign For Food Safety: Monsanto Watch
www.purefood.org/monlink.htm

Consumer Attitudes Toward Food Biotechnology: A Summary
http://ificinfo.health.org/press/questsummary.htm

Diane Rehm Program: Agricultural Biotechnology
www.nal.usda.gov/bic/Audio/DRehmtext.htm

FDA/CFSAN: Policy For Foods Developed By Biotechnology
http://vm.cfsan.fda.gov/~lrd/bioeme.html

Genetically Modified Foods
www.healthyeating.org/general/gmf.htm

IFIC: Food Biotechnology
http://ificinfo.health.org/backgrnd/bkgr14.htm

IFIC: Food Insight: Food Biotechnology: Benefits for Developing Countries
http://ificinfo.health.org/insight/janfeb99/foodbiotechnology.htm

IFIC: What The Experts Say About Food Biotechnology
http://ificinfo.health.org/foodbiotech/whatexpertssay.htm

IFIC: U.S. Consumer Attitudes Toward Food Biotechnology
http://ificinfo.health.org/press/quest.htm

Monsanto: A Life Sciences Company
www.monsanto.com

USDA: Biotechnology Information Center
www.nal.usda.gov/bic

USFDA Backgrounder: Biotechnology of Food
http://vm.cfsan.fda.gov/~lrd/biotechn.html

Food Handling

Once you are up to speed on the bugs in your food and water supply, visit these web sites to learn how to keep them out of your kitchen. Safe food handling must be a part of our daily existence.

All About Shell Eggs
www.fsis.usda.gov/OA/pubs/shelleggs.htm

American Dietetic Association: Home Food Safety - It's In Your Hands
www.eatright.org/feature/060199.html

American Dietetic Association: Safe Cooking Temperatures
www.eatright.org/cookingtemps.html

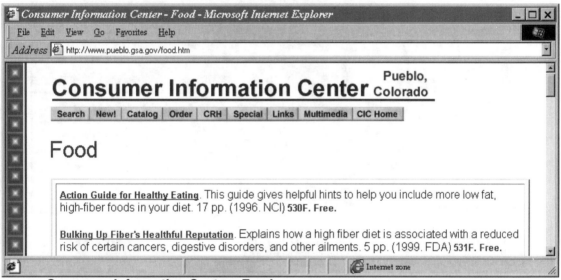

Consumer Information Center - Food
www.pueblo.gsa.gov/food.htm

Cooking Ground Beef Safely
www.fsis.usda.gov/OA/topics/gb.htm

drkoop.com: The Food Safety Guide
www.drkoop.com/wellness/nutrition/healthyliving/index.asp?id=29

FDA Consumer: Home Cookin' - Consumers' Kitchens Fail Inspections
http://vm.cfsan.fda.gov/~dms/fdcookin.html

FDA/CFSAN: Can Your Kitchen Pass the Food Safety Test?
http://vm.cfsan.fda.gov/~dms/fdkitchn.html

FDA/CFSAN: Seniors & Food Safety
http://vm.cfsan.fda.gov/~dms/seniors.html

FDA/CFSAN: Seniors & Food Safety - Preventing Food-borne Illness
http://vm.cfsan.fda.gov/~dms/seniorse.html

FDA: All About Cooking Thermometers
http://vm.cfsan.fda.gov/~dms/fdtherm.html

FDA: Center For Food Safety & Applied Nutrition
http://vm.cfsan.fda.gov/~dms/wh-food.html

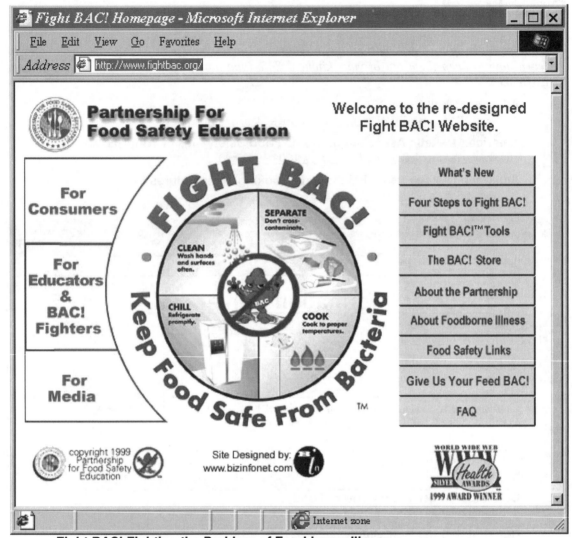

Fight BAC! Fighting the Problem of Food-borne Illness
www.fightbac.org

FOOD Files: Kitchen Practices
http://library.advanced.org/11960/handling/kitchen.htm

FOOD Files: Preparing & Cooking Food
http://library.advanced.org/11960/handling/prepcook.htm

FOOD Files: Storing Food
http://library.advanced.org/11960/handling/storing.htm

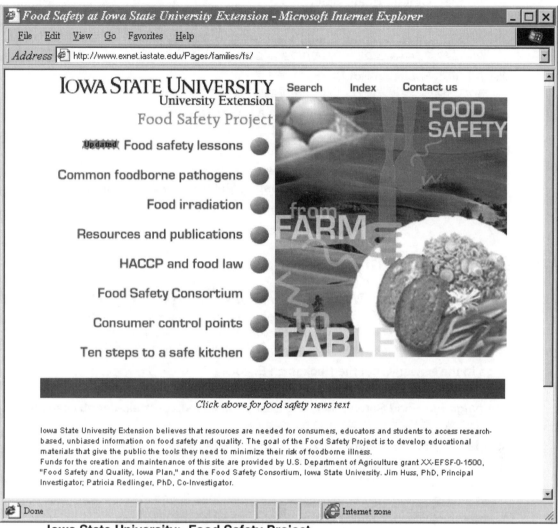

IOWA STATE UNIVERSITY
University Extension
Food Safety Project

Search   Index   Contact us

FOOD SAFETY

Updated Food safety lessons
Common foodborne pathogens
Food irradiation
Resources and publications
HACCP and food law
Food Safety Consortium
Consumer control points
Ten steps to a safe kitchen

from FARM to TABLE

Click above for food safety news text

Iowa State University Extension believes that resources are needed for consumers, educators and students to access research-based, unbiased information on food safety and quality. The goal of the Food Safety Project is to develop educational materials that give the public the tools they need to minimize their risk of foodborne illness.
Funds for the creation and maintenance of this site are provided by U.S. Department of Agriculture grant XX-EFSF-0-1500, "Food Safety and Quality, Iowa Plan," and the Food Safety Consortium, Iowa State University. Jim Huss, PhD, Principal Investigator; Patricia Redlinger, PhD, Co-Investigator.

Iowa State University: Food Safety Project
www.exnet.iastate.edu/Pages/families/fs

Mayo Clinic Health Oasis: E. coli Bacteria -
Protecting Yourself From Food-borne Illness
www.mayohealth.org/mayo/9511/htm/ecoli.htm

Mayo Clinic Health Oasis: Food Storage -
Knowing When to Toss or Keep Shelf Goods
www.mayohealth.org/mayo/9610/htm/storage.htm

Mayo Clinic Health Oasis: Guide to Food Storage
www.mayohealth.org/mayo/9610/htm/stor_sb.htm

National Food Safety Database: Bacteria on Cutting Boards
www.foodsafety.org/il/il114.htm

USDA Food-borne Illness Education Information Center
www.nal.usda.gov/fnic/foodborne/wais.shtml

USDA/FSIS: Barbecue Food Safety
www.fsis.usda.gov/OA/pubs/cibarbecue.htm

USDA/FSIS: Cutting Board Safety
www.fsis.usda.gov/OA/pubs/cutboard.htm

USDA/FSIS: Does Washing Food Promote Food Safety?
www.fsis.usda.gov/OA/pubs/washing.htm

USDA/FSIS: Focus on Hot Dogs
www.fsis.usda.gov/OA/pubs/focushotdog.htm

USDA/FSIS: Keeping Food Safe During a Power Outage ·
www.fsis.usda.gov/OA/pubs/pofeature.htm

USDA/FSIS: Microwave Food Safety
www.fsis.usda.gov/OA/pubs/cimwave.htm

USDA/FSIS: The Big Thaw - Safe Defrosting Methods for Consumers
www.fsis.usda.gov/OA/pubs/bigthaw.htm

Germs: A Primer

Have you ever thought that you had the flu when it wasn't even flu season? There's a good chance that you experienced some form of food poisoning. It seems that it is with alarming frequency that we read about a massive outbreak of E. Coli, Listeria, or Salmonella in our food or water supply. Get up to speed on what's happening, and why, by visiting these sites.

Bugs in the News: What the Heck is an E. coli?
http://falcon.cc.ukans.edu/~jbrown/ecoli.html

Campaign For Food Safety: Mad Pig & Cow Disease/Creutzfeld-Jacob Disease
www.purefood.org/meatlink.html

Campaign For Food Safety: Toxic & Contaminated Food
www.purefood.org/toxiclink.html

Campylobacter
www.cdc.gov/ncidod/diseases/bacter/campyfaq.htm

Centers for Disease Control & Prevention: Food-borne Illnesses
www.cdc.gov/health/foodill.htm

Centers For Disease Control: Escherichia coli 0157:H7
www.cdc.gov/ncidod/diseases/foodborn/e_coli.htm

Emerging Food-borne Diseases
www.cdc.gov/ncidod/EID/vol3no4/tauxe.htm

FDA's Bad Bug Book: E. coli
http://vm.cfsan.fda.gov/%7Emow/chap15.html

FDA/CFSAN: Bad Bug Book
http://vm.cfsan.fda.gov/~mow/intro.html

FDA/CFSAN: Bad Bug Book: Clostridium Botulinum
http://vm.cfsan.fda.gov/~mow/chap2.html

FDA/CFSAN: Bad Bug Book: Salmonella
http://vm.cfsan.fda.gov/~mow/chap1.html

FDA/CFSAN: Bad Bug Book: Staphylococcus aureus
http://vm.cfsan.fda.gov/~mow/chap3.html

FDA: Center For Food Safety & Applied Nutrition
http://vm.cfsan.fda.gov/~dms/wh-food.html

Food-borne Bacterial Diseases
www.cdc.gov/ncidod/diseases/bacter/foodborn.htm

FoodNet
www.cdc.gov/ncidod/dbmd/foodnet/98surv.htm

Iowa State University: Food Safety Project
www.exnet.iastate.edu/Pages/families/fs

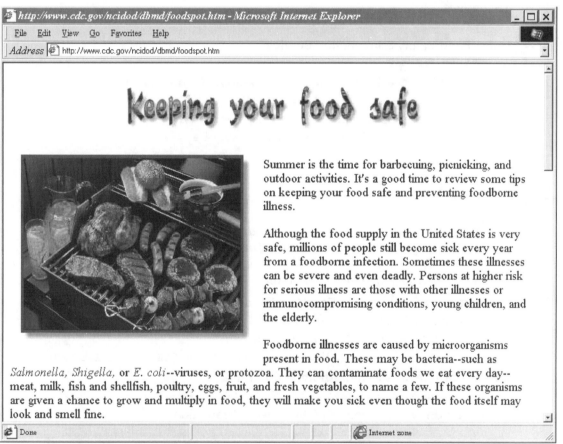

Keeping your food safe

Summer is the time for barbecuing, picnicking, and outdoor activities. It's a good time to review some tips on keeping your food safe and preventing foodborne illness.

Although the food supply in the United States is very safe, millions of people still become sick every year from a foodborne infection. Sometimes these illnesses can be severe and even deadly. Persons at higher risk for serious illness are those with other illnesses or immunocompromising conditions, young children, and the elderly.

Foodborne illnesses are caused by microorganisms present in food. These may be bacteria--such as *Salmonella, Shigella,* or *E. coli*--viruses, or protozoa. They can contaminate foods we eat every day-- meat, milk, fish and shellfish, poultry, eggs, fruit, and fresh vegetables, to name a few. If these organisms are given a chance to grow and multiply in food, they will make you sick even though the food itself may look and smell fine.

Keeping Your Food Safe
www.cdc.gov/ncidod/dbmd/foodspot.htm

Listeriosis
www.cdc.gov/ncidod/diseases/foodborn/lister.htm

Mayo Clinic Health Oasis: Listeria - A Deadly Bacteria
www.mayohealth.org/mayo/9902/htm/listeria.htm

Mayo Clinic Health Oasis: The "Bug" That Made Milwaukee Famous
www.mayohealth.org/mayo/9606/htm/cryptosp.htm

National Food Safety Database
www.foodsafety.org/index.htm

National Food Safety Database: Germs, Chemicals, & Other Hazards
www.foodsafety.org/conthome.htm

National Food Safety Database: The Bugs Within Us
www.foodsafety.org/sf/sf033.htm

Official Mad Cow Disease Home Page
http://mad-cow.org

Pure-food.com: Facts About Herbicides & Pesticides
www.pure-food.com/pesticid.htm

Salmonellosis
www.cdc.gov/ncidod/diseases/foodborn/salmon.htm

Trichinosis
www.cdc.gov/ncidod/dpd/trichino.htm

USDA Food Safety & Inspection Service
www.fsis.usda.gov

USDA Food Safety & Inspection Service: Listeria Monocytogenes
www.fsis.usda.gov/OA/pubs/listeria.htm

USDA/FSIS: Food-borne Illness Peaks in Summer--Why?
www.fsis.usda.gov/OA/pubs/illpeaks.htm

Irradiation

They're zapping our food now with radiation to kill germs. What does that mean to us -- the consumers? Some argue that it depletes vitamins and nutrients from the products, others deny it. Right now the FDA is trying to decide if irradiated food should be labelled as such. Decide for yourself after checking out a few of these sites.

Campaign For Food Safety: Food Irradiation - News, Articles, Links, Books
www.purefood.org/irradlink.html

IAEA/ICGFI: Facts About Food Irradiation
www.iaea.or.at/worldatom/inforesource/other/food/index.html

IFIC: Questions & Answers About Food Irradiation
http://ificinfo.health.org/qanda/qairradi.htm

Iowa State University: Food Safety Project: Irradiation
www.extension.iastate.edu/foodsafety/rad/irradhome.html

Irradiation: A Safe Measure For Safer Food
www.fda.gov/fdac/features/1998/398_rad.html

Mayo Clinic Health Oasis: Food Irradiation: The Answer to E. coli?
www.mayohealth.org/mayo/9709/htm/food_irr.htm

Pure-food.com
www.pure-food.com/food.htm

Pesticides

Health concerns over the use of pesticides has resulted in a growing "organic" produce industry. How do pesticides affect what you eat? Are there alternatives to pesticides? The answers to these questions and more can be found at sites listed here.

A Consumer's Guide to Pesticides & Food Safety
http://ificinfo.health.org/brochure/cgfs&p.htm

National Coalition Against the Misuse of Pesticides (NCAMP)
http://www.ncamp.org

Northwest Coalition for Alternatives to Pesticides (NCAP)
http://www.pesticide.org

Pesticide Action Network of North America (PANNA)
http://www.panna.org/panna

Pesticide Information Services Database (PESTIS)
http://www.panna.org/resources/pestis.html

Pesticides, Human Health & the Environment
http://www.pmac.net/pestenv.htm

Pesticides News Index
http://www.gn.apc.org/pesticidestrust/pnindex.htm

PICOL - Pesticide Information Center OnLine
http://picol.cahe.wsu.edu/

Safe & Effective Use of Pesticides on Agricultural Crops
http://www.vtpp.ext.vt.edu/htmldocs/safety_regs.html

Safe Use of Pesticides in Agriculture
http://www.ext.vt.edu/pubs/safety/442-036/442-036.html

US Environmental Protection Agency: Office of Pesticide Programs
http://www.epa.gov/pesticides

Virginia Tech Programs: Pesticide Site Locator
http://www.vtpp.ext.vt.edu:8080/catlist.html

News Updates & Alerts

Get the latest news on food recalls and food poisoning outbreaks from these sites. You can subscribe to some of them to receive free, e-mail updates.

Campaign For Food Safety
www.purefood.org

Campaign For Food Safety News
www.purefood.org/listserv.htm

Center For Science in the Public Interest
www.cspinet.org

National Food Safety Database: Critical Issues in Food Safety
www.foodsafety.org/hothome.htm

Special Considerations

People who have been around for awhile are less apt to change their eating habits. Others who are immunocompromised have special considerations as well. These web sites serve to increase awareness of food safety.

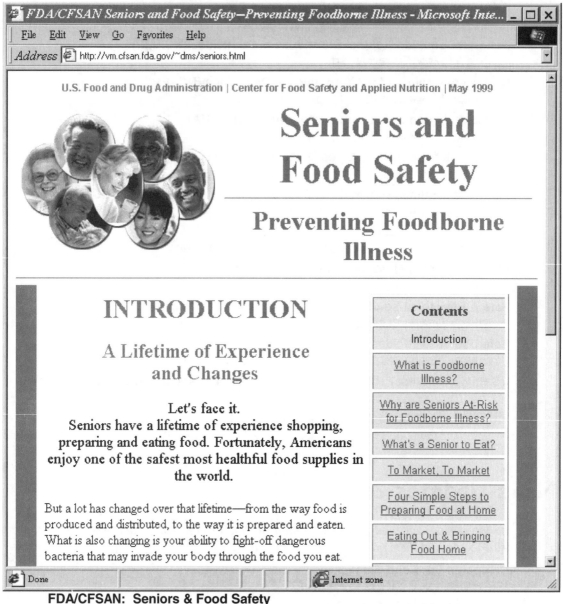

FDA/CFSAN: Seniors & Food Safety
http://vm.cfsan.fda.gov/~dms/seniors.html

FDA/CFSAN: Seniors & Food Safety - Preventing Food-borne Illness
http://vm.cfsan.fda.gov/~dms/seniorse.html

FDA/CFSAN: Seniors & Food Safety - What's a Senior to Eat?
http://vm.cfsan.fda.gov/~dms/seniorsc.html

FDA/CFSAN: Seniors & Food Safety -
Why Are Seniors at Risk for Food-borne Illness?
http://vm.cfsan.fda.gov/~dms/seniorsb.html

Understanding the Issues

Visit these sites to get a feeling for current issues in food safety. The broad political spectrum is represented, from the government to various consumer watchdog agencies such as the Center for Science in the Public Interest.

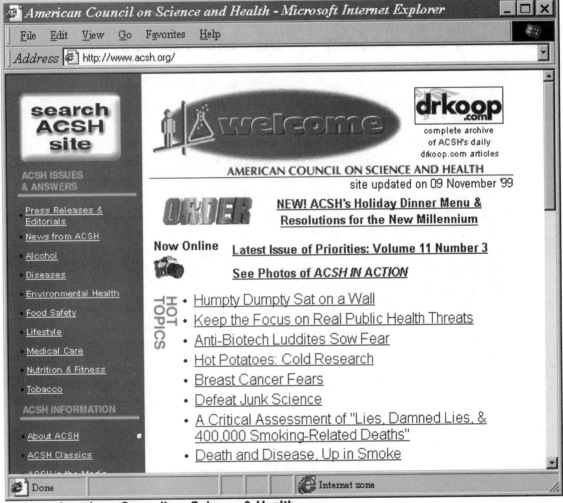

American Council on Science & Health
www.acsh.org

American Council on Science & Health: Food Safety
www.acsh.org/food/index.html

American Council on Science & Health: Nutrition & Fitness
www.acsh.org/nutrition/index.html

Campaign For Food Safety
www.purefood.org

Campaign For Food Safety News
www.purefood.org/listserv.htm

Campaign For Food Safety: Bovine Growth Hormone Controversy
www.purefood.org/rbghlink.html

Center For Science in the Public Interest
www.cspinet.org

USDA/FSIS: Additives in Meat & Poultry Products
www.fda.gov/fdac/features/1998/398_rad.html

USDA/FSIS: The Facts About Ground Poultry
www.fsis.usda.gov/OA/pubs/grndpoul.htm

More on Food Safety - Directories & Links

Use these directories and links to learn more about food safety issues.

Campaign For Food Safety: Bovine Growth Hormone Controversy
www.purefood.org/rbghlink.html

FDA: Center For Food Safety & Applied Nutrition
http://vm.cfsan.fda.gov/~dms/wh-food.html

Pure-food.com: Alerts - What Can I Do?
www.pure-food.com/alerts.htm

USDA Food Safety & Inspection Service
www.fsis.usda.gov

USDA/FSIS: Food Safety Publications for Consumers
www.fsis.usda.gov/OA/pubs/consumerpubs.htm

USFDA: Center for Food Safety & Applied Nutrition
http://vm.cfsan.fda.gov

Combating Fraud Online

As consumers in a free market society, we must assume some responsibility for our buying decisions. It is up to each of us to combat fraud, fallacies, myths, and fads. It is too easy to throw our hard-earned money down the drain. Whether we are searching for a definitive and final diet that will really work, searching for that magic pill, or looking for that cure for cancer or heart disease, we must practice vigilance. Thankfully, there are consumer and government organizations that can help us separate myth from reality. Be an informed consumer and seek help from some of these sources. Check out the credibility of what you read or hear, and verify those credentials.

Identifying Fraud on the Web

There are many places on the World Wide Web that want our money. To help us find the facts, these sites are designed to give us guidelines to follow before buying. Whether it's a new diet plan, an incredible energy supplement, or a highly touted cure for cancer, check these sites out for a bit of advice.

American Heart Association: Phony AMA Diet
www.americanheart.org/Heart_and_Stroke_A_Z_Guide/pahad.html

Colorado State University Cooperative Extension: Nutrition Quackery
www.colostate.edu/depts/CoopExt/PUBS/FOODNUT/09350.html

drkoop.com: Spotting Nutrition Quackery
www.drkoop.com/wellness/nutrition/healthyliving/index.asp?id=214

Internet Scambusters
www.scambusters.com

Mayo Clinic Health Oasis: Buyer Beware
    www.mayohealth.org/mayo/9707/htm/me_5sb.htm

National Council Against Health Fraud
    www.ncahf.org

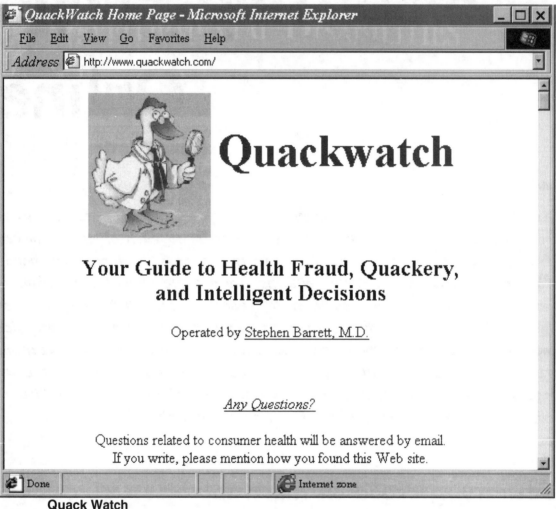

Quack Watch
    www.quackwatch.com

Quack Watch: Appropriate Use of Supplements
    www.quackwatch.com/03HealthPromotion/supplements.html

Quack Watch: DHEA: Ignore the Hype
    www.quackwatch.com/01QuackeryRelatedTopics/dhea.html

Quack Watch: Don't Buy Phony Ergogenic Aids
    www.quackwatch.com/01QuackeryRelatedTopics/ergo.html

Going Offline

A frequent sign of a scam is the reluctance by a company to reveal its contact information. If you can't easily find a phone number or address for a company that is willing to take your credit card number online, you may be in for trouble.

However, in order to purchase and use a domain name (the short version of a web address - such as www.quackwatch.com*), one must provide contact information (including name, e-mail, mailing address, and phone number). This information is stored in a central database that may be accessed by the public for free. One spot where you can access this information is iNet's WhoIs Gateway, located at* www.inet.net/cgi-bin/whoisqw*. Simply type in the domain name in the search field and hit enter. The contact information should appear on the next screen.*

License Verification

The Internet has revolutionized society. Almost every aspect of life has gone "online," and employment is no exception. Health-related occupations often require certification of some kind. Unfortunately, a piece of paper framed on a wall does not always mean that a person is licensed to practice. Therefore, jobs which require licensing require verification, and the Internet is fast becoming a way of facilitating the verification process.

Presented here are various health-related occupations as well as URLs (or e-mail addresses) which may be used to verify the licensure of the professions listed. Not all health-related professions may be verified online, but as time passes more and more government agencies will venture into cyberspace.

The information provided in this section comes from BRB Publications' The Sourcebook to Public Record Information. If you need to verify occupations in addition to those in the health-related industries, The Sourcebook to Public Record Information is strongly recommended. Call BRB Publications at 1-800-929-3811 for more information.

Alabama

Medical Doctor
www.mindspring.com/~bmedixon

Alaska

Dental Hygienist
www.commerce.state.ak.us/com/owa/comdata.occlic

Dentist
www.commerce.state.ak.us/com/owa/comdata.occlic

Nurse (RN & LPN)-Nurse Anesthetist
www.commerce.state.ak.us/com/owa/comdata.occlic

Nurse Practitioner (Advanced)
www.commerce.state.ak.us/com/owa/comdata.occlic

Optician
www.commerce.state.ak.us/com/owa/comdata.occlic

Arizona

Hearing Aid Dispenser
www.hs.state.az.us/als/databases/index.html

Medical Doctor
www.docboard.org/az/df/azsearch.htm

Physician Assistant
www.docboard.org/az/df/azsearch.htm

Professional Counselor
http://aspin.asu.edu/~azbbhe/directory/listing.html

Psychologist
www.goodnet.com/~azbpe/dir.html

Social Worker
http://aspin.asu.edu/~azbbhe/directory/listing.html

Substance Abuse Counselor
http://aspin.asu.edu/~azbbhe/directory/listing.html

Arkansas

Dental Hygienist
www.asbde.org/hygenist.htm

Dentist
www.asbde.org/dentists.htm

Nurse
www.state.ar.us/nurse/database/search.html

California

Medical Doctor/Surgeon
www.docboard.org/ca/df/casearch.htm

Optometrist
www.iabopt.org/cal/search.asp

Optometry Branch Office
www.iabopt.org/cal/search.asp

Podiatrist
www.docboard.org/ca/df/casearch.htm

Colorado

Acupuncturist
www.dora.state.co.us/real/owa/ARMS_Search.Disclaimer_Page

Medical Doctor
www.dora.state.co.us/real/owa/ARMS_Search.Disclaimer_Page

Colorado

Chiropractor
www.dora.state.co.us:81/real/owa/ARMS_Search.Disclaimer_Page

Clinical Social Worker
www.dora.state.co.us:81/real/owa/ARMS_Search.Disclaimer_Page

Dental Hygienist
www.dora.state.co.us:81/real/owa/ARMS_Search.Disclaimer_Page

Dentist
www.dora.state.co.us:81/real/owa/ARMS_Search.Disclaimer_Page

Family Therapist
www.dora.state.co.us:81/real/owa/ARMS_Search.Disclaimer_Page

Hearing Aid Dealer/Dispenser
www.dora.state.co.us:81/real/owa/ARMS_Search.Disclaimer_Page

Medical Doctor
www.dora.state.co.us:81/real/owa/ARMS_Search.Disclaimer_Page

Nurse
www.dora.state.co.us:81/real/owa/ARMS_Search.Disclaimer_Page

Nurses' Aide
www.dora.state.co.us:81/real/owa/ARMS_Search.Disclaimer_Page

Nursing Care Facility
www.hfd.cdphe.state.co.us/criter.asp

Optometrist
www.dora.state.co.us:81/real/owa/ARMS_Search.Disclaimer_Page

Pharmacist
www.dora.state.co.us:81/real/owa/ARMS_Search.Disclaimer_Page

Pharmacy
www.dora.state.co.us:81/real/owa/ARMS_Search.Disclaimer_Page

Physical Therapist
www.dora.state.co.us:81/real/owa/ARMS_Search.Disclaimer_Page

Podiatrist
www.dora.state.co.us:81/real/owa/ARMS_Search.Disclaimer_Page

Professional Counselor
www.dora.state.co.us:81/real/owa/ARMS_Search.Disclaimer_Page

Psychologist
www.dora.state.co.us:81/real/owa/ARMS_Search.Disclaimer_Page

Connecticut

Acupuncturist
www.state.ct.us/dph/scripts/hlthprof.asp

Alcohol/Drug Counselor
www.state.ct.us/dph/scripts/hlthprof.asp

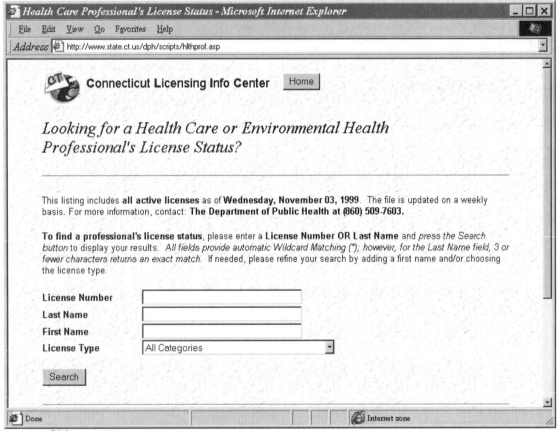

Chiropractor
www.state.ct.us/dph/scripts/hlthprof.asp

Dentist/Dental Hygienist
www.state.ct.us/dph/scripts/hlthprof.asp

Hearing Aid Dealer
www.state.ct.us/dph/scripts/hlthprof.asp

Homeopathic Physician
www.state.ct.us/dph/scripts/hlthprof.asp

Massage Therapist
www.state.ct.us/dph/scripts/hlthprof.asp

Medical Doctor
www.state.ct.us/dph/scripts/hlthprof.asp

Naturopathic Physician
www.state.ct.us/dph/scripts/hlthprof.asp

Nurse
www.state.ct.us/dph/scripts/hlthprof.asp

Nurse Midwife
www.state.ct.us/dph/scripts/hlthprof.asp

Nurse, Advance Registered Practice
www.state.ct.us/dph/scripts/hlthprof.asp

Occupational Therapist/Assistant
www.state.ct.us/dph/scripts/hlthprof.asp

Optical Shop
www.state.ct.us/dph/scripts/hlthprof.asp

Optician
www.state.ct.us/dph/scripts/hlthprof.asp

Optometrist
www.state.ct.us/dph/scripts/hlthprof.asp

Osteopathic Physician
www.state.ct.us/dph/scripts/hlthprof.asp

Paramedic
www.state.ct.us/dph/scripts/hlthprof.asp

Physical Therapist
www.state.ct.us/dph/scripts/hlthprof.asp

Physician Assistant
www.state.ct.us/dph/scripts/hlthprof.asp

Podiatrist
www.state.ct.us/dph/scripts/hlthprof.asp

Practical Nurse
www.state.ct.us/dph/scripts/hlthprof.asp

Professional Counselor
www.state.ct.us/dph/scripts/hlthprof.asp

Psychologist
www.state.ct.us/dph/scripts/hlthprof.asp

Radiographer
www.state.ct.us/dph/scripts/hlthprof.asp

Respiratory Care Practitioner
www.state.ct.us/dph/scripts/hlthprof.asp

Social Worker
www.state.ct.us/dph/scripts/hlthprof.asp

Georgia

Chiropractor
www.sos.state.ga.us/ebd-chiro/search.htm

Counselor
www.sos.state.ga.us/ebd-counselors/search.htm

Dental Hygienist
www.sos.state.ga.us/ebd-dentistry/search.htm

Dentist
www.sos.state.ga.us/ebd-dentistry/search.htm

Dietitian
www.sos.state.ga.us/ebd-dieticians/search.htm

Dispensing Optician
www.sos.state.ga.us/ebd-opticians/search.htm

Family Therapist
www.sos.state.ga.us/ebd-counselors/search.htm

Hearing Aid Dealer/Dispenser
www.sos.state.ga.us/ebd-hearingaid/search.htm

Medical Doctor
www.sos.state.ga.us/ebd-medical/medsearch.htm

Nurse (Registered)
www.sos.state.ga.us/ebd-rn/search.htm

Occupational Therapist
www.sos.state.ga.us/ebd-ot/search.htm

Occupational Therapist Assistant
www.sos.state.ga.us/ebd-ot/search.htm

Optometrist
www.sos.state.ga.us/ebd-optometry/search.htm

Paramedic
www.sos.state.ga.us/ebd-medical/medsearch2.htm

Pharmacist
www.sos.state.ga.us/ebd-pharmacy/search.htm

Physical Therapist
www.sos.state.ga.us/ebd-pt/search.htm

Physical Therapist Assistant
www.sos.state.ga.us/ebd-pt/search.htm

Physician Assistant
www.sos.state.ga.us/ebd-medical/medsearch2.htm

Podiatrist
www.sos.state.ga.us/ebd-podiatry/search.htm

Practical Nurse
www.sos.state.ga.us/ebd-lpn/search.htm

Psychologist
www.sos.state.ga.us/ebd-psych/search.htm

Respiratory Care Practitioner
www.sos.state.ga.us/ebd-medical/medsearch2.htm

Social Worker
www.sos.state.ga.us/ebd-counselors/search.htm

Idaho

Dental Hygienist
www.state.id.us/isbd/isbdqry.htm

Dentist
www.state.id.us/isbd/isbdqry.htm

Illinois

Chiropractor
www.state.il.us/dprapp

Dentist/Dental Hygienist
www.state.il.us/dprapp

Dietitian/Nutrition Counselor
www.state.il.us/dprapp

Medical Doctor/Physician's Assistant
www.state.il.us/dprapp

Nurse
www.state.il.us/dprapp

Occupational Therapist
www.state.il.us/dprapp

Optometrist
www.state.il.us/dprapp

Osteopathic Physician
www.state.il.us/dprapp

Pharmacist/Pharmacy
www.state.il.us/dprapp

Physical Therapist
www.state.il.us/dprapp

Podiatrist
www.state.il.us/dprapp

Psychologist
www.state.il.us/dprapp

Social Worker
www.state.il.us/dprapp

Iowa

Medical Doctor
www.docboard.org/ia/find_ia.htm

Kansas

Chiropractor
www.docboard.org/ks/df/kssearch.htm

Medical Doctor
www.docboard.org/ks/df/kssearch.htm

Occupational Therapist/Assistant
www.docboard.org/ks/df/kssearch.htm

Physician Assistant
www.docboard.org/ks/df/kssearch.htm

Podiatrist
www.docboard.org/ks/df/kssearch.htm

Respiratory Therapist
www.docboard.org/ks/df/kssearch.htm

Maine

Medical Doctor
www.docboard.org/me/df/mesearch.htm

Maryland

Medical Doctor
www.docboard.org/md/df/mdsearch.htm

Massachusetts

Acupuncturist
www.docboard.org/ma/df/masearch.htm

Chiropractor
http://license.reg.state.ma.us/pubLic/licque.asp?color=red&Board=CH

Dental Hygienist
http://license.reg.state.ma.us/pubLic/licque.asp?color=red&Board=DN

Dentist
http://license.reg.state.ma.us/pubLic/licque.asp?color=red&Board=DN

Dispensing Optician
http://license.reg.state.ma.us/pubLic/licque.asp?color=red&Board=DO

Medical Doctor
www.docboard.org/ma/df/masearch.htm

Mental Health Counselor
http://license.reg.state.ma.us/pubLic/licque.asp?query=personal&color=red&board=MH

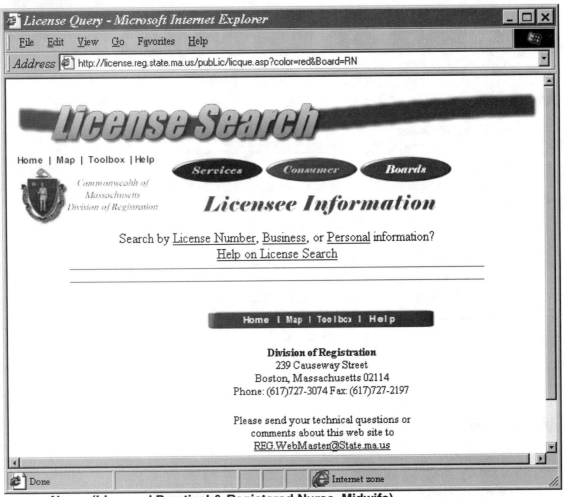

Nurse (Licensed Practical & Registered Nurse, Midwife)
http://license.reg.state.ma.us/pubLic/licque.asp?color=red&Board=RN

Occupational Therapist
http://license.reg.state.ma.us/pubLic/licque.asp?color=red&Board=AH

Occupational Therapist Assistant
http://license.reg.state.ma.us/pubLic/licque.asp?color=red&Board=AH

Optometrist
http://license.reg.state.ma.us/pubLic/licque.asp?color=red&Board=OP

Pharmacist
http://license.reg.state.ma.us/pubLic/licque.asp?color=red&Board=PH

Physical Therapist
http://license.reg.state.ma.us/pubLic/licque.asp?color=red&Board=AH

Physical Therapist Assistant
http://license.reg.state.ma.us/pubLic/licque.asp?color=red&Board=AH

Physician Assistant
http://license.reg.state.ma.us/pubLic/licque.asp?color=red&Board=AP

Podiatrist
http://license.reg.state.ma.us/pubLic/licque.asp?color=red&Board=PD

Respiratory Care Therapist
http://license.reg.state.ma.us/pubLic/licque.asp?color=red&Board=RC

Social Worker
http://license.reg.state.ma.us/pubLic/licque.asp?color=red&Board=SW

Michigan

Hearing Aid Dealer
www.cis.state.mi.us:8020/public/lic_reg$.startup

Social Worker
www.cis.state.mi.us:8020/public/lic_reg$.startup

Acupuncturist
www.docboard.org/mn/df/mndf.htm

Medical Doctor
www.docboard.org/mn/df/mndf.htm

Physical Therapist
www.docboard.org/mn/df/mndf.htm

Physician Assistant
www.docboard.org/mn/df/mndf.htm

Respiratory Care Practitioner
www.docboard.org/mn/df/mndf.htm

Missouri

Chiropractor
www.ecodev.state.mo.us/pr/ftp4.htm

Dental Hygienist
www.ecodev.state.mo.us/pr/ftp4.htm

Dentist
www.ecodev.state.mo.us/pr/ftp4.htm

Hearing Instrument Specialist
www.ecodev.state.mo.us/pr/ftp4.htm

Medical Doctor
www.ecodev.state.mo.us/pr/ftp4.htm

Occupational Therapist
www.ecodev.state.mo.us/pr/ftp4.htm

Occupational Therapist Assistant
www.ecodev.state.mo.us/pr/ftp4.htm

Optometrist
www.ecodev.state.mo.us/pr/ftp4.htm

Osteopathic Physician
www.ecodev.state.mo.us/pr/healarts/listings.html

Pharmacist/Pharmacy Intern
www.ecodev.state.mo.us/pr/pharmacy/search.htm

Pharmacy
www.ecodev.state.mo.us/pr/pharmacy/phesearch.htm

Physical Therapist
www.ecodev.state.mo.us/pr/ftp4.htm

Physician Assistant
www.ecodev.state.mo.us/pr/ftp4.htm

Podiatrist
www.ecodev.state.mo.us/pr/ftp4.htm

Professional Counselor
www.ecodev.state.mo.us/pr/ftp4.htm

Psychologist
www.ecodev.state.mo.us/pr/ftp4.htm

Respiratory Care Practitioner
www.ecodev.state.mo.us/pr/ftp4.htm

Social Worker (Clinical)
www.ecodev.state.mo.us/pr/ftp4.htm

Montana

Nurse, RN/LPN
compolnur@state.mt.us

Nursing
compolnur@state.mt.us

Pharmacist
compolpha@state.mt.us

Respiratory Care Practitioner
compolrcp@state.mt.us

Nebraska

Chiropractor
www.hhs.state.ne.us/lis/lis.asp

Dental Hygienist
www.hhs.state.ne.us/lis/lis.asp

Dentist
www.hhs.state.ne.us/lis/lis.asp

Health Clinic & Emergency Medical Care
www.hhs.state.ne.us/lis/lis.asp

Hearing Aid Dispenser/Fitter
www.hhs.state.ne.us/lis/lis.asp

Massage Therapy School
www.hhs.state.ne.us/lis/lis.asp

Medical Nutrition Therapy
www.hhs.state.ne.us/lis/lis.asp

Mental Health Center
www.hhs.state.ne.us/lis/lis.asp

Nurse
www.hhs.state.ne.us/lis/lis.asp

Nursing Home
www.hhs.state.ne.us/lis/lis.asp

Occupational Therapist
www.hhs.state.ne.us/lis/lis.asp

Optometrist
www.hhs.state.ne.us/lis/lis.asp

Pharmacist
www.hhs.state.ne.us/lis/lis.asp

Pharmacy
www.hhs.state.ne.us/lis/lis.asp

Physical Therapist
www.hhs.state.ne.us/lis/lis.asp

Physician
www.hhs.state.ne.us/lis/lis.asp

Physician Assistant
www.hhs.state.ne.us/lis/lis.asp

Podiatrist
www.hhs.state.ne.us/lis/lis.asp

Psychologist
www.hhs.state.ne.us/lis/lis.asp

Radiographer
www.hhs.state.ne.us/lis/lis.asp

Nevada

Chiropractor
www.state.nv.us/chirobd/dcactive.htm

New Jersey

Chiropractor
www.state.nj.us/lps/ca/chirofrm.htm

Optometrist
www.state.nj.us/lps/ca/optometry/optomet.htm

Physician
www.state.nj.us/lps/ca/bme/medfrm.htm

Podiatrist
www.state.nj.us/lps/ca/bme/podfrm.htm

Psychologist
www.state.nj.us/lps/ca/psyfrm.htm

New Mexico

Optometrist
OptometryBd@state.nm.us

Psychologist
www.rld.state.nm.us/b&c/psychology/lcnssrch.asp

New York

Acupuncturist
www.nysed.gov/dpls/opnme.html

Chiropractor
www.nysed.gov/dpls/opnme.html

Dental Assistant
www.nysed.gov/dpls/opnme.html

Dental Hygienist
www.nysed.gov/dpls/opnme.html

Dentist
www.nysed.gov/dpls/opnme.html

Dietitian
www.nysed.gov/dpls/opnme.html

Massage Therapist
www.nysed.gov/dpls/opnme.html

Medical Doctor
www.nysed.gov/dpls/opnme.html

Midwife
www.nysed.gov/dpls/opnme.html

Nurse
www.nysed.gov/dpls/opnme.html

Nurse Practitioner
www.nysed.gov/dpls/opnme.html

Nutritionist
www.nysed.gov/dpls/opnme.html

Occupational Therapist/Assistant
www.nysed.gov/dpls/opnme.html

Optometrist
www.nysed.gov/dpls/opnme.html

Pharmacist
www.nysed.gov/dpls/opnme.html

Physical Therapist/Assistant
www.nysed.gov/dpls/opnme.html

Physician
www.nysed.gov/dpls/opnme.html

Physician Assistant
www.nysed.gov/dpls/opnme.html

Podiatrist
www.nysed.gov/dpls/opnme.html

Practical Nurse
www.nysed.gov/dpls/opnme.html

Psychologist
www.nysed.gov/dpls/opnme.html

Social Worker
www.nysed.gov/dpls/opnme.html

North Carolina

Chiropractor
www.ncchiroboard.org/public/licensed_chiros.html

Medical Doctor
www.docboard.org/nc/df/ncsearch.htm

Nurse
www.docboard.org/nc/df/ncsearch.htm

Osteopathic Physician
www.docboard.org/nc/df/ncsearch.htm

Physician Assistant
www.docboard.org/nc/df/ncsearch.htm

Practical Nurse
www.docboard.org/nc/df/ncsearch.htm

Ohio

Counselor
www.state.oh.us/scripts/csw/query.asp

Dental Assistant Radiologist
www.state.oh.us/scripts/den/query.stm

Dental Hygienist
www.state.oh.us/scripts/den/query.stm

Dentist
www.state.oh.us/scripts/den/query.stm

Medical Doctor
http://207.136.232.45/oh/df

Optometrist
www.state.oh.us/scripts/opt/query.asp

Optometrist-Diagnostic
www.state.oh.us/scripts/opt/query.asp

Optometrist-Therapeutic
www.state.oh.us/scripts/opt/query.asp

Social Worker
www.state.oh.us/scripts/csw/query.asp

Oklahoma

Health Spa
www.state.ok.us/~okdcc/database.htm

Medical Doctor
www.osbmls.state.ok.us/physrch.html

Osteopathic Physician
www.docboard.org/ok/df/oksearch.htm

Oregon

Acupuncturist
www.docboard.org/or/df/search.htm

Medical Doctor/Surgeon
www.docboard.org/or/df/search.htm

Osteopathic Physician
www.docboard.org/or/df/search.htm

Physician Assistant
www.docboard.org/or/df/search.htm

Podiatrist
www.docboard.org/or/df/search.htm

Pennsylvania

Nurse
nursing@pados.dos.state.pa.us

Rhode Island

Medical Doctor
www.docboard.org/ri/df/search.htm

Osteopathic Physician
www.docboard.org/ri/df/search.htm

South Carolina

Chiropractor
www.llr.state.sc.us/dss/chirop.asp

Medical Doctor
www.llr.state.sc.us/dss/lu2.asp

Nurse
www.llr.state.sc.us/dss/nurs.asp

Occupational Therapist
www.llr.state.sc.us/dss/occup.asp

Pharmacist/Pharmacy Store
www.llr.state.sc.us/dss/pharm.asp

Practical Nurse
www.llr.state.sc.us/dss/nurs.asp

Respiratory Care Practitioner
www.llr.state.sc.us/dss/respir.asp

Social Worker
www.llr.state.sc.us/dss/social.asp

Tennessee

Pharmacist
www.state.tn.us/cgi-bin/commerce/roster2.pl

Pharmacy
www.state.tn.us/cgi-bin/commerce/roster2.pl

Texas

Dietitian
www.tdh.state.tx.us/hcqs/plc/dtrost.txt

Emergency Medical Technician
www.tdh.state.tx.us/hcqs/ems/certqury.htm

Health Facility
www.ecptote.state.tx.us/serv/verification/ftverif.taf

Medical Doctor
www.docboard.org/tx/df/txsearch.htm

Occupational Therapist/Assistant
www.ecptote.state.tx.us/serv/verification/otverif.taf

Paramedic
www.tdh.state.tx.us/hcqs/ems/certqury.htm

Pharmacist
www.tsbp.state.tx.us/dbsearch/pht_search.asp

Pharmacy
www.tsbp.state.tx.us/dbsearch/phy_search.asp

Physical Therapist/Assistant
www.ecptote.state.tx.us/serv/verification/ptverif.taf

Professional Counselor
www.tdh.state.tx.us/hcqs/plc/lpcrost.txt

Radiologic Technologist
www.tdh.state.tx.us/hcqs/plc/mrtrost.txt

Respiratory Care Practitioner
www.tdh.state.tx.us/hcqs/plc/rcrost.txt

Social Worker
www.tdh.state.tx.us/hcqs/plc/lsw_list.txt

Utah

Acupuncturist
www.commerce.state.ut.us/web/commerce/DOPL/current/1201.htm

Chiropractor
www.commerce.state.ut.us/web/commerce/DOPL/current/1202.htm

Clinical Social Worker
www.commerce.state.ut.us/web/commerce/DOPL/current/3501.htm

Dental Hygienist
www.commerce.state.ut.us/web/commerce/DOPL/current/0701.htm

Dental Hygienist with Local Anesthesia
www.commerce.state.ut.us/web/commerce/DOPL/current/9920.htm

Dentist
www.commerce.state.ut.us/web/commerce/DOPL/current/9900.htm

Dietitian
www.commerce.state.ut.us/web/commerce/DOPL/current/4901.htm

Health Care Assistant
www.commerce.state.ut.us/web/commerce/DOPL/current/6201.htm

Hearing Aid Specialist
www.commerce.state.ut.us/web/commerce/DOPL/current/4601.htm

Hospital Pharmacy
www.commerce.state.ut.us/web/commerce/DOPL/current/1705.htm

Massage Apprentice
www.commerce.state.ut.us/web/commerce/DOPL/current/4702.htm

Massage Technician
www.commerce.state.ut.us/web/commerce/DOPL/current/4701.htm

Medical Doctor/Surgeon
www.commerce.state.ut.us/web/commerce/DOPL/current/1205.htm

Naturopathic Physician
www.commerce.state.ut.us/web/commerce/DOPL/current/7100.htm

Nurse
www.commerce.state.ut.us/DOPL/current/nurse.htm

Nurse Midwife
www.commerce.state.ut.us/DOPL/current/nurse.htm

Occupational Therapist
www.commerce.state.ut.us/web/commerce/DOPL/current/4201.htm

Occupational Therapist Assistant
www.commerce.state.ut.us/web/commerce/DOPL/current/4202.htm

Optometrist
www.commerce.state.ut.us/web/commerce/DOPL/current/1600.htm

Osteopathic Physician
www.commerce.state.ut.us/web/commerce/DOPL/current/1204.htm

Pharmacist
www.commerce.state.ut.us/web/commerce/DOPL/current/1701.htm

Pharmacy Technician
www.commerce.state.ut.us/web/commerce/DOPL/current/1717.htm

Physical Therapist
www.commerce.state.ut.us/web/commerce/DOPL/current/2401.htm

Physician Assistant
www.commerce.state.ut.us/web/commerce/DOPL/current/1206.htm

Podiatrist
www.commerce.state.ut.us/web/commerce/DOPL/current/0501.htm

Practical Nurse
www.commerce.state.ut.us/DOPL/current/nurse.htm

Professional Counselor
www.commerce.state.ut.us/web/commerce/DOPL/current/6004.htm

Psychologist
www.commerce.state.ut.us/web/commerce/DOPL/current/2501.htm

Radiology Practical Technician
www.commerce.state.ut.us/web/commerce/DOPL/current/5402.htm

Radiology Technologist
www.commerce.state.ut.us/web/commerce/DOPL/current/5401.htm

Respiratory Care Practitioner
www.commerce.state.ut.us/web/commerce/DOPL/current/5701.htm

Social Worker
www.commerce.state.ut.us/web/commerce/DOPL/current/3502.htm

Substance Abuse Counselor
www.commerce.state.ut.us/web/commerce/DOPL/current/6006.htm

Vermont

Acupuncturist
www.sec.state.vt.us/seek/lrspseek.htm

Chiropractor
www.sec.state.vt.us/seek/lrspseek.htm

Dental Assistant
www.sec.state.vt.us/seek/lrspseek.htm

Dental Hygienist
www.sec.state.vt.us/seek/lrspseek.htm

Dentist
www.sec.state.vt.us/seek/lrspseek.htm

Dietitian
www.sec.state.vt.us/seek/lrspseek.htm

Hearing Aid Dispenser
www.sec.state.vt.us/seek/lrspseek.htm

Medical Doctor/Surgeon
www.docboard.org/vt/df/vtsearch.htm

Mental Health Counselor, Clinical
www.sec.state.vt.us/seek/lrspseek.htm

Naturopathic Physician
www.sec.state.vt.us/seek/lrspseek.htm

Nurse/Nurse Practitioner/LNA
www.sec.state.vt.us/seek/lrspseek.htm

Occupational Therapist
www.sec.state.vt.us/seek/lrspseek.htm

Optician
www.sec.state.vt.us/seek/lrspseek.htm

Optometrist
www.sec.state.vt.us/seek/lrspseek.htm

Osteopathic Physician
www.sec.state.vt.us/seek/lrspseek.htm

Pharmacist
www.sec.state.vt.us/seek/lrspseek.htm

Pharmacy
www.sec.state.vt.us/seek/lrspseek.htm

Physical Therapist
www.sec.state.vt.us/seek/lrspseek.htm

Physician Assistant
www.docboard.org/vt/df/vtsearch.htm

Podiatrist
www.docboard.org/vt/df/vtsearch.htm

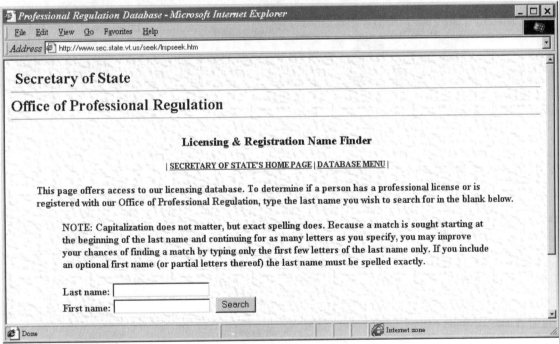

Psychologist
www.sec.state.vt.us/seek/lrspseek.htm

Radiologic Technologist
www.sec.state.vt.us/seek/lrspseek.htm

Social Worker, Clinical
www.sec.state.vt.us/seek/lrspseek.htm

Virginia

Nurse Aide
www.dhp.state.va.us/nurse/nuraide.htm

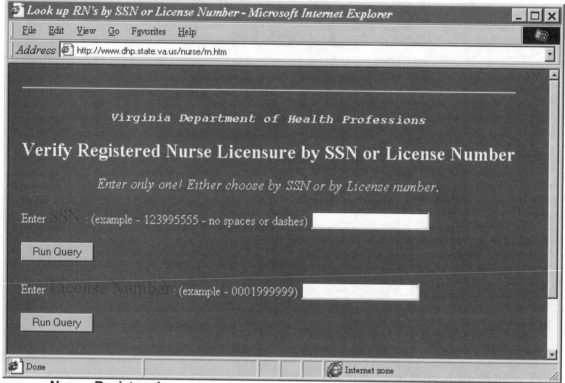

Nurse, Registered
www.dhp.state.va.us/nurse/rn.htm
Practical Nurse
www.dhp.state.va.us/nurse/lpn.htm

DIETS & NUTRITION
Site Profiles

Not sure where you want to start? Here you will find full descriptions of some of the web pages that appear in this book. Along with the description, you will see various icons that are designed to help you size up the sites before you visit them. For instance, sites that are considered "must see" material are marked with an ☞ icon. By "browsing" here, you can determine if these sites have content that is of interest to you __before__ going online.

24 Carrot Press: Nutrition for Kids $

www.nutritionforkids.com

> Getting kids to eat right has never been this much fun! 24 Carrot Press publishes materials that take a positive, fun approach to the more serious issues that affect children today, including poor eating habits, obesity and inactivity. You can order "How to Teach Nutrition to Kids," and a leader/activity guide as a companion to the book. Looks like cool stuff if you're a teacher, parent, or a health professional.

3 Day Diet

www.dietnutrition.com/3daydiet.html

> Psst! Want to lose 10 pounds real fast?

 MUST SEE!   VIDEO   AUDIO   SELLS STUFF

 CHAT ROOMS   MAILING LISTS   MESSAGE BOARDS   ADULT CONTENT

 FREE REGISTRATION REQUIRED   MEMBERS ONLY CONTENT   SEARCHABLE

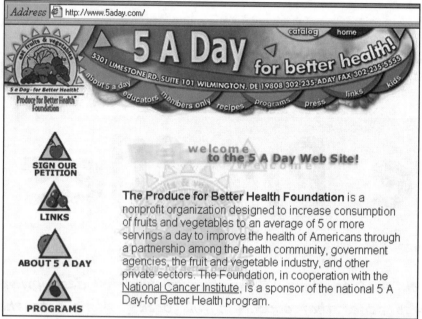

5 A Day

www.5aday.com

> This site is sponsored by the Produce for Better Health Foundation. Its mission is to raise awareness of the health benefits of consuming at least five servings of produce a day, improve our nation's health, and of course ultimately sell more fruits and veggies. Really, it's a win/win situation.

A Good Start: Nutrition During Pregnancy

www.beef.org/nut_libr/preg_index.htm

> The National Cattlemen's Beef Association has placed this web site on the net to help you choose the proper foods during your pregnancy. Can you guess what's good for you? Under "Achieving a Well-Balanced Diet," check out the snack suggestions. (Cubes of ham on toothpicks, squares of lunchmeat??)

About.com: Vegetarian Cuisine

http://vegetarian.about.com

> About.com can direct you to further vegetarian articles, news, and recipes. A good place to begin your search for vegetarian information.

Academy of Bariatric Surgeons

www.obesityhelp.com/abs

> This a good place to get useful information about surgical obesity, to find qualified surgeons, and to meet other people who have been through these procedures.

Academy of Bariatric Surgeons: FAQs

www.obesityhelp.com/abs/faq.htm

> Listed are about twenty questions and answers relating to the surgical treatment of extreme obesity.

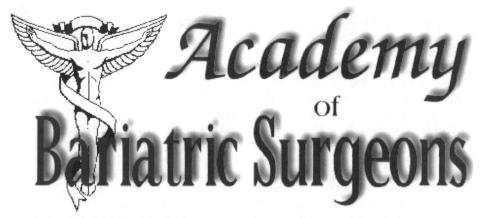

Academy of Bariatric Surgeons: Meet Patients

www.obesityhelp.com/abs/patients.htm

> Meet three patients who have undergone surgery and see before and after pictures. They've gone through some pretty dramatic changes rather quickly.

Academy of Bariatric Surgeons: Types of Surgery

www.obesityhelp.com/abs/surgerytypes.htm

> Various categories of surgery are discussed, with illustrations. Benefits and risks are an important part of this page.

Active Living Canada

http://activeliving.ca/activeliving/alc.html

> Active Living Canada is a program that strives for nothing less than to make active living a visible and important expression of Canadian culture. Active living is a way of life in which physical activity is valued and integrated into daily life, not to mention that it is extremely effective in disease prevention. Check out this initiative, and how it's working.

Aerobics & Fitness Association of America

www.afaa.com

> If you're looking for aerobics certification, a personal trainer, or just some fitness facts, this is the place to be. The AFAA is the world's largest fitness educator, with over 145,000 instructors in 73 countries.

Aerobics & Fitness Association of America: FitTown

www.afaa.com/10010.ASP?1=&1=12

> Check out this work in progress, where you can visit the café for recipes, the town hall for discussion, the library for references, and go to the health club, or to the town square where you can be connected to the world of fitness.

 MUST SEE!   VIDEO   AUDIO   SELLS STUFF

 CHAT ROOMS   MAILING LISTS   MESSAGE BOARDS   ADULT CONTENT

 FREE REGISTRATION REQUIRED   MEMBERS ONLY CONTENT   SEARCHABLE

AIDS Project LA: Positive Living Newsletter: Good Nutrition & HIV

www.thebody.com/apla/sep98/nutrition.html

AIDS treatment centers estimate that the rate of malnutrition is as high as 50%. This is a summary of a symposium on metabolism and wasting which was held during the 12th World Conference on AIDS. A major challenge of fighting AIDS is maintaining body weight. Although it's lengthy, it is packed with up-to-date information on wasting, body shape changes, and various treatments. Long term survivors of HIV seem to be those who are current with up-to-date treatment; it's worth reading.

AIDS-Related Quackery & Fraud

www.quackwatch.com/01QuackeryRelatedTopics/aids.html

Stephen Barrett, M.D. wrote this article to help you make informed decisions about treatment options. Because AIDS is still a deadly disease, and there is yet a proven cure, it has generated a mass of unsubstantiated claims including vitamin and supplement therapies, cures, and herbal extracts. Usually, the "cure" does nothing but empty your wallet.

Alchemy Pages: An Introduction

www.creative.net/~kaareb/index.html/intro.html

"The intent of a macrobiotic way of eating and lifestyle is to become a free, independent human being. In the endeavor to fulfill this intent it is considered a necessity that one knows how to take care of oneself, physically, emotionally, mentally and spiritually." - from The Alchemy Pages Introduction. Read on about yin and yang, and "abnormal discharges."

Alchemycal Pages: General Dietary Recommendations

www.creative.net/~kaareb/index.html/dietrec.html

This page is intended primarily for those people who are unfamiliar with a macrobiotic practice. The dietary recommendations are essentially those given to anyone who wishes to allow their body to heal; that is, restore itself to vitality and well-being.

Alchemycal Pages: What is Macrobiotics?

www.creative.net/~kaareb/index.html/qa.html

Macrobiotics is an approach to living which also places a great deal of emphasis on a proper dietary practice in daily life. This is a good starting spot to answer questions from the curious. This isn't just a diet, it's a way of life.

All About Shell Eggs

www.fsis.usda.gov/OA/pubs/shelleggs.htm

Everything, and I mean everything, you need to know about eggs is right here. Most importantly, read up on salmonella, how it gets in your egg, how to prevent it, and who's at risk.

All Raw Times: E-mail Resources ⌐📭

www.rawtimes.com/email.html

Do you want to talk to or contact others who eat it raw? Here you can find support, get help, or relate your experiences. It's also a short list of other good Internet resources.

All Raw Times: Juicers
www.rawtimes.com/index.html

> Before you buy your juicer you should visit this site. From All Raw Times comes reviews, experiences, and recommendations from real live people who juice. You'll also find out where to order your machine.

Allco Group - Independent Metabolife Distributors $
www.allcogroup.com/metabolife/index.html

> This product's claim is that it can raise the body's metabolism and create what they call a thermogenic response, so that you burn fat, not lean muscle tissue. Go ahead, get your credit card out.

allHealth.com: Never Say Diet
www.allhealth.com/neversaydiet

> Plenty of good support can be found here where you'll find new ways about thinking about food, exercise, and self image.

AM-300 Natural Herbal Energizer $
www.angelfire.com/biz2/am300herbal/index.html

> Another thermogenic product which contains chromium picolonate and other herbs. Lose fat, not muscle. Order online, send money, and get a free brochure.

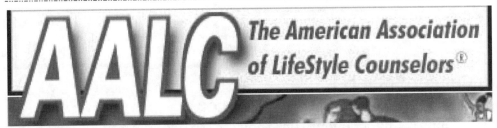

American Association of Lifestyle Counselors
www.AALC.org

> The American Association of Lifestyle Counselors aim is to improve the health of the American population by promoting healthy lifestyles that reduce the risks of preventable diseases through education directed toward the population and its healthcare providers. Here you can check into becoming a certified lifestyle counselor specializing in weight control or in stress management. You can also inquire about membership.

American Association of Lifestyle Counselors: Forum
www.AALC.org/experts.htm

> Ask the Experts' is a new public forum where individuals can ask questions and receive responses from experts in weight control and stress management.

MUST SEE!	VIDEO	AUDIO	SELLS STUFF
CHAT ROOMS	MAILING LISTS	MESSAGE BOARDS	ADULT CONTENT
FREE REGISTRATION REQUIRED	MEMBERS ONLY CONTENT	SEARCHABLE	

American Cancer Society:
Alternative & Complementary Methods
www.cancer.org/alt_therapy/index.html

Alternative and complementary medicine is a major factor in healthcare today. This article, which appeared in "Cancer," explores the alternatives, their rationale, and their methods of treatment.

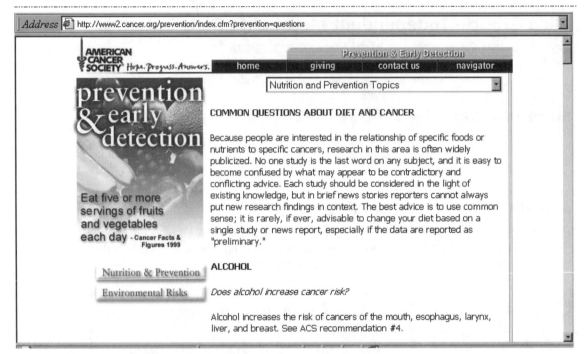

American Cancer Society:
Common Questions About Diet & Cancer
http://www2.cancer.org/prevention/index.cfm?prevention=questions

"Do fluorides cause cancer? Should I avoid nitrite preserved meats? Do artificial sweeteners cause cancer?" These and many other questions about diet and cancer are answered here.

American Cancer Society: Dietary & Herbal Remedies
www.cancer.org/alt_therapy/index.html

If you've considered fighting cancer with shark cartilage, herbal therapy, pau d'arco, or with fasting and juice therapies, make sure you visit here. The ACS recommends that you discuss with your doctor any alternative and complementary methods you may be considering.

American Cancer Society:
Fat Consumption & Breast Cancer Risk
http://www2.cancer.org/zine/dsp_SecondaryStories.cfm?sc=001&archiveLink=001_04261999_0

The American Cancer Society's web site has a news section where recent research news is discussed. When I visited this site there was an article about how two different studies on fat intake and breast cancer produced different results. A discussion of how that can happen and how studies are undertaken shows you the methodology used in these particular instances.

American Cancer Society: Healthy Eating Cookbook $

www.cancer.org/bookstore/cook_exc.html

> The ACS's cookbook is available through this site by either calling their toll free number or by ordering online.

American Cancer Society:
Importance of Nutrition in Cancer Prevention

http://www2.cancer.org/prevention/index.cfm?prevention=1

> The American Cancer Society says that of the 500,000 cancer deaths that occur each year, one third are due to dietary factors. Sounds to me that one third of these deaths could have been avoided with some lifestyle changes. Read the ACS Guidelines on Diet, Nutrition, and Cancer Prevention.

American Cancer Society: Prevention

http://www2.cancer.org/prevention/index.cfm?prevention=factors

> Diet and activity factors that affect risks for the most common cancers are listed here. The bottom line seems to be what Mom always said: "Eat your vegetables!"

American Cancer Society: Recommendations ☞

http://www2.cancer.org/prevention/index.cfm?prevention=recommendations

> Greater consumption of fruits and vegetables reduces the risk of cancer. Read the official statement from the ACS.

American Cancer Society: Top Stories ☞

http://www2.cancer.org/zine/dsp_StoryIndex.cfm?sc=001&fn=001_07151999_0.html

> This web site should be bookmarked if your interests lie in cancer news, research, and prevention. When I checked in, the lead article was also in my newspaper and on TV. The news of the day related to the "virtues" of the soybean in its purported role in cancer prevention. It's a nicely done section, and there are other stories as well. All are presented in layman's terms, so you don't need a medical dictionary at your side.

American College of Sports Medicine

www.acsm.org

> "The American College of Sports Medicine promotes and integrates scientific research, education, and practical applications of sports medicine and exercise science to maintain and enhance physical performance, fitness, health, and quality of life." That is their mission statement; this site is primarily aimed at membership, although you can click on "Media Room," and read some fairly recent news releases. If you click on "Public Arena," you'll just learn that the links between fitness and well-being are firmly established. Wow.

 MUST SEE!   VIDEO   AUDIO   SELLS STUFF

 CHAT ROOMS   MAILING LISTS   MESSAGE BOARDS   ADULT CONTENT

 FREE REGISTRATION REQUIRED   MEMBERS ONLY CONTENT   SEARCHABLE

American Council on Exercise
www.acefitness.org

ACE is a source of education and certification for fitness professionals, and for the evaluation of fitness products. At this site you can purchase a home study kit to become a certified personal trainer, and even take your tests online. But if you're not interested in that, click onto "Fit Facts," then click on the bottom of the page where it says "Want to see all the fitfacts?" and you'll be taken to an extensive list of articles on exercise and nutrition.

American Council on Science & Health
www.acsh.org

The American Council on Science and Health, Inc. (ACSH) is a consumer education consortium concerned with issues related to food, nutrition, chemicals, pharmaceuticals, lifestyle, the environment and health. ACSH is an independent, nonprofit, tax-exempt organization. Their top priority is to help Americans distinguish between real and hypothetical health risks. Its funding list is highly diversified, so the appearance of bias is supposed to be absent. Although I found a list of advisors, I could not find online a list of major donors.

American Council on Science & Health: Food Safety
www.acsh.org/food/index.html

The ACSH gives us science based information on food safety at this site. Its job is to separate fact from fiction, so as to help us make informed decisions. Read their press releases, editorials, and check out their links. In a quick scan of their press releases, it seems they like irradiation of our food for safety, nothing's wrong with Olestra, biotechnology on our farms is great, and Sucralose is just fine. They take on the Physicians Committee for Responsible Medicine (PCRM), and take issue with the Center for Science in the Public Interest (CSPI) on many fronts. I guess it's up to us to make our choices.

American Council on Science & Health: Nutrition & Fitness
www.acsh.org/nutrition/index.html

The ACSH serves up a diet of press releases that are directed at clearing up food scares and preventing us from pushing the panic button. This group gives a very shaky OK to vegetarianism, says that Alar on apples was safe for kids, really likes the beef industry, decries the decline of egg consumption, and called "foul" when the USDA decided to disallow irradiated foods or biogenetically altered foods to be called "organic." I couldn't find out who their main sources of funding came from, but I am suspicious that the beef and dairy industry, food processors, and Monsanto kind of like these guys. Or maybe they're just Republicans. Bottom line? You gotta decide.

American Diabetes Association:
FAQs About Nutrition & Diabetes
www.diabetes.org/nutrition/faqs.asp

"What foods can I eat a lot of?" Now that would be my first question, and it's here in this web page along with other frequently asked questions. By the way, the answer wasn't the one I was looking for, but I guess it was the right one.

American Diabetes Association: Feed Your Brain:
Nutrition Quiz
www.diabetes.org/nutrition/i_quiz.asp

I took this 10 question multiple choice quiz and scored 50%. I guess I better start doing my homework. I still had the old ideas about diabetes, and how people had to avoid so many kinds of foods. Go ahead, take it, but make sure you hang around to learn more.

American Diabetes Association:
Healthy Restaurant Eating: Is It Possible?
`www.diabetes.org/nutrition/restauranteating.asp`

Eating healthy restaurant foods is always a challenge. Here you can discover strategies for healthful eating in any restaurant, tips on drinking alcohol, delayed meals, and how to get nutrition information from a restaurant. This information is excerpted from the book, "The American Diabetes Association Guide to Healthy Restaurant Eating," by Hope Warshaw, MMSc, RD, CDE, who is a nationally recognized expert on nutrition and diabetes, and author of several other best-selling books. You can order the book in the ADA Bookstore.

American Diabetes Association: Nutrition
`www.diabetes.org/nutrition`

The American Diabetes Association has a huge web site packed with lots of information you can use. This page is the beginning of your diabetic nutrition search. Anyone with an interest in diabetic nutrition should bookmark this. You'll find advice, recipes, quizzes, and games, all in a very navigable site.

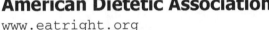

American Dietetic Association
`www.eatright.org`

The beginning page of the American Dietetic Association, its membership of professional dieticians promote optimal nutrition and health. It includes a "Tip of the Day," and a feature article. It's a great place to begin your search for nutritional truth, whether you are a professional or a consumer. It's a huge sight, and the more you navigate through this labyrinth, the more you'll find. At first, it didn't look like there was much there, but if you poke around "In the News," and in "Nutrition Resources," you'll soon find what you're looking for.

American Dietetic Association:
Antioxidant Vitamins for Optimal Health
`www.eatright.org/nfs/nfs84.html`

Bone up on the antioxidants here. Until I read this, I thought carotenoids were aliens.

American Dietetic Association: Athletes Fuel Up For Fitness
`www.eatright.org/nfs/nfs0.html`

The ADA says that nutrition is fundamental to fitness. Read their recommendations on how variety, moderation, and balance fit into your sports diet.

MUST SEE!	VIDEO	AUDIO	SELLS STUFF
CHAT ROOMS	MAILING LISTS	MESSAGE BOARDS	ADULT CONTENT
FREE REGISTRATION REQUIRED	MEMBERS ONLY CONTENT	SEARCHABLE	

American Dietetic Association:
Facts About Acesulfame Potassium
www.eatright.org/nfs/nfs69.html

Quick, what's 200 times sweeter than sugar and doesn't promote tooth decay? Check out the ADA's thoughts about this artificial sweetener.

American Dietetic Association:
Fats & Oils in the Diet - The Great Debate
www.eatright.org/nfs/nfs82.html

Once upon a time we just knew we should choose a low-fat diet, but now the debate rages on regarding what type of fat is good and what kind is bad, and how much is enough. I'll let the ADA figure it out while I work on this macadamia nut brownie.

American Dietetic Association: Fitness & Bone Health
www.eatright.org/nfs/nfs38.html

Strength training is known to help bone health, no matter what age you are. Read what the ADA says about exercise and osteoporosis.

American Dietetic Association: Food Biotechnology
www.eatright.org/nfs/nfs9.html

Is genetic engineering of your food safe? The ADA gives us their definitive and authoritative and unequivocal answer. You have to go read it here.

American Dietetic Association:
Gaining Weight - A Healthy Plan For Adding Pounds
www.eatright.org/nfs/nfs10.html

Believe it or not, some people have trouble gaining weight. Here's practical and safe advice on how to get started. Getting in touch with a registered dietician is highly recommended.

American Dietetic Association:
Home Food Safety - It's In Your Hands
www.eatright.org/feature/060199.html

Very often, when you feel like you've got a case of "flu," it very likely could be a food-borne illness, or food poisoning. And it's often due to mishandling of food right at home. Read up on how to decrease the risks.

American Dietetic Association: Journal Highlights
www.eatright.org/pr/highlights.html

Check out monthly highlights of interesting articles and research studies from the Journal of The American Dietetic Association.

American Dietetic Association: News: Using Diet Drugs
www.eatright.org/newsusingdd

Read what the ADA thinks about prescription diet drugs, and how they should fit it in your diet plans.

American Dietetic Association: Nutrition & Health Campaign For Older Americans

www.eatright.org/olderamericans

You can buy the ADA's Food Guide Pyramid for persons over 50 years old. There is one here but it's fuzzy and doesn't print very well. Order it here, or read about it.

American Dietetic Association: Nutrition & Health Campaign for Women

www.eatright.org/womenshealth

While women recognize the relationship between nutrition and health, they are barraged with confusing, contradictory and often misleading information that is the result of fads or promotions rather than solid science. This ongoing campaign seeks to help women make informed decisions that can help them decrease their risk for heart disease, breast cancer, osteoporosis, obesity, and diabetes. The ADA continues to advocate for nutrition research on women's health issues.

American Dietetic Association: Nutrition & Health Campaign for Women: Breast Cancer & Nutrition

www.eatright.org/womenshealth/breastcancer.html

Breast cancer kills 46,000 women each year in America. The ADA's campaign for nutrition and health for women discusses what is known and what is unknown. You'll learn what things you can do to reduce your risk based on what is known.

American Dietetic Association: Nutrition & Health for Older Americans: Antioxidants

www.eatright.org/olderamericans/antioxidants.html

If you live in New England, you know what oxidation does to your car over time. We call it "road cancer." Although we don't rust, antioxidants help us keep going and possibly decrease our risk of cancer. Where do we get them? How much do we need to keep from "rusting"?

American Dietetic Association: Nutrition & Health for Older Americans: Calcium

www.eatright.org/olderamericans/calcium.html

Calcium isn't just a woman's thing. If you're an older American, this mineral needs your attention, too. See how certain medications can interfere with calcium absorption, and check out which foods give you a good dose of the stuff.

 MUST SEE!   VIDEO   AUDIO $ SELLS STUFF

 CHAT ROOMS   MAILING LISTS   MESSAGE BOARDS   ADULT CONTENT

 FREE REGISTRATION REQUIRED   MEMBERS ONLY CONTENT   SEARCHABLE

American Dietetic Association:
Nutrition & Health for Older Americans: Fiber
`www.eatright.org/olderamericans/fiber.html`

Eat your beans. They're good for you. Actually, there's a lot to know about fiber, and you'll learn how to get your recommended 35 grams a day. There's a lot more to it than "roughage."

American Dietetic Association:
Nutrition & Health for Older Americans: Grains
`www.eatright.org/olderamericans/grains.html`

Think you're getting enough grains from your bowl of cereal? The trick here is to think "whole grains," and eat your spelt.

American Dietetic Association:
Nutrition & Health for Older Americans: Water
`www.eatright.org/olderamericans/waterhydration.html`

Did you know that you could live for weeks without food, but you wouldn't last a week without water? Visit this site, but take your water bottle along.

American Dietetic Association:
Nutrition Care of Your Loved One With Alzheimer's Disease
`www.eatright.org/nfs/nfs61.html`

People with Alzheimer's Disease often have a number of problems that affect their ability to eat. The ADA gives you some tips on caring for someone who may depend on you.

American Dietetic Association:
Nutrition for Physical Fitness & Athletic Performance
`www.eatright.org/afitperform.htmlwww.eatright.org/afitperform.html`

This position paper was written with the Canadian Dietetic Association.

American Dietetic Association:
Nutrition Intervention in the Care of Persons With HIV
`www.eatright.org/ahivinter.html`

Nutrition issues, including wasting and nutritional deficiencies, are among the many aspects of this position paper of the ADA. You'll find it helpful whether you are caring for someone or you are a healthcare provider.

American Dietetic Association: Position on Vegetarian Diets
`www.eatright.org/adap1197.html`

This position statement discusses health implications of vegetarianism, nutritional concerns, and recommendations for supplementation.

American Dietetic Association:
Questions Men Ask About Nutrition & Fitness
`www.eatright.org/nfs/nfs51.html`

Do men have special dietary needs? (Besides beer and chips, they mean.)

American Dietetic Association: Safe Cooking Temperatures
www.eatright.org/cookingtemps.html

> The ADA has posted this chart of recommended safe cooking temperatures.

American Dietetic Association: Search Daily Tips
www.eatright.org/cgi/searchtemp.cgi?dir=erm&template=searcherm.htm

> Search the American Dietetic Association's Daily Tips.

American Dietetic Association: Seniors - Eat Well for Good Health
www.eatright.org/nfs/nfs62.html

> The ADA says that as you age your nutritional needs change. Read up on what it is you need to do to stay healthy.

American Dietetic Association: Soluble Fiber & Heart Disease
www.eatright.org/nfs/nfs88.html

> Soluble fiber has been scientifically proven to reduce blood cholesterol levels, which may help reduce your risk of heart disease. Read more about the wonders of fiber, its sources, and how much is enough.

American Dietetic Association: Straight Answers About Vitamin & Mineral Supplements
www.eatright.org/nfs/nfs66.html

> For the most part we get all the nutrients we need if we are following the food guide pyramid; however, there are many reasons why a vitamin or mineral supplement may be needed. Read this and seek help from a registered dietician (900-225-5267).The cost of the call will be $1.95 for the first minute and $.95 for each additional minute.

American Dietetic Association: The Proof Is In The Tea Leaves
www.eatright.org/nfs/nfs87.html

> Folk medicine has long valued tea as a remedy for a variety of ailments. And many tea drinkers find the beverage soothing. Currently researchers are studying the possibility that tea reduces the risk of certain types of cancer and heart disease, when consumed as part of a healthful eating plan.

American Dietetic Association: Tip of the Day
www.eatright.org/erm.html

> Search the archives of the ADA's daily tips; they're brief, and useful.

 MUST SEE!   VIDEO   AUDIO   SELLS STUFF

 CHAT ROOMS   MAILING LISTS   MESSAGE BOARDS   ADULT CONTENT

 FREE REGISTRATION REQUIRED   MEMBERS ONLY CONTENT   SEARCHABLE

American Dietetic Association:
Tip: Sports Nutrition Game Plan
www.eatright.org/erm/erm012699.html

From the archives of the ADA comes this sports nutrition tip. Choosing the right foods helps you energize muscles for your main event, and helps to rebuild them for the next competition.

American Dietetic Association: Weight Management
www.eatright.org/adap0197.html

"It is the position of The American Dietetic Association that successful weight management for adults requires a life-long commitment to healthful lifestyle behaviors emphasizing eating practices and daily physical activity that are sustainable and enjoyable." Read the entire position statement on weight management from the ADA - before you go on a diet plan or spend money.

American Dietetic Association: What Are Triglycerides?
www.eatright.org/nfs/nfs13.html

Aren't they just 3 glycerides? Why complicate matters. But you just better make sure you know how high yours are. Your doctor will know when he checks your total blood cholesterol. Read up on what they are, and what they do, and why you've got to watch them.

American Dietetic Association: What Is Olestra?
www.eatright.org/nfs/nfs18.html

I'm confused. The ADA says that Olestra is OK, even if it does reduce your body's ability to absorb the fat-soluble vitamins and carotenoids; but the International Food Information Council (IFIC) says that if you eat it, it'll stain your shorts. The truth must lie in moderation, but I'm not one to open up a bag of chips and eat "just a couple." Pass the fat and I'll walk an extra mile.

American Dietetic Association: Whole - Grain Goodness
www.eatright.org/nfs/nfs30.html

Nutrition experts recommend we eat at least three servings of whole-grain foods daily. Apparently, white bread and hot dog buns don't really count.

American Dietetic Association: Catch the Calcium Craze
www.eatright.org/nfs/nfs72.html

Is calcium available in anything else besides dairy products? Got kale? Time to bone up on the whys and wheres of calcium.

American Dietetic Association: Diabetes Meal Planning
www.eatright.org/nfs/nfs37.html

There's no one diet for diabetes. General guidelines exist, such as "eat less fat and saturated fat" and "eat more whole grains, fruits, and vegetables." See what the ADA suggests for a diabetic meal plan.

American Dietetic Association: Nutrition & Health Campaign for Women: Diabetes & Nutrition
www.eatright.org/womenshealth/diabetes.html

Diabetes occurs in more than 13 million persons in the United States, and approximately 60 percent of the new cases are diagnosed in women. Find out what is known and what is unknown about diabetes, and how it is now treated.

American Dietetic Association: Nutrition & Health Campaign for Women: Good News Guide For Healthy Women

`www.eatright.org/womenshealth/guide.html`

> It's the little things that you do that can make big differences to your health. Find out in this good news guide.

American Dietetic Association: Nutrition & Health Campaign for Women: Heart Disease & Nutrition

`www.eatright.org/womenshealth/heartdisease.html`

> Bad News: This year heart disease will kill over 500,000 women according to the ADA. Good News: Nutrition intervention can lower risk factors for many women. Take a minute to visit this ADA site for more good news, and take charge.

American Dietetic Association: Nutrition & Health Campaign for Women: Osteoporosis & Nutrition

`www.eatright.org/womenshealth/osteoporosis.html`

> 1.5 million bones will break this year alone as a result of osteoporosis. Although many factors contribute to this breakdown, find out what role good nutrition plays in decreasing the risk of a fracture.

American Dietetic Association: Nutrition & Health Campaign for Women: Weight Management & Nutrition

`www.eatright.org/womenshealth/weightmanagement.html`

> 27% of American women are overweight, 52% of women consider themselves to be overweight, 40% are trying to lose weight, and 70% of obese children will become obese adults. Want more startling facts? Visit this ADA site to learn more about what we know, and what we don't know about weight management.

American Dietetic Association: Position Paper: Promotion of Breastfeeding

`www.eatright.org/adap0697.html`

> "It is the position of The American Dietetic Association (ADA) that public health and clinical efforts to promote breast-feeding should be sustained and strengthened. ADA strongly encourages the promotion and advocacy of activities that support longer duration of successful breast-feeding, in order to optimize the indisputable nutritional, immunological, psychological, and economic benefits." (from the ADA position paper on Promotion of Breastfeeding) Read up on the benefits here.

 MUST SEE!   VIDEO   AUDIO   SELLS STUFF

 CHAT ROOMS   MAILING LISTS   MESSAGE BOARDS   ADULT CONTENT

 FREE REGISTRATION REQUIRED   MEMBERS ONLY CONTENT   SEARCHABLE

American Dietetic Association:
The ABCs of Fats, Oils, & Cholesterols

www.eatright.org/nfs/nfs2.html

This is a good primer on fats.

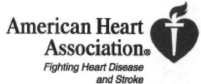

American Heart Association

www.americanheart.org

The AHA's site is loaded with information relating to heart disease and stroke. It's an excellent directory.

American Heart Association:
An Eating Plan For Healthy Americans

www.americanheart.org/catalog/Health_catpage5.html

Better food habits can help you reduce one of the major risk factors for heart attack — high blood cholesterol. This eating plan from the American Heart Association describes the latest advice of medical and nutrition experts. The best way to help lower your blood cholesterol level is to eat less saturated fatty acids and cholesterol, and control your weight. The AHA Diet gives you an easy-to-follow guide to eating with your heart in mind.

American Heart Association: Body Composition Tests

www.americanheart.org/Heart_and_Stroke_A_Z_Guide/body.html

Obesity is a major risk factor for heart disease. The AHA lists measurements used in assessing overall physical fitness. Learn how to measure your waist circumference and body mass index.

American Heart Association: Cholesterol

www.americanheart.org/Heart_and_Stroke_A_Z_Guide/choldi.html

A soft, waxy substance? It's not only in my heart; that must be what's in my ears, too! This story could be good; there's good guys and bad guys in this site. It's a short page, but of great importance to us all. I especially like the part where alcohol is linked to good cholesterol.

American Heart Association:
Commercial Weight Reduction Programs

www.americanheart.org/Heart_and_Stroke_A_Z_Guide/commw.html

When choosing a weight loss program the AHA recommends that you look for these features before you show them the money.

American Heart Association: Diet & Nutrition

www.americanheart.org/catalog/Health_catpage4.html

Choosing the right foods to eat and preparing them in a healthy way can reduce your risk of heart attack. Start here for eating with your heart in mind.

American Heart Association: Dietary Guidelines For Healthy Children

www.americanheart.org/Heart_and_Stroke_A_Z_Guide/dietgk.html

These guidelines are for kids and adolescents over the age of two.

American Heart Association: Dietary Recommendations

www.americanheart.org/catalog/Health_catpage5.html

Start here for your journey through this huge and authoritative web site where you'll find information on dietary guidelines for healthy adults and children, managing your weight, menu planning, vegetarian diets, and much more.

American Heart Association: Dietary/Lifestyle Interventions & the AHA Diet

www.americanheart.org/Heart_and_Stroke_A_Z_Guide/dietlife.html

People with coronary heart disease should be managed by their physicians, who can also assess other risks. The AHA is particularly concerned with people who may have inherited cholesterol metabolism defects.

American Heart Association: Dietary/Weight Loss Supplements

www.americanheart.org/Heart_and_Stroke_A_Z_Guide/dietw.html

Read the position statement here of the AHA regarding supplements and drugs for weight loss.

American Heart Association: Fad Diets

www.americanheart.org/Heart_and_Stroke_A_Z_Guide/fad.html

AHA recommends: "The American Heart Association has declared "war" on fad diets. American Heart Association nutrition experts recommend adopting healthful eating habits permanently, rather than impatiently pursuing crash diets in hopes of losing unwanted pounds in a few days." Read more here about fad diets before you take out your credit card and load your shopping cart.

American Heart Association: Guidelines for Weight Management Programs for Healthy Adults

www.americanheart.org/Heart_and_Stroke_A_Z_Guide/commw.html

Things to look for when choosing a weight loss/management program should include these essential components listed by the AHA.

 MUST SEE!   VIDEO   AUDIO $ SELLS STUFF

 CHAT ROOMS   MAILING LISTS   MESSAGE BOARDS   ADULT CONTENT

 FREE REGISTRATION REQUIRED   MEMBERS ONLY CONTENT   SEARCHABLE

American Heart Association: Managing Your Weight 👁

www.americanheart.org/Heart_and_Stroke_A_Z_Guide/obesity.html

> Obesity can contribute to heart disease, and managing your weight can be smart for your heart. Start with a healthful diet and an active lifestyle. Begin here for suggestions and guidelines before you go anywhere.

American Heart Association: Phony AMA Diet

www.americanheart.org/Heart_and_Stroke_A_Z_Guide/pahad.html

> "The AHA warns that the public should be wary of any diet (including fad diets) purporting to be the AHA diet that gives specific menus or suggests that the diet should be followed for a specific length of time. The true AHA diet gives recommended servings per day of various food categories, not of specific foods. The AHA diet is a nutritionally adequate eating plan for lifetime use. While it can help healthy people lose excess weight or maintain ideal body weight, quick weight loss is not its purpose." (from the AHA). Read more about phony claims and misuse of the AHA sanctions before you send money or follow any diet.

American Heart Association: Trans Fatty Acids

www.americanheart.org/Heart_and_Stroke_A_Z_Guide/tfa.html

> Find out if butter is better, and learn what the heck trans fatty acids really are right here. Saturated, monounsaturated, and polyunsaturated fats are defined. Then see what their relationship to cholesterol is. And what about hydrogenation? Do I really need to know all this?

American Heart Association: Vegetarian Diets

www.americanheart.org/Heart_and_Stroke_A_Z_Guide/vegdiet.html

> Vegetarian diets are healthful and nutritionally adequate when properly planned, according to the AHA. Some basic questions are answered here, and some suggestions for menu planning are offered.

American Heart Association:
Women, Heart Disease & Stroke

www.americanheart.org/Heart_and_Stroke_A_Z_Guide/women.html

> Many women believe that cancer is more of a threat, but they're wrong. Nearly twice as many women in the United States die of heart disease and stroke as from all forms of cancer, including breast cancer.

American Heart Association:
Women, Heart Disease & Stroke Statistics

www.americanheart.org/Heart_and_Stroke_A_Z_Guide/womens.html

> These statistics are mind-boggling.

American Heart Association:
Dietary Guidelines for Healthy American Adults

www.americanheart.org/Heart_and_Stroke_A_Z_Guide/dietg.html

> OK, we all know we have to eat our vegetables, but what else? Any chance it might be chocolate? Visit American Heart and see if there's anything good to eat that's good for you.

American Medical Association Health Insight:
Developing Your Fitness Program

www.ama-assn.org/insight/gen_hlth/trainer/index.htm

The human body is designed for motion and requires regular exercise to stay functional and avoid disease. With this site, you can begin with the fitness questionnaire, and begin to move. I suspect we know we need to move, but it's the time thing, or the motivation thing. This could give you a bit of a boost.

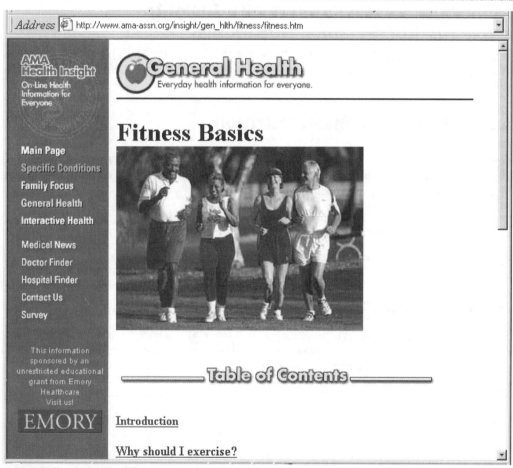

American Medical Association Health Insight:
Fitness Basics

www.ama-assn.org/insight/gen_hlth/fitness/fitness.htm

"We are the most physically inactive generation that ever lived." Thus begins fitness basics from the AMA. Check out their fitness tips and goals.

 MUST SEE!   VIDEO   AUDIO $ SELLS STUFF

 CHAT ROOMS   MAILING LISTS   MESSAGE BOARDS   ADULT CONTENT

 FREE REGISTRATION REQUIRED   MEMBERS ONLY CONTENT   SEARCHABLE

American Medical Association Health Insight: Interactive Health 👁

www.ama-assn.org/consumer/interact.htm

> Check out these health assessments that are interactive; the personal nutritionist will rate your nutritional habits, the personal trainer will help you to develop a personalized exercise program, and healthy weight will give you a personal evaluation. There are other interactive tools to try as well.

American Medical Association Health Insight: Interactive Health: Personal Nutritionist

www.ama-assn.org/insight/yourhlth/pernutri/pernutri.htm

> This is a quick online eating assessment to see how your eating habits are. The you can read their suggestions for you to begin a healthy lifestyle.

American Society for Clinical Nutrition

www.faseb.org/ascn

> The American Society for Clinical Nutrition is a professional organization whose purpose is to promote the application of nutrition science in health promotion and disease prevention, and to participate in public policy. Requires membership.

American Sports Nutrition $

www.fitness-connection.com/American_Sports_Nutrition.htm

> They carry a LOT of brands. Do your homework. Buy stuff here.

Aoqili Fat Loss Soap $

www.dfwbiznet.com/Soap.htm

> Go no further; we've found THE magic bullet. By using this seaweed-based soap, people have lost an average of 33 pounds! Read more of these amazing claims, then fill your shopping cart, empty your wallet, and lather up.

Arbor Nutrition Guide 👁

www.arborcom.com

> This is an extensive tool to help you through the nutrition maze. It can lead you to hospitals, universities, and government sites. You can search clinical and applied nutrition sites as well. This is a great starting point for your nutrition search with credible sources. These sites aren't selling stuff, either. This is the most thorough nutrition resource I've found. Although it's primarily aimed at health professionals, you too can wade through this and chances are you'll find what you're looking for.

Arizona Health Sciences Center: Nutrition Information & Your Health 👁

www.ahsc.arizona.edu/~lei/nutrition

> Here's a great resource to help you search the Web. If you are looking for info on nutrients, additives, consumer info, or recipes, this guide will link you to where you want to go. There's a wealth of resource information here. Bookmark this site.

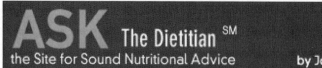

Ask the Dietician 👁

www.dietitian.com

Scroll down an alphabetical list ranging from "alcohol" to "zinc," click and read answers on the subject which have been previously asked. The site is maintained by Joanne Larsen, a registered dietician, whose web site has garnered many top awards in the nutrition category. All answers include many links on any subject, and most end up with the recommendation that you consult a registered dietician in your local area. There are no fancy graphics here, but questions are answered within 3 days.

Ask the Dietician: Allergies

www.dietitian.com/allergie.html

Questions from people who have concerns regarding food allergies are answered here. Ask the Dietician has links to help you learn more or suggestions on where to go or what to get for help.

Ask the Dietician: Cancer

www.dietitian.com/cancer.html

Vitamin B17 can cure cancer? That's an airplane, and not a vitamin. Read up on diet and cancer here from Joanne Larsen.

Ask the Dietician: Diabetic Exchange & Carbo Counting

www.dietitian.com/diabexch.html

I hate counting and I hate getting in the exchange line. But if you're a diabetic, you have to do both every day. Go visit the dietician here to see what it's all about.

Ask the Dietician: Fad Diets

www.dietitian.com/faddiet.html

The dietician is "in," and she's answering your questions about The Sacred Heart Diet, adaptogens, and anabolic diets.

Ask the Dietician: Fatty Acids & Trans Fat

www.dietitian.com/fattyaci.html

Polyunsaturated, cholesterol, omega 3, omega 6, ratios, and trans fat. I'm getting a new vocabulary, and more confused. Better find a registered dietician.

Ask the Dietician: Headaches & Migraines

www.dietitian.com/headaches.html

Food triggers that can set off migraines are discussed here with reference to other sources to help you.

 MUST SEE!   VIDEO   AUDIO $ SELLS STUFF

 CHAT ROOMS   MAILING LISTS   MESSAGE BOARDS   ADULT CONTENT

 FREE REGISTRATION REQUIRED   MEMBERS ONLY CONTENT   SEARCHABLE

Ask the Dietician: Sports Nutrition

www.dietitian.com/sportnut.html

Ask the Dietician gets questions from her E-mail and answers them online. Questions are answered and recommendations are usually made to see a dietician or certified trainer or exercise physiologist. But information is concise and answers are linked to other useful sites in specific areas.

Ask the Dietician: Underweight

www.dietitian.com/underwei.html

Here are questions from people who are underweight and trying to gain some. Subjects range from protein powders to "what should I eat to pack it on" type questions. The topics of calories, fats, and protein are discussed.

Ask the Dietician: Vitamin Supplements

www.dietitian.com/vitamins.html

Do you really need to be buying all those pricey vitamins and supplements? Joanne Larsen says that you just might be sending your money down the toilet in some cases.

Association for Morbid Obesity Support ⬇ 🗣

www.obesityhelp.com/morbidobesity

This is a peer support group of over 1,300 people whose aim is to reduce the frustration and isolation often associated with morbid obesity. You can find a surgeon or a list of peers in your area if you want, or join a chat room. Ask a question about weight loss surgery, and get an answer on their message board.

AST Sports Science $

www.ast-ss.com

Get your vitamins, supplements, DHEA, andro, and a testosterone saliva test kit right here.

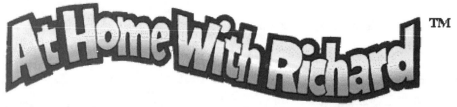

At Home With Richard Simmons ⬇$🗣🎬

www.richardsimmons.com

This is huge. Join Richard's Clubhouse for only $9.95 a month, and enter this very busy web site. Last time I looked, well over three million hits were recorded. You can also go shopping and buy his stuff. "Move, groove, and Lose" your pounds and your money. But if it works for you, go for it. Video downloads require Micosoft Newshow. Create your own web page here, or get an e-mail address that ends in @richardsimmons.com.

Atkins Diet

www.atkinscenter.com/diet101.html

Dr. Atkins is the best-selling author/biochemist who espouses a lifetime nutritional philosophy of consuming nutrient dense, unprocessed foods and vita-nutrient supplementation. He finds fault with the current food pyramid, questioning the emphasis on carbohydrates especially. Although highly controversial, he has sold over 5 million diet books.

Atlantic Surgery Associates: Gastric Surgery Information

www.stomachstapling.com/surgery.html

Discussion of things to consider before and after the operation.

Australian School of Macrobiotics

www.comcen.com.au/~safe77/index.html

The Australian School of Macrobiotics was established in Melbourne 5 years ago.. The center has 4 practitioner's rooms, a large seminar room that will accommodate up to a 100 persons for lectures and a well equipped kitchen where they teach whole foods cooking. The role of the center is to boost an awareness to the general public to take better care of themselves, understand how to handle stress and use the services provided at the center. To learn a teeny bit about the macrobiotic philosophy, go to Natalie Jung's Cooking School and read about the 7 Principles of the Infinite Universe and the 12 Laws of Diversity.

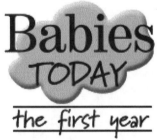

Babies Today Online: Breastfeeding Articles & Resources

Breastfeeding basics, articles, FAQs, and suggested books to help you.

Barbara's Obesity Meds & Research News

www.obesity-news.com

Subscribe to this and you get up-to-date news on obesity research from journals and medical conferences. There's really a lot of stuff here that does not require subscription and tons of links to help you find what you need. You can also check into Barbara's phen/fen diary and see pictures of her before and after her 100 pound weight loss.

Battling Boredom

http://primusweb.com/fitnesspartner/library/activity/battleboredom.htm

Having trouble getting motivated for your daily walk, or finding excuses not to stop by the gym after work? Here's what to do.

Benefits of Fasting

www.healthpromoting.com/articles/benefit.doc

"Fasting is the complete abstinence from all substances except pure water, in an environment of total rest," begins this treatise on fasting, from Alan Goldhamer, D.C.

 MUST SEE!   VIDEO   AUDIO $ SELLS STUFF

 CHAT ROOMS   MAILING LISTS   MESSAGE BOARDS   ADULT CONTENT

 FREE REGISTRATION REQUIRED   MEMBERS ONLY CONTENT   SEARCHABLE

BeTrim Too $

www.betrimtoo.com

Does weight loss without diet, drugs, exercise, or hunger sound like the road you want to go down? With claims of losses up to 50 pounds in a month, why not place your order, then order a couple of pizzas? Delivered, of course.

Better Health: Dean Ornish M.D.

www.betterhealth.com/ornish

Dr. Dean Ornish is a leading researcher who demonstrated that comprehensive lifestyle changes may reverse coronary heart disease without surgery or drugs. He is also the author of five bestsellers. This site is updated daily. Sign up for his weekly E-mail bulletin. Here you can learn about his program, search the archives, and even chat with him on occasion.

Better Health: Dean Ornish M.D.:
Key Elements of His Program

www.betterhealth.com/ornish/articles/gen/0,4260,6754_125300,00.html

This is a very brief overview of Dr. Ornish's program, giving you a tiny insight into components of his program including diet, stress management, exercise, and group support. There's also a list of participating providers who supervise the program.

Better Health: Never Say Diet

www.betterhealth.com/neversaydiet

The Never Say Diet Center is not about traditional dieting; it's about new ways of thinking about food, exercise and self-image. This seems to be a place for everyone - from those who have lots of weight to lose to those who want to put on weight. You choose a goal - specific community, and go from there. Better Health is a division of iVillage.com, The Women's Network.

Beyond Dieting

www.beyonddieting.com

Beyond Dieting is a support group in Calgary, Alberta. This is not a diet program, but rather a program that discusses and encourages healthy lifestyle choices.

BigFitness.com $

www.bigfitness.com

Inside this site you will find quality fitness equipment, both new and reconditioned. They have commercial, light commercial, and stuff for home use. Order online.

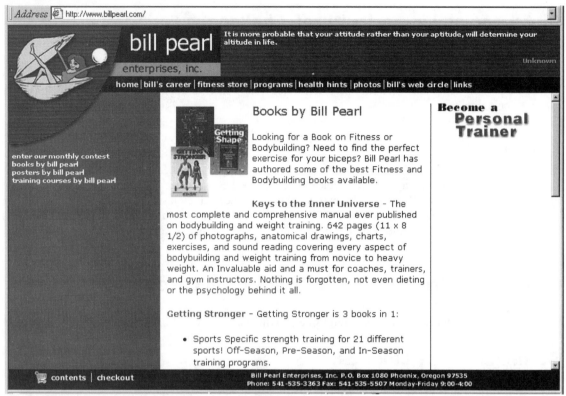

Bill Pearl Enterprises, Inc. $

www.billpearl.com

Bill Pearl has been training and competing for over 55 years, and I certainly wouldn't be one to tell him he's an old guy, but he has an incredible web site for anyone interested in strength training, from beginner to champion. Check out "20 Months to a Champion Physique," which is the finest strength training you can get for free on the web. Each month has information, charts, pictures, and everything you need to do to become a Bill Pearl clone. You can stop anytime if you're afraid you might get too big! Bill also is a storekeeper where you can buy books, courses, videos, posters, vitamins and supplements. Try "Health Hints" for exercising your brain. And his web circle will keep you so busy that you might just have to skip today's exercise session.

Bionomic Nutrition Forum

http://venus.nildram.co.uk/veganmc/forum.htm

You can join, or you can lurk. It's designed to be an ongoing scientific discussion of natural hygiene. If you're interested in the natural living philosophy, jump right in!

 MUST SEE!   VIDEO   AUDIO $ SELLS STUFF

 CHAT ROOMS   MAILING LISTS   MESSAGE BOARDS   ADULT CONTENT

 FREE REGISTRATION REQUIRED   MEMBERS ONLY CONTENT   SEARCHABLE

Biotechnology in Agriculture: Challenges For The Future
www.nal.usda.gov/bic/Audio/BT-MD.html

On March 19,1999, Dan Glickman, Secretary of Agriculture, hosted this "Millenium Discussion." Listen to these audio segments with RealPlayer, which you can download. There's an interesting discussion of "terminator" (sterile) seed technology, as well as the major impact biotechnology may have on agriculture.

Body Positive
www.bodypositive.com

BodyPositive looks at ways we can feel good in the bodies we have. "Remember, your body hears everything you think." Body Positive explores taking up occupancy inside your own skin, rather than living above the chin until you're thin. It is a set of ideas that may help you find greater well-being in the body you have. The underlying philosophy of this site is "Change your mind, change your culture, and let your body be."

Bugs in the News: What the Heck is an E. coli? 👁
http://falcon.cc.ukans.edu/~jbrown/ecoli.html

This is reader friendly; that is, it's in English and written at my level of understanding - seventh grade.

Burning Holiday Calories
http://primusweb.com/fitnesspartner/library/activity/holicals.htm

You're eating your way through the Holidays, and you don't have time for your exercise program. The calorie calculator alarm is ringing, but wait; you may be burning more calories than you think. Here's an interesting list of holiday activities, and the energy they can consume. Kissing under the mistletoe looks like it's only good if you do it repeatedly. Don't bother counting the reps.

Buying Equipment For a Home Gym
http://primusweb.com/fitnesspartner/library/features/0298hmgym.htm

There's a lot of junk out there. This site will give you some good background info from the American Council on Exercise. Read up on these five steps before venturing out.

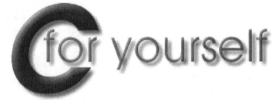

C For Yourself
www.cforyourself.com

The Vitamin C controversy rages on. Here's an extensive site with lots of prestigious links to presumably give itself some credibility.

Cabbage Soup Diet: Mayo Clinic
www.mayohealth.org/mayo/9704/htm/wabout1.htm

The miracle of the cabbage soup diet is explained in a nutshell by the dieticians at the Mayo Clinic. Please continue the search for the magic bullet; it's not here.

CADIS Information

www.toon.org/~cadis/info/cadis.html

This Carbohydrate Addict Diet group is not part of Dr. Heller's, but is a forum for discussion of hyperinsulinism and it's symptoms.

CADIS: Carbohydrate Addict's Diet Information & Support

www.toon.org/~cadis/info/subscribe.html

CADIS is the Carbohydrate Addict's Diet Information and Support mailing list. It is a private discussion group designed to give support, advice, and share successes and failures.

California Dietetic Association

www.dietitian.org

CDA is a state association of the American Dietetic Association. Over 7,000 professionals practice in California. Their web site is filled with short tips on everything nutrition. I found easy to read information in the "Food for Thought" section, including short articles on margarine products that lower cholesterol, the new DRI's (formerly RDA's), and breakfast of champions. Also check out their archives in that same section. You'll find lots of good links to other sites if what they give you seems like just a tease.

Calorie Control Council

Calorie Control Council

www.caloriecontrol.org

The Calorie Control Council, established in 1966, is an international association representing the low-calorie and reduced-fat food and beverage industry. Today it represents 60 manufacturers and suppliers of low-calorie, low-fat and light foods and beverages, including the manufacturers and suppliers of more than a dozen different dietary sweeteners, fat replacers and other low-calorie ingredients. Although they obviously have an axe to grind, their pages are informative and helpful.

Calorie Control Council: Calorie Calculator

www.caloriecontrol.org/caloriecontrol/cgi-bin/calorie_calculator.cgi

Just enter a food item and it calculates how much fat and how many calories are in it; for instance, I entered "brownie," and it told me that there were 3 grams of fat and 160 calories. So I figured I had room for six brownies today.

 MUST SEE!   VIDEO   AUDIO $ SELLS STUFF

 CHAT ROOMS   MAILING LISTS   MESSAGE BOARDS   ADULT CONTENT

 FREE REGISTRATION REQUIRED   MEMBERS ONLY CONTENT   SEARCHABLE

Calorie Control Council: Enhanced Calorie Calculator
www.caloriecontrol.org/cgi-
bin/Enhanced_calcalc/enhanced_calcalc.cgi

This calculator kind of works like an online shopping cart; you can scroll through all the things you've eaten, check the proper servings off, and it totals your fat and calorie intake. You can add, delete, and enter serving sizes.

Calorie Control Council: Exercise Calculator
www.caloriecontrol.org/exercalc.html

Answer some simple questions such as what you are going to do ("play hockey" or "mop up after the guests leave"), how long you'll do it, and how much you weigh, and this nifty calculator tell you how many calories you will burn. They say it should only be used as an estimate.

Calorie Control Council: Fat Replacers
www.caloriecontrol.org/fatrepl.html

This seems to be the place to get the skinny on this subject. Lots of questions here regarding fat: what it is, the kinds of fat, reduced fat, fat replacers, labels, and glossaries.

Calorie Control Council: Low Calorie Sweeteners
www.caloriecontrol.org/lowcal.html

Any questions about artificial sweeteners, their safety, their makeup, and their uses are answered here.

Calorie Control Council: Winning Weights
www.caloriecontrol.org/winweigh.html

Here's some commonsense approaches mixed with interesting trivia. Of course, they do toot their own horn, and sing praises of fat replacers and low-cal sweeteners at times.

Campaign For Food Safety 👁
www.purefood.org

The Campaign for Food Safety is a public interest organization dedicated to building a healthy, safe, and sustainable system of food production and consumption. They are a global clearinghouse for information and grassroots technical assistance, and are affiliated with the Organic Consumers Association. Their site is filled with news about food safety, and if you have any concerns regarding such areas as use of bovine growth hormone, irradiation, mad cow disease, or genetically engineered food, check this out. Read their Campaign for Food Safety News.

Campaign For Food Safety News
www.purefood.org/listserv.htm

Campaign for Food Safety maintains this page of past issues of their electronic newsletter concerning genetic engineering, factory farming and organics. You can also sign up to receive the newsletter in your E-mail. See the bottom of the page for instructions.

Campaign For Food Safety:
Bovine Growth Hormone Controversy
www.purefood.org/rbghlink.html

Bovine growth hormone has been given to up to 30% of America's dairy cows for about 5 years to make them produce more milk. There is indirect evidence that BGH may contribute to breast and prostate cancer, and the issue is being hotly debated in Canada and in Europe. However, the FDA says it's harmless, basing much of their information on studies supposedly done by Monsanto, who coincidentally produce the suspect. So, are Americans currently unwittingly participating in a huge nationwide study of BGH and its effects? And now, America's dairy farmers are suing the FDA, saying more studies should have been done. Sounds to me like somebody's going to get caught with their hand in the cookie jar. I'm going to buy my own cow, and have cookies and milk. This site has links galore to help you understand what's going on.

Campaign For Food Safety:
Dangers of Genetic Engineered Food
www.purefood.org/gelink.html

Europe requires labeling of gene altered foods, so does Australia. But the US says it's not necessary. Food processors and retailers are adamantly opposed, saying the FDA doesn't see any need for labeling. Observers say that labeling genetically altered foods would be tantamount to imprinting a skull and crossbones on the package, and it could be a fatal blow to biotechnology. I'm beginning to feel like I may be like one of those rats in a study, and that I'm not in the control group.

Campaign For Food Safety:
Food Irradiation - News, Articles, Links, Books
www.purefood.org/irradlink.html

Are you looking for a wealth of information on irradiation? The Campaign for Food Safety hands it over to you so you can be an informed consumer, as well as a healthy consumer. At this visit to this web site, the FDA was proposing to eliminate all irradiation labeling from your food, and the CFS was actively seeking your help in writing to the FDA and your congressperson. Seems there's something fishy going on among the FDA, Department of Energy, and the meat industry. If you feel you should be able to choose foods that haven't been zapped, and you'd rather just have the processors clean up their slaughterhouses and processing plants, write your letters now, and bookmark this site.

Campaign For Food Safety:
Mad Pig & Cow Disease/Creutzfeld-Jacob Disease
www.purefood.org/meatlink.html

Get up to speed here, where you can find all the news and links you ever wanted. Click on a few of these links, and after reading them, you'll be following me to the organic/vegetarian farm.

 MUST SEE!   VIDEO   AUDIO   SELLS STUFF

 CHAT ROOMS   MAILING LISTS   MESSAGE BOARDS   ADULT CONTENT

 FREE REGISTRATION REQUIRED   MEMBERS ONLY CONTENT   SEARCHABLE

Campaign For Food Safety: Monsanto Watch
www.purefood.org/monlink.htm

Terminator seeds, suicide seeds, gene giants, genetically modified seeds, call it what you want, it's controversial. Brazil, Europe, Japan all don't want their seeds. What's a giant to do? Campaign for Food Safety maintains the Monsanto Watch, and it does make one wonder whether American consumers have been blindfolded and muzzled. Where's the truth?

Campaign For Food Safety: Toxic & Contaminated Food
www.purefood.org/toxiclink.html

Current news on pesticides, dioxin, toxic sludge, antibiotics, and other food contaminants can be found here, along with articles and links to other areas of food safety.

CancerGuide: Bovine Cartilage
http://cancerguide.org/btc.html

Bovine tracheal cartilage has been around longer than shark cartilage and has its following of fans, apparently. Although this is not to be confused with conventional therapy, the author, Steve Dunn, suggests that BTC can be used with conventional treatment.

CancerGuide: PSK
http://cancerguide.org/psk.html

Derived from a common edible mushroom, Coriolus Versicolor, PSK has been shown to have modest to moderate benefit when used in combination with chemotherapy. If you're investigating alternative therapy in conjunction with standard therapy, this may be of interest to you.

CancerNet: Eating Hints For Cancer Patients 👁
http://cancernet.nci.nih.gov/eating_hints

This is a huge site put together by the National Institutes of Health and the National Cancer Institute with the help of many health professionals and cancer patients as well. Because eating well is an important part of fighting disease, the NCI wants you to learn about your diet needs and how to manage eating problems.

CancerNet: Eating Well During Cancer Treatment
http://cancernet.nci.nih.gov/eating_hints/eatwell.htmlanchor29017

What kind of foods should you eat? Can good nutrition treat cancer? These are some of the topics found under "Eating Well." There's also a sample menu for good nutrition.

CancerNet: Managing Eating Problems During Treatment
http://cancernet.nci.nih.gov/eating_hints/eatmanage.htmlanchor55967

Coping with the side effects of cancer treatments is the hardest part of maintaining good nutrition. Consideration is given to dry mouth, change of sense of taste and smell, nausea, loss of appetite, and many others.

CancerNet: Special Diets For Special Needs
http://cancernet.nci.nih.gov/eating_hints/eatdiets.htmlanchor47914

Here's some guidelines for common special diets such as clear liquid, soft, low lactose, and others.

Carbohydrate-Addicted Kids
www.carbohydrateaddicts.com/cakidsindex.html
>According to Richard and Rachael Heller, the authors of the carbohydrate addict series, carbohydrate addiction affects up to 74% of youngsters who struggle with their weight and an untold number of children and teens who have been diagnosed with behavior, motivation, concentration, and learning problems as well as mood swings. This page explains their premise, and tells about their book, "Carbohydrate-Addicted Kids."

Carbohydrate Addict's Official Home Page
www.carbohydrateaddicts.com
>Drs. Richard and Rachael Heller explain The Carbohydrate Addict's Network here.

Carbohydrate Addiction Defined
www.carbohydrateaddicts.com/cadfnd.html
>After you read the definition you will most likely find that you fit the profile. You'll be treated with sensitivity and compassion because your addiction is real. The Drs. Heller say they know what causes it, and how to treat it.

Carbohydrate Addiction Support Online
www.carbohydrateaddicts.com/caonline.html
>CA-Online® is a fellowship of carbohydrate addicts of all ages, along with their friends and family, who come together to share their strategies, support, and strength, as well as their stories of challenge and success. They say it is important to read on of the Heller's books before preceding to chat, however. From here you can go to a chat room or get in on an Email support group

Carbohydrate-Addicted Kids: A Definition
www.carbohydrateaddicts.com/cakidsdef.html
>Their definition seems to fit every kid I know: "A compelling hunger, craving, or desire for carbohydrate-rich foods; an escalating, recurring need or drive for starches, snack foods, junk food, or sweets. It sounds like an epidemic to me.

Carbondale Center for Macrobiotic Studies
www.macrobiotic.org
>This site is managed by Fred Pulver. Fred is a Macrobiotic consultant, educator and free lance writer who lives in Carbondale, Colorado, USA. His knowledge of Macrobiotics comes from life-long study and application. The center was founded in 1979, and its purpose is to disseminate information about macrobiotics and the restoration, preservation, and continuation of natural health for life in general.

MUST SEE!	VIDEO	AUDIO	$ SELLS STUFF
CHAT ROOMS	MAILING LISTS	MESSAGE BOARDS	ADULT CONTENT
FREE REGISTRATION REQUIRED	MEMBERS ONLY CONTENT	SEARCHABLE	

Carbondale Center: Marcobiotic Center
www.macrobiotic.org/CCMS_Classes.htm

If you want to go to Carbondale, here's the scoop: It's in the Roaring Fork Valley, between Aspen and Glenwood Springs, Colorado. If there is such a place as heaven on earth, this area is it! You might as well just buy a one-way ticket, because you're not going to leave. This site lists the courses offered, along with tuition and payment terms.

Carbondale Center: The Importance of Chewing
www.macrobiotic.org/health16.html

I've always wondered why macrobiotics chew so much. At last the answer! Mahatma Ghandi condensed all wisdom about health into just one admonition: "Chew your drink, and drink your food." That is, chew your food until it turns to liquid in your mouth. More about this here.

Cardiovascular Exercise Principles & Guidelines: Part I
http://primusweb.com/fitnesspartner/library/activity/gf_guide1.htm

Warm-up, stretching, cool-down, frequency, and duration: it's all part of cardiovascular exercise, and it's important to know why you need to do these things.

Cardiovascular Exercise Principles & Guidelines: Part II
http://primusweb.com/fitnesspartner/library/activity/gf_guide2.htm

Monitoring exercise intensity and heart zone training are all part of understanding and getting the most out of your cardiovascular workout. This is informative and an easy to read page.

Cardiovascular Machine Workouts
http://primusweb.com/fitnesspartner/library/activity/cardiowork.htm

Does looking inside a gym look practically frightening? Here's some beginning workouts on those machines that are meant to help you, not scare you.

Carrot & Stick News Articles
www.goldfever.com/fatbrat/Page2.htm

Here's some news about vegetarianism that ranges from symptoms to expect if you make the change to a vegetarian diet to why pro athletes are turning vegetarian.

Catabolic Diet
www.catabolic.com/index2.htm

The catabolic diet claims that it works three times faster than starvation! It simply requires more calories to digest than the actual caloric value of the food you eat. Send for the book here; I'm not sure, but I guess you eat the book.

Causes of Obesity from Michael D. Myers M.D. Inc.
www.weight.com/causes.html

Here's a discussion of the factors that contribute to obesity, including hereditary factors.

Caution: Approaching the Zone
www.cyberveg.org/navs/voice/zone.html

An excellent article debunks the myths surrounding Barry Sears' ideas regarding "The Zone." Good reading if you're thinking of entering the zone.

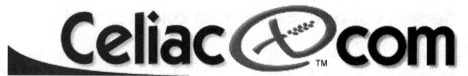

Celiac Disease - Safe & Forbidden List - A Gluten Free Diet
www.celiac.com/forbiden.html

Here's a very in-depth list of safe food and additives, as well as an extensive list of forbidden foods for the gluten free diet.

Celiac Support Page 👁
www.celiac.com/index.htmltoc

Marked by a gluten intolerance, celiac disease may affect as many as 1 in 300 people. Find out more here, and get lots of links for help and information.

Center For Science in the Public Interest 👁
www.cspinet.org

The Center for Science in the Public Interest seeks to promote health through educating the public about nutrition and alcohol; it represents citizens' interests before legislative, regulatory, and judicial bodies; and it works to ensure that advances in science are used for the public's good. It is supported by over 1,000,000 subscribers to Nutrition Action Newsletter, foundation grants, and sales of educational materials. This site will bring you up to date on the latest on food safety and nutrition.

Center for Science in the Public Interest: Problems With Olestra
www.cspinet.org/olestra/11cons.html

Besides removing fat soluble nutrients, read the many reasons why you should probably avoid products with Olestra, according to this group.

Centers for Disease Control & Prevention: Foodborne Illnesses
www.cdc.gov/health/foodill.htm

This is the starting point for food-borne illnesses listed by the CDC. It looked to me like it was written in Latin at first, but then I remembered this is science. I'd rather see a pathogen named "Ralph," instead of cryptosporidium; it's a lot easier to say. This stuff is scary.

 MUST SEE!   VIDEO   AUDIO $ SELLS STUFF

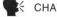 CHAT ROOMS   MAILING LISTS   MESSAGE BOARDS   ADULT CONTENT

 FREE REGISTRATION REQUIRED   MEMBERS ONLY CONTENT   SEARCHABLE

Centers for Disease Control: Escherichia coli 0157:H7 👁

www.cdc.gov/ncidod/diseases/foodborn/e_coli.htm

It's time to bone up on E.coli, because it sounds like it's going to be around for a while. Most illnesses related to this bug seem to come from undercooked, contaminated beef; it's also contracted from swimming in, and drinking, yucky water. I know one thing after reading this: I'm getting a meat thermometer today. Read this to find out how it's spread, what the symptoms are, and most importantly, how to treat it.

Challenges to Vegetarianism

http://vegetarian.about.com/library/weekly/aa080299.htm?pid=2757&cob=home

If you are a vegetarian, you've no doubt been challenged countless times by questions like, "where do you get your protein?" and you've been told that "God gave us animals to eat!" Read some of the answers that people give when confronted with their eating habits.

Chickertarian Information Page

www.newveg.av.org/animals/chicketarian.htm

Be careful, this isn't sponsored by KFC, Tyson, or Perdue. In fact, there are some graphic pictures form previous newscasts about the process.

Childhood Obesity

www.healthyeating.org/general/childhood_obesity.htm

From Eat Well, Live Well down under in Australia comes this well researched article on childhood obesity. Their statistics for prevalence of obesity in adolescents are remarkably close to ours, and the social and health implications of course are the same in either society.

Children With Diabetes: Carbohydrate Counting

www.childrenwithdiabetes.com/d_08_d00.htm

When I think of diabetes, I think of not being able to eat sweets. This web page from Children with Diabetes will introduce you to the concept of carbohydrate counting and show you that it isn't that complicated. Let them walk you through it.

Children With Diabetes: Computerized Meal Planning

www.childrenwithdiabetes.com/d_08_400.htm

Children with Diabetes maintains this site which lists and reviews meal planning software, with links to each site. Many have evaluation software to download for free.

Children With Diabetes: Fast Food Facts

www.childrenwithdiabetes.com/d_08_700.htm

A table on this page gives you nutrition and exchange information for some fast food products. Although not fully comprehensive, it did contain info on five major restaurants, and adds items occasionally.

Children With Diabetes: Meal Planning Aids

www.childrenwithdiabetes.com/d_08_430.htm

Children with Diabetes maintains a frequently updated list of meal planning aids to help you plan proper diets, especially if you're just getting started. Find books, booklets, and software to help you understand and plan.

Children's Nutrition Research Center

www.bcm.tmc.edu/cnrc/newsletter/spr99let.html

Baylor College of Medicine is responsible for this site. Click on the Nutrition and your Child Newsletter for some up-to-date reading. For good kid nutrition information click on "What's News?" and go to "Nutrition Tips."

Choose to Lose Weight Loss/Healthy Eating Program $

www.choicediets.com

See if there's a location near you, or go it alone using their participant materials. Order the book by Dr. Ron and Nancy Goor.

Circle of Hope - Free Weight Loss Support Group

www.swlink.net/~colonel/coh.html

For people with 100 or more pounds to lose, this support group will send you E-mail to help you along the path.

Circulation:
Summary of a Scientific Conference on Preventive Nutrition

http://circ.ahajournals.org/cgi/content/full/100/4/450

In the July 27th, 1999, issue of "Circulation," there's a summary of a scientific conference in which the American Heart Association, American Cancer Society, American Dietetic Association, American Academy of Pediatrics, the National Institutes of Health, and the American Society for Clinical Nutrition participated. Through years of research and by citing multiple studies, they found common threads that point to dietary recommendations to reduce the risk of heart disease, cancer, obesity, and diabetes. Unfortunately, longevity is not dependent upon increased intake of potato chips and chocolate, but upon more fruits and veggies, less fat and cholesterol, and whole grains. Looks like "variety, balance, and moderation" are the keys to good living. Get it here straight from the horse's mouth, so to speak.

Club Veg

www.clubveg.org

Club Veg is a regional, nonprofit, vegetarian education group whose goal is to spread the news about the benefits of a healthy vegetarian lifestyle, and is a good resource to those who may be thinking about changing their diets.

Colorado State University Cooperative Extension:
Nutrition & Aging

www.colostate.edu/depts/CoopExt/PUBS/FOODNUT/09322.html

This is a good discussion of aging; it covers sensory and structural changes we undergo, and the nutritional requirements of the aging body.

 MUST SEE!　　 VIDEO　　 AUDIO　　$ SELLS STUFF

 CHAT ROOMS　　 MAILING LISTS　　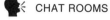 MESSAGE BOARDS　　 ADULT CONTENT

 FREE REGISTRATION REQUIRED　　 MEMBERS ONLY CONTENT　　 SEARCHABLE

Colorado State University Cooperative Extension: Nutrition Quackery 👁

www.colostate.edu/depts/CoopExt/PUBS/FOODNUT/09350.html

If it sounds too good to be true and if it promises a quick fix you should send up red flags and hold on to your credit card. This is a must read for nearly everyone. Targets of fraud range from adolescents to athletes to seniors.

Colorado State University Cooperative Extension: Osteoporosis

www.colostate.edu/depts/CoopExt/PUBS/FOODNUT/09359.html

Here's an informative discussion that provides background and the therapies available for treatment and prevention of osteoporosis.

Colorado State University Cooperative Extension: Weight Loss Diets & Books 👁

www.colostate.edu/depts/CoopExt/PUBS/FOODNUT/09364.html

Diet programs from the Atkins to the Zone are reviewed, showing strengths, weaknesses, and dangers of each. The bottom line? Yep: variety, balance, moderation, plus exercise. Didn't we hear that before?

Colorado State University Cooperative Extension: Weight Loss Programs & Products 👁

www.colostate.edu/depts/CoopExt/PUBS/FOODNUT/09363.html

Here's a nice review of weight loss programs and products, what they like about them, and especially what they don't like about them. There's a few programs they really do like, but you have to visit this site to see which ones they are.

Colorado State University Cooperative Extension: Women's Health Issues 👁

www.colostate.edu/depts/CoopExt/PUBS/FOODNUT/09360.html

How to achieve bone strength, how to ward off heart disease, and many other women's health issues are discussed here.

Combating Alzheimer's Disease With Diet

www.awesomelibrary.org/alzheimer.html

Magnesium and thiamine? What's that got to do with Alzheimer's? Check here for interesting summaries of recent research on diet and Alzheimer's.

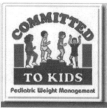

Committed To Kids
Pediatric Weight Management
www.committed-to-kids.com

Committed to Kids Pediatric Weight Management Program

www.committed-to-kids.com

> Learn about the program, where they're located, and even find out how to start a program in your area if you are an investor or physician.

Comprehensive Obesity Treatment
by Michael Myers M.D. Inc.

www.weight.com/comprehensive.html

> The most effective weight loss programs are comprehensive: they combine diet, behavior modification (lifestyle change), nutritional education, exercise, medication (where appropriate) and long-term maintenance support. Although Dr. Myers is located in Los Alamitos, CA., if you Email him, he will try to refer you to a physician or a program in your area.

Consumer Attitudes Toward Food Biotechnology: A Summary

http://ificinfo.health.org/press/questsummary.htm

> In February, 1999, the International Food Information Council commissioned a survey. They asked 1,000 Americans about their attitude toward food biotechnology. Here's a brief summary of what they found.

Consumer Information Center - Food

www.pueblo.gsa.gov/food.htm

> You can order or read online any of the publications from the CIC. Subjects range from safe seafood to healthy eating to food safety in the kitchen.

Cooking Ground Beef Safely

www.fsis.usda.gov/OA/topics/gb.htm

> 160 degrees, and not a degree less. Here's some news releases from the USDA pertaining to the safe cooking of ground beef. With E. coli around, say goodbye to those medium rare burgers. And wash that thermometer!

 MUST SEE!   VIDEO   AUDIO   SELLS STUFF

 CHAT ROOMS   MAILING LISTS   MESSAGE BOARDS   ADULT CONTENT

 FREE REGISTRATION REQUIRED   MEMBERS ONLY CONTENT   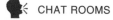 SEARCHABLE

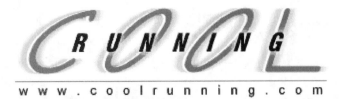

w w w . c o o l r u n n i n g . c o m

Cool Running 👁

www.coolrunning.com

> Looking for an event? If it isn't here, it isn't happening from what I can see. You'll find a calendar of events, results of previous races, and lots of training help, health and fitness articles. It's a cool site!

Cool Running: A Walking & Running Program for All Abilities

www.coolrunning.com/major/97/training/swit0214.htm

> Just get out and begin walking, because before you can run you have to walk! Makes sense to me. The advice is simple, but not condescending.

Cool Running: Basic Training Site 👁

www.coolrunning.com/training/indexbegin.shtml

> Cool Runnings tells us that even the best runners had a time when they were just starting out, so be cool, get the right shoes, and get started. This is a very helpful site.

Cool Running: Sole Searching

www.coolrunning.com/training/shoes.shtml

> Here's how to find the shoe that's right for you. If the shoe fits, wear it.

CSPI: A Brief History of Olestra

www.cspinet.org/olestra/history.html

> Olestra, a "sucrose polyester," was produced by Proctor & Gamble scientists in 1968. At one point it was hailed as the greatest development in P&G's history. But critics have lambasted P&G for inadequate testing before pressuring the FDA to approve its use. Read the history of this fat replacer before you buy your own bag of "WOW"s. CSPI would like to see this polyester go the way of the leisure suit, I suspect.

CSPI: Additives to Avoid

www.cspinet.org/reports/food.htm

> Check out this list of additives to avoid, and you'll want to update your will. On the other hand, if you looked up some of these additives from the IFIC pages, your head will be spinning too wildly to do anything. Relax, have a coolatta, and call your registered dietician.

CSPI: Olestra Adverse Effects Report Form

www.cspinet.org/olestraform

> If you've ever had a strange reaction to a product containing Olestra, you're invited to fill out this form, and send it to CSPI, who will evaluate it and forward it to the FDA.

CSPI: Rate Your Diet Quiz
www.cspinet.org/quiz/quiz_diet1.html

Here's 39 questions that you don't have to know the answers to. It's about what you eat, not what you know.

CSPI: Statement of Ilene Ringel Heller on CSPI's DESHEA Recommendations
www.cspinet.org/reports/diet_supplement.html

CSPI is a non-profit consumer organization supported by more than 1,000,000 members that has worked since 1971 to improve national health policies. The Dietary Supplement Health and Education Act was supposed to help us with choosing dietary supplements by ensuring product safety and that product claims were valid. Unfortunately, the Congress didn't allocate any funds to give the law any teeth! So the FDA only has the resources to issue warnings to the public and request voluntary recalls. These are the recommendations of the CSPI to beef up the Act.

CSPI: The Facts About Olestra
www.cspinet.org/olestra/index.html

This web site, from the Center for Science in the Public Interest, has lots of information and older news about the fat replacer, Olestra. It's mostly from news releases from 1996 to 1998, but it's enough to make you think about avoiding this invention.

Cyberdiet

Cyberdiet
www.cyberdiet.com

This is the self-proclaimed "best place to go to answer all your questions about adopting a healthy lifestyle." The site is loaded with assessment tools and good advice. They sell nothing, but do have sponsors.They do, however, have Cyberdiet Health Club that you can join for a more personal aid to lifestyle changes. This all encompassing page is one of the best organized and user friendly places to visit on the web.

Cyberdiet's Assessment Tools
www.cyberdiet.com/tools/assess.html

Want to find out what your waist/hip ratio is? Target heart rate? Body fat distribution? Body mass index? Or do you want to know how many calories you might burn if you go for a moderately paced walk? You'll find lots of useful information here. What'll really count, though, is what you do with that newfound knowledge.

 MUST SEE!   VIDEO   AUDIO   SELLS STUFF

 CHAT ROOMS   MAILING LISTS   MESSAGE BOARDS   ADULT CONTENT

 FREE REGISTRATION REQUIRED   MEMBERS ONLY CONTENT   SEARCHABLE

Cyberdiet's Awards
www.cyberdiet.com/awards/awards.html

If you're curious about Cyberdiet's credentials, look here to see the awards and accolades they've garnered from both diet authorities and web directories.

Cyberdiet's Daily Food Planner ☞
www.cyberdiet.com/dfl

Incredible! Just enter what you ate, or plan to eat, for the day, or week. Enter meals, snacks, and beverages, and you caloric intake is calculated. You then get nutritional info, shopping list for your choices, as well as recipes for your choices. Some of the menu choices include fast foods (along with nutritional info). This is a very comprehensive planner!

Cyberdiet's E-mail Newsletter
www.cyberdiet.com/subscribe

Get on Cyberdiet's mailing list and you can receive a free newsletter to your E-mail address. You'll receive the latest news on weight loss, exercise, and often some recipes. Try it out.

Cyberdiet's Eating Right
www.cyberdiet.com/ni/htdocs

Select a food category, follow the links to it, and you can see a food label. I entered "hamburger," and over 30 different kinds came up, from a simple burger to a Wendy's Triple Cheeseburger. It's fast and easy to use.

Cyberdiet's Exercise & Fitness Tips
www.cyberdiet.com/exer/exercise.html

Here's a whole list of timely articles that are quick to read. Subjects are related to exercise, and cover everything from walking tips to kickboxing to choosing exercise machines.

Cyberdiet's Food Facts
www.cyberdiet.com/foodfact/f_food.html

"The Uses of Juices" and "What's That on my Apple?" are among the topics you'll discover as you peruse this site. Phytochemicals and the latest on Calcium are included. Very informative and up-to-date news, from anti-aging diets to "Moods and Foods."

Cyberdiet's Forums ♨
www.cyberdiet.com/messages

At least ten different message boards are listed here. If you are looking for a group that's aiming to lose more than 100 pounds, a group of dieters over 50 years old, or even teen talk, this is the place.

Cyberdiet's Health Club ♨ 🗣 ☞ ✍
www.cyberdiet.com/new_healthclub_site/health_club

Sign up as a member of their Health Club and you'll get personalized meal plans, counseling and weight loss advice, as well as exercise and motivational support. You'll get interactive tools, and one on one advice with a registered dietician. Enter the Member's Lounge for starters, and jump into other areas from the Locker Room to Chat Rooms to Exercise Rooms. Just don't spend so much time here that you forget to go for a walk! There once was a charge to enter the Health Club, but the fees have been deleted. You'll still need to register, but it might be just the boost you need to get started.

Cyberdiet's Low Fat Recipes

www.cyberdiet.com/recipe_index/recipe_index.html

Here you will find lots of recipes for good health. There's even a shopping list for you to check off. Print it out, and your on your way to the grocery store!

Cyberdiet's Nutritional Profile

www.cyberdiet.com/profile/profile.cgi

Answer a few simple questions about yourself (age, height, weight), and your Body Mass Index is calculated. From there, a nutritional profile based on your current weight or your target weight shows your recommended caloric intake each day. They are broken out into proteins, carbs, and fats. You can also choose the percentage of fat you want in your diet.

Cyberdiet's Over 50 & Going Strong

www.cyberdiet.com/seniors/over50.html

You'll find lots of articles that are quick reads regarding exercise and fitness for the over 50 group. Everything from posture and osteoporosis to stretching and competitive exercise can be found here.

Cyberdiet's Success Stories

www.cyberdiet.com/success/s197.html

Read some of these many journal entries written by people who have been up and down, up and down, the diet path. Most likely you have been down that path, but what is most inspiring is that these people have not just lost weight, but have adopted lifestyle changes that support good health.

Cyberdiet's Vitamins & Minerals

www.cyberdiet.com/foodfact/vitmins/vitmins.html

Did you ever wonder why selenium is on a nutrition label? This is a great primer on why things are listed, and what they do to your body. Not only do they tell you what they're for, they tell you what happens if you're deficient, and what symptoms you'll experience if you've got too much on board.

Cyberdiet: Succeeding at Weight Loss - A Program

www.cyberdiet.com/modules/wl/outline.html

From Cyberdiet comes this interactive weight loss module that is aimed to help you on your journey to weight loss and a healthy lifestyle. The program contains a road map that will take you through areas of healthy eating, exercise, and emotional support. Filled with helpful hints, charts, and graphs, this road to success is fun and easy to use. It's free, too.

 MUST SEE!   VIDEO   AUDIO   SELLS STUFF

 CHAT ROOMS   MAILING LISTS   MESSAGE BOARDS   ADULT CONTENT

 FREE REGISTRATION REQUIRED   MEMBERS ONLY CONTENT   SEARCHABLE

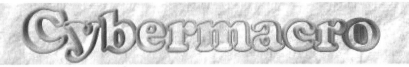

Cybermacro 📫

`www.cybermacro.com`

An interesting site sponsored by Marcobiotic Times, you'll be able to navigate to articles, calendars, forums, recipes, and links.

Cybermacro: Articles

`www.cybermacro.com/articles11.html`

Browse through a list of articles that first appeared in Macrobiotic Times

Cybermacro: Chat 🗣

`www.cybermacro.com/chat.html`

This chat room is hosted Sundays at 1:00 PM Eastern Time, same time the NFL kicks off.

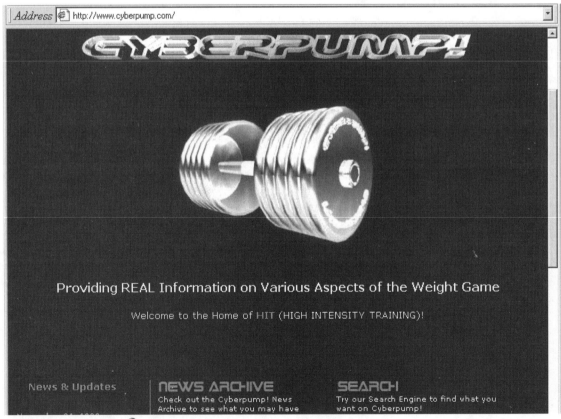

Cyberpump! 🔑 👁

`www.cyberpump.com`

This is the home of HIT (high intensity training). It's hard, brief, intense, infrequent, and must be safe. (Wait a minute, this sounds like sex ed.) There are lots of FAQs here if you want to go down this road. The site is well organized, and there's a lot of help for anyone who's in the weight game.

Cyerdiet's Fast Food Quest 🔊👁

www.cyberdiet.com/ffq/index.html

> You can compare food items among fast food restaurants, or just look up to see how much fat really is in an Egg McMuffin, for example. This is a very helpful interactive display complete with obnoxious music. It's a real eye-opener even with the sound off.

DASH Diet Navigation Page

http://dash.bwh.harvard.edu./dashdiet.html

> This page provides links to information which will help you understand and follow the diet. Click on a topic to get more information. Items in green are geared towards the general public with easy to understand information about the DASH diet. Items in red are of a more scientific nature for those who wish to dig a little deeper into the DASH diet.

DASH Diet: Salt & Losing Weight

http://dash.bwh.harvard.edu./dashdietsalt.html

> If you have high blood pressure and are overweight, weight loss as well as the DASH diet may have a beneficial effect on your blood pressure. Watching your sodium intake has also been recommended for good blood pressure control.

DASH Diet: Sample Menus

http://dash.bwh.harvard.edu./dashdietsamplemenus.html

> Check out the sample menus. Nice pictures, too, but there were none of brownies. This diet really cuts down on the sugars.

Delicious Decisions from the American Heart Association 👁

www.deliciousdecisions.org

> This web site is nicely put together. It looks like a spiral bound cookbook with side tabs which you can open to. Six chapters take you from understanding a well-balanced plan to recipes, shopping, eating out, and tips on physical activity. It has a lot of good information and tips, and it's not as stodgy as its sister AHA site.

Delicious Decisions from the AHA: Approved Diets

www.deliciousdecisions.org/ff/tsd_diets_main.html

> From providing reliable dietary guidelines for healthy adults and children to developing the Step I and Step II Diet programs, the American Heart Association is your trustworthy source for healthy dieting advice. Here you'll find more on vegetarian diets, and the AHA Step I and Step II Diet Programs.

Delicious Decisions from the AHA: Cookbook 🔍 👁

www.deliciousdecisions.org/cb/index.html

> Delectable AHA recipes, professional preparation and cooking advice, and satisfying, nutritious eating are just a heartbeat and a click of the mouse away! This easy-to-use cookbook is searchable: just type in an ingredient you want to use, or browse by category.

 MUST SEE!   VIDEO   AUDIO $ SELLS STUFF

CHAT ROOMS   MAILING LISTS   MESSAGE BOARDS   ADULT CONTENT

 FREE REGISTRATION REQUIRED   MEMBERS ONLY CONTENT   SEARCHABLE

Delicious Decisions from the AHA: Enjoy Eating
www.deliciousdecisions.org/ee/index.html

Here you will find the most current AHA nutrition recommendations and guidelines. You'll also find dependable advice and friendly guidance that makes eating a low-fat, healthful diet a cinch.

Delicious Decisions from the AHA: Fit Forever
www.deliciousdecisions.org/ff/index.html

The features in Fit Forever give you reliable AHA diet, weight and exercise advice you can count on and easily work into your improved healthy lifestyle!

Delicious Decisions from the AHA:
Heart Healthy Chef's Tour 👁
www.deliciousdecisions.org/cb/hhc.html

In this cookbook from the American Heart Association you will learn the best methods for low-fat cooking, the super substitutions that save your heart while pleasing your taste buds, and the sodium secrets and tips that make low-sodium dining a pleasure.

Delicious Decisions from the AHA: Non AHA Approved Diets
www.deliciousdecisions.org/ff/tsd_nondiets_main.html

Before you buy into a fad diet plan, be sure to look into the facts. Everything you'll need to know about "diet traps" is here. Beware the hype and the before and after stories. The magic bullet just may be that there is no magic bullet.

Delicious Decisions from the AHA: Out & About
www.deliciousdecisions.org/oa/index.html

Today many restaurants offer fantastic, low-fat, low-cholesterol options. If you're in the know, the menu from any type of restaurant - from Cajun to Vietnamese - is open to you. This section of Delicious Decisions also contains information on healthful snacking and has a "Snack-Attack Selector." Just point and click to your craving - sweet, crunchy, munchy, hot, or thirst quencher.

Delicious Decisions from the AHA: Step by Step
www.deliciousdecisions.org/ss/index.html

The primary aim of this dietary therapy is to reduce the risk for coronary heart disease, which causes heart attack. The diets help patients decrease their intakes of saturated fat and cholesterol and restore appropriate calorie balance. Take the Step Diet Quiz here, and your score will tell you which diet you'll need to adopt.

Delicious Decisions from the AHA: Supermarket
www.deliciousdecisions.org/sm/index.html

Here at the Delicious Decisions Supermarket, you'll discover the secrets that make you the smartest shopper in your grocery store. You'll not only save money, you'll save your heart.

Delicious Decisions from the AHA: Supplement Your Knowledge

www.deliciousdecisions.org/ff/tsd_supp_main.html

Take a trip down the vitamin aisle of your local grocery or drug store, and you'll probably be amazed by the selection of vitamins and minerals on display. Read here what the American Heart Association recommends before you load your cart.

Delicious Decisions from the AHA: The Skinny on Dieting

www.deliciousdecisions.org/ff/tsd.html

Get off that diet roller-coaster! From absurd, single-food diets to those unsatisfying liquid diet shakes, fad diets are often un-nutritious, ineffective and even dangerous. If you are interested in losing weight while maintaining healthy nutrition and eating a delicious variety of foods, then the Skinny on Dieting is the right place for you.

Delicious! Online: Your Guide to Natural Living 👁

www.delicious-online.com

To inspire health-conscious men and women to take responsibility for their health and well-being by providing the latest medical and scientific research in a practical, easy-to-understand format is the purpose of this web site. There are lots of good cooking ideas, along with healthy living and herbal healing news. You'll find information on dieting, nutrition, vegetarianism, herbs, vitamins, and minerals. Visit here to see this nicely presented site.

Designer Protein

www.designerprotein.com

The home page of the self-proclaimed ultimate whey protein powder, they do not sell stuff online, but give you a toll free number so you can find your closest retail outlet.

Dexfenfluramine

www.rxlist.com/cgi/generic/dexfen.htm

Removed from the US market 9/15/97, this drug was also known as Redux. Lawsuits abound for alleged heart valve damages.

Diabetes.com: Healthy Diet & Exercise 👁

www.diabetes.com/health_library/diet_and_exercise.html

"You can live a long, healthy life, savor all the foods you ever dreamed of, go anywhere, and do anything you're capable of -- despite diabetes." So begins this upbeat web site which is part of Diabetes.com. There's lots of helpful information here about managing your condition.

 MUST SEE!   VIDEO    AUDIO $ SELLS STUFF

 CHAT ROOMS   MAILING LISTS   MESSAGE BOARDS   ADULT CONTENT

 FREE REGISTRATION REQUIRED   MEMBERS ONLY CONTENT   SEARCHABLE

Diabetes.Store $ ⚲ ☞

http://merchant.diabetes.org/adabooks/Default.asp

This is THE place to come to if you want to buy books on diabetes. It is sponsored by the American Diabetes Association, and offers books, CDs, and more, all at a discount. There are educational resources, meal planners, cookbooks, and self-care guides.

Diane Rehm Program: Agricultural Biotechnology 🔊

www.nal.usda.gov/bic/Audio/DRehmtext.htm

Today agricultural bioengineers working for seed companies are using technology to limit the way farmers work, including creating plant varieties that are sterile. American innovation isn't going over very well in Europe, where concerns about the long-term effects of consuming bioengineered fruits and vegetables has contributed to trade tensions. A panel talks about bioengineered plants and seeds: how safe they are and how they're changing American agriculture and trade. This is a recording of this PBS radio show that aired May 20, 1999. You'll need RealPlayer, which you can download.

Diet & Nutrition Resource Center - Quizzes

www.mayohealth.org/mayo/common/htm/dietquiz.htm

Are you ready for a test? There are quizzes here on fat, fast food, alcohol, sodium, diet and nutrition, and others. They're quick and if you don't know it all, you can learn the right answers with background after the test. The good news is that if you flunk, you don't have to stay back or go to summer school.

Diet & Weight Loss News Wire Summaries

http://www1.mhv.net/~donn/wire.html

Listed here are very short summaries of news related to diet and weight loss.

Diet & Weight Loss Tips Collection 🔊

http://www1.mhv.net/~donn/tips.html

Here's a very lengthy collection of tips from readers to help you move along the diet trail.

Diet & Weight Loss/ Fitness Home Page

http://www1.mhv.net/~donn/diet.html

Here's a comprehensive resource page that is aimed to give you information, knowledge, and resources. There are no fancy graphics but a ton of links that can lead you to any information you may need regarding weight loss and fitness. But be careful: Donn must be selling something, so do your homework!

Diet Analysis Web Page

http://dawp.anet.com

A diet analysis lets you enter the foods you've eaten for one day and then reports a complete nutritional review of your diet based on the Recommended Dietary Allowances for your demographic. After entering your intake for a meal, or a day's worth of meals, you can get an analysis in text or bar graph. Just follow the instructions.

Diet Depot: Digital Market $

https://secure.gcci.com/cgi-bin_001/web_store.cgi

Find all the products you need for the Atkins Diet, as well as vitamins, supplements, and books.

Diet Doctor

http://thedietdoctor.itool.com

> For $45.00, the Diet Doctor will act as your personal diet consultant. Just download a daily diet record, fill it out, and send it to him. You'll get a dietary analysis, suggestions to help you reach your goal, and ways to improve your diet. Not sure if this is legit. Be careful.

Diet Magic Now!

Diet Magic Now! $

www.dietmagicnow.com/4frame.htm

> Maybe this is the magic bullet. Body sculpting and fat burning herbal supplements are available, and they work while you sleep! Spend about $200 and wake up looking and feeling great.

Dietary Approaches to Stop Hypertension

Official World Wide Web Site

Dietary Approaches to Stop Hypertension (DASH)

http://dash.bwh.harvard.edu

> The official site of the DASH diet (Dietary Approaches to Stop Hypertension), you'll find out how the research was carried out, the results, as well as lots of help to try it out yourself.

Dietary Treatment of Obesity

www.weight.com/diets.html

> A discussion of dietary options, both good and bad, appears here. Dr. Myers writes in layman terms, and the bottom line basically is that low-cal, low-fat, and behavior modification are the primary keys to success. Didn't we hear that before?

Dietsite.com ⬇ 👁

www.dietsite.com

> This site has it all. From alternative nutrition to sports nutrition to weight loss, it's all here. One of the best features is its diet analysis page. Check it out.

Dietsite.com: Calorie Controlled Diet

www.dietsite.com/Diets/WeightManagement/Calorie%20Controlled%20Diet.htm

> The calorie-controlled diet may be adapted for weight reduction and weight maintenance. It is also used for persons with elevated serum cholesterol levels or those who are high-risk candidates for heart disease.

 MUST SEE!   VIDEO   AUDIO $ SELLS STUFF

 CHAT ROOMS   MAILING LISTS   MESSAGE BOARDS   ADULT CONTENT

 FREE REGISTRATION REQUIRED   MEMBERS ONLY CONTENT   SEARCHABLE

Dietsite.com: Creatine & Sports Performance

www.dietsite.com/SportsNutrition/Creatine%20and%20Sports%20Performance.htm

Creatine is an amino acid is made in your body and stored in your muscles. It's a powerful ergogenic aid. Are you a candidate to use this supplement? How do you take it? How will it work? What will it do to you? How much do you take? This Q&A sheet will help you learn a bit about it.

Dietsite.com: Diabetes

www.dietsite.com/Diets/Diabetes/diabetesfs.htm

Diet, exercise and medication are important factors that must be coordinated for diabetes to be kept in control. Unless the diet plan is followed carefully no method of treatment will be effective. By eating the right foods in the right amounts diet can actually help control the basic problem of diabetes.

Dietsite.com: Diet & Recipe Analysis

www.dietsite.com/nutr/index.htm

This web site will analyze your diet, menus, recipes, or a specific food. It will also assess your calorie and nutrient needs so you know what your nutrient goals are for each day. They can also track your weight over time for you. You can get a nutritional breakdown of your diet after you've entered some personal information. It seemed a little slow, but the results were worth the wait. Give it a try if you're counting something.

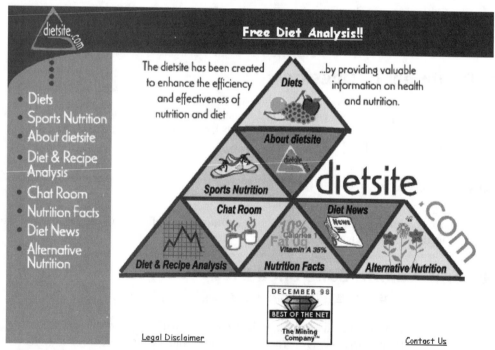

Dietsite.com: Diet to Improve Performance

www.dietsite.com/SportsNutrition/improved%20Performance%20Diet.htm

Proper nutrition during training will help you during competition. Here you can find just what your body needs for maximal efficiency.

Dietsite.com: Dietary Goals for Improved Performance
www.dietsite.com/SportsNutrition/Performance%20Diet's%20Goals.htm

Nutritional factors can conceivably influence performance at almost any stage during training or competition. If you want to prevent muscle fatigue, tiredness, and decreased performance, read here about appropriate nourishment before, during, and after exercise.

Dietsite.com: Ergogenic Aids
www.dietsite.com/SportsNutrition/Ergogenic%20Aids.html

Nutritional ergogenic aids are foods or supplements that supposedly have the potential to increase work output. The following are ergogenic aids that have not been scientifically proven to be effective.

Dietsite.com: Food Additive Labeling Terms
www.dietsite.com/NutritionFacts/FoodAdditives/Labeling/Labeling%20content.htm

Did you ever wonder what sulfites, nitrates, and nitrites were? Here's a list of additive label terms, what they are, and what they do.

Dietsite.com: Gluten Free Diet
www.dietsite.com/Diets/FoodSensitivities/Gluten%20Free%20Diet.htm

This diet is designed to provide adequate nutrition while eliminating foods that contain gliadin (gliadin is the alcohol soluble fraction of gluten), the protein found in wheat, rye, oats and barley. The gluten-restricted, gliadin-free diet will help prevent uncomfortable side effects such as: weight loss, abdominal cramping and bloating, intestinal gas, diarrhea, and fatigue. It is used for people with non-tropical sprue (celiac syndrome or gluten-induced enteropathy), and dermatitis herpetiformis. A gluten-restricted, gliadin-free diet is used if you are unable to digest gliadin, one of the proteins that make up gluten. The gluten-free diet should be continued for life.

Dietsite.com: Grades of Obesity
www.dietsite.com/Diets/WeightManagement/Grades%20Of%20Obesity.htm

Grades of Obesity range from "not obese" to "super morbid;" it's based on the BMI chart.

Dietsite.com: High Calorie & Protein Diet
www.dietsite.com/SportsNutrition/high_calorie_and_protein_diet.htm

When higher amounts of nutrients are needed, check out these diet recommendations. This diet can also be used when you need to gain weight or help your body heal.

Dietsite.com: Hyperglycemia
www.dietsite.com/Diets/Diabetes/SickDayManagement/HYPERglycemia.htm

Hyperglycemia is the condition that happens when your blood glucose level rises and stays too high—240 mg/dl or above. When hyperglycemia happens, it means that your diabetes is out of control. Learn what the warning signs are, how it happens, how to treat it, and most importantly, how to avoid it.

 MUST SEE!   VIDEO   AUDIO   SELLS STUFF

 CHAT ROOMS   MAILING LISTS   MESSAGE BOARDS   ADULT CONTENT

 FREE REGISTRATION REQUIRED   MEMBERS ONLY CONTENT   SEARCHABLE

Dietsite.com: Hypoglycemia or Insulin Reaction
www.dietsite.com/Diets/Diabetes/SickDayManagement/HYPOglycemia.htm

If untreated, it can be deadly; but the good news is that it's fairly easy to treat. Learn what causes hypoglycemia, how to treat it, and how to prevent it.

Dietsite.com: No Concentrated Sweets, Low Fat Diet
www.dietsite.com/Diets/Diabetes/DiabeticDiets/No%20Concentrated%20Sweets%20Low%20Fat%20Diet.htm

This diet is for people who find the exchange system too confusing or restricting to follow.

Dietsite.com: Nutrients for Athletes
www.dietsite.com/SportsNutrition/NutrientsAthletes/nutrients_2.htm

This is a basic and understandable article for athletes who desire peak performance and want information on nutrition. The role of carbohydrates, fats, protein and amino acids, as well as fluids are all necessary to understand peak performance.

Dietsite.com: Ranking the Sports Drinks
www.dietsite.com/SportsNutrition/Ranking%20the%20Sports%20Drinks.html

Here's a great chart which gives you the nutritional values of various sports drinks from water to Powerade; most importantly, this chart shows you what to look for in a drink.

Dietsite.com: Sports Drinks
www.dietsite.com/SportsNutrition/Sports%20Drinks.htm

Sports drinks are recommended for activities that exceed 60 minutes. Here you'll find recommendations on how to choose a sports drink, and when to take them.

Dietsite.com: Sports Nutrition 👁
www.dietsite.com/SportsNutrition/index.htm

Many athletes are trying to find that magic bullet that will help take them "to the next level." If you're looking to improve physical performance and stamina, this is a great place to start. Learn about high performance diets, fluid recommendations before and after training, and find out about those sports drinks and energy bars. This web site is authored by Traci Van Der Vorste-Kaufman, Registered Dietitian, who received her bachelor's degree in dietetics and nutrition from the University of Wisconsin-Madison. She has worked as a clinical nutritionist at UCI Medical Center-Irvine in Orange California, and served as team nutritionist for the Los Angeles Rams.

Dietsite.com: Sports Performance & Caffeine
www.dietsite.com/SportsNutrition/Caffeine%20and%20Sports%20Performance.htm

Caffeine use in sports has been controversial. Some studies show that it can enhance performance while others show the opposite can be true. The Olympics have banned high doses and you must be aware that it acts as a diuretic. Read more about it in this article.

Dietsite.com: The Exchange System

www.dietsite.com/Diets/Diabetes/exchange_system.htm

The main goal of the diabetic diet is to keep the carbohydrate intake constant throughout the day. The exchange system is used to plan meals with controlled amounts of nutrients throughout the day and can be used in order to provide variety and flexibility in meal planning.

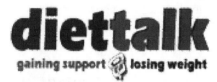

Diettalk

www.diettalk.com/index.shtml

You'll find lots of links to diet and nutrition information.

Dilip's Vegetarian Resource Page

www.cs.unc.edu/~barman/vegetarian.html

There's a link list here with some slightly off-Main Street links that look like fun: check out Vegan Bikers, or Feminists for Animal Rights. There are also many Main Street sights like Physicians Committee for Responsible Medicine. A few newsgroups are listed, too.

Dole 5 A Day

www.dole5aday.com

Here's an interactive kid's web site loaded with catchy jingles, puzzles, and yes, dancing elephants.

Dr. Brad's Calorad $

www.caloradnet.com/drbrad/index.htm

Click here and you can spend $200 on five bottles of this "revolutionary wellness product"; not only that, but you too can become a distributor. "Calorad® nutritionally feeds the body, which allows it to support itself in maintaining lean muscle tissue, which helps the body to utilize fat and sugar effectively." They claim that it's even good if you're underweight, or in good physical condition. This must be THE magic bullet..

Drink Up!

http://primusweb.com/fitnesspartner/library/nutrition/fluids.htm

The American College of Sports Medicine reminds us that not only are a balanced diet and physical exercise crucial to good health, but also that adequate hydration is important for peak performance and injury avoidance. The ACMS recommends these tips to enhance performance, safety, and good health.

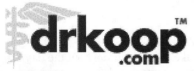

drkoop.com: 10 Basic Stretches
http://drkoop.com/wellness/fitness/exercise/stretch.asp

Stretching should be part of your daily activity. Here's ten basic stretches to improve flexibility and mobility. Be sure your muscles are warmed up before you start.

drkoop.com: A Growing Problem
www.drkoop.com/wellness/nutrition/healthyliving/index.asp?id=192

"Type 2 diabetes affects more than 16 million people in North America, and an estimated 5.4 million are undiagnosed. Though the disease previously was seen only in adults in their 40s or 50s, doctors are now seeing more young people, even teen-agers, develop the disease. People who develop type 2 diabetes are usually overweight, and treatment always involves diet management." Read more from this informative page, and see how diet, exercise, and maybe medication can help.

drkoop.com: Aerobics
http://drkoop.com/wellness/fitness/facts/aerobics.asp

Are you curious about aerobics? Think you might want to try it as a form of exercise? Drkoop.com tells you all about it, including advantages, disadvantages, and even what to wear when you show up.

drkoop.com: Bicycling
http://drkoop.com/wellness/fitness/facts/bicycling.asp

Here's an introduction to the sport of bicycling. This sport takes place outdoors, requires good equipment, good weather, and can be a good workout. Read up on this brief introduction to the sport.

drkoop.com: DASH Away High Blood Pressure
www.drkoop.com/wellness/nutrition/healthyliving/index.asp?id=216

About 25% of American adults have high blood pressure. In addition to decreased sodium intake, weight loss, and use of prescribed medication, the DASH diet is being shown to be an effective tool in reducing risks associated with hypertension.

drkoop.com: Exercise & Diabetes
http://drkoop.com/wellness/fitness/facts/exercise-diabetes.asp

Diabetics who stay physically active usually do a whole lot better than their inactive counterparts. Drkoop.com explains how good nutrition and a program of exercise helps you to better manage this disease.

drkoop.com: Exercise & Heart Disease
http://drkoop.com/wellness/fitness/facts/exercise-heart-disease.asp

A consistent program of exercise reduces the risk for heart disease, and can improve your fitness after a bout with heart failure. The bottom line in this site is to check in with your doctor, and begin a supervised program. Check the details.

drkoop.com: **Exercise & Obesity**

http://drkoop.com/wellness/fitness/facts/exercise-obesity.asp

Do you want to feel better? Visit here to help understand the features and benefits, as well as the risks, of structuring a good exercise and nutrition plan to help achieve a healthy person. Check out that list of ailments that are often associated with obesity, and consider a lifestyle change to be a ticket to improved health and well-being.

drkoop.com: **Exercise & Pregnancy**

http://drkoop.com/wellness/fitness/facts/exercise-pregnancy.asp

Choosing to exercise while exercise while pregnant can enhance your health and your child's as well. Follow the guidelines you'll see at this site.

drkoop.com: **Exercise & the Elderly**

http://drkoop.com/wellness/fitness/facts/exercise-elderly.asp

If you are over 65, you may find more changes going on with your body than when you were an adolescent; however, these have nothing to do with growing pains. Visit this site to see how you can keep the wolves away, so to speak.

drkoop.com: **Exercise & Your Child**

http://drkoop.com/wellness/fitness/facts/exercise-child.asp

Flexibility, balance, mobility, endurance, and stamina are but a few reasons to encourage your children to get away from the video games and the TV. Showing them a lifestyle of fitness and activity by your example will ensure the probability of a healthy adulthood for all. OK, so you have to get up and get out too. Read up on some ideas for getting started and some considerations for their safety.

drkoop.com: **Exercising to Lose Weight**

www.drkoop.com/wellness/fitness/files/ex2-lose-wght.asp

Did you ever try a new diet and find that it wasn't worth the trouble? Are you really practicing variety, balance, and moderation, but not losing any discernable weight? Take it up a notch and begin an exercise program. Read here the many reasons to add exercise to your program, and look at the simple math involved to lose one pound. There's some easy, great, and logical suggestions here.

drkoop.com: **Fitness Center**

www.drkoop.com/wellness/fitness

Dr. Koop has a great site for fitness-related information. You'll find a section on up-to-date fitness news, an ask the expert section, a message board, and lots of fitness facts to look up. And guess what? He doesn't sell anything! Not even a treadmill; however, his advertisers will sell you one if you like. After all, someone has to pay for this great site.

MUST SEE!	VIDEO	AUDIO	SELLS STUFF
CHAT ROOMS	MAILING LISTS	MESSAGE BOARDS	ADULT CONTENT
FREE REGISTRATION REQUIRED	MEMBERS ONLY CONTENT		SEARCHABLE

drkoop.com: **Fitness Facts For Older Americans**

http://drkoop.com/wellness/fitness/facts/exercise-older.asp

If you think that just because you're getting older, you should take it easy and park yourself in your recliner, take a look here. Drkoop.com will convince you to get up and take a hike over to this site if you want to increase your chances of living long and living well.

drkoop.com: **Four Get Fit** 👁

http://drkoop.com/wellness/fitness/four_fit

Look in on 4 people from 26 to 47 years of age who have decided to undergo lifestyle changes. You'll be able to read their initial assessments, the treatment plans from the dietician and from the trainer. Each week David, Lisa, Ryan, and Jennifer send in their journal entries. For example, David is starting off at 280 pounds, and wants to drop weight and get fit. Drop by weekly or so and see how they're doing.

drkoop.com: **How to Kick Start Your Exercise Program**

www.drkoop.com/wellness/fitness/files/exercise-program.asp

There comes a time when your exercise routine becomes a real drag after you've lost some weight, you've gained some endurance, and you feel stronger. It's just boring. Here's some good ideas on how to get out of the doldrums, and take it to another level.

drkoop.com: **Jogging**

http://drkoop.com/wellness/fitness/facts/jogging.asp

If you are thinking of joining the millions of Americans who run and jog, visit this site for an introduction to the pros and cons of this sport, and you'll find out what you may need for clothing and shoes. There's also a glossary that contains some of the terminology associated with this workout.

drkoop.com: **Muscular Fitness Exercise**

http://drkoop.com/wellness/fitness/facts/muscular-fitness.asp

This exercise is not just for body sculpting or competition anymore. If you're interested in losing some body fat and increasing your metabolism, improving your posture, and preventing the ravages of osteoporosis, you might want to check this form of exercise out. Working your muscles against an externally-applied resistance, such as free weights, weight machines, water, rubber tubing or your body weight is muscular fitness exercise. Its advantages and disadvantages are discussed at this site.

drkoop.com: **Nutrition Center** 👁

www.drkoop.com/wellness/nutrition

Dr. Koop, the former surgeon general, hosts this ambitious web site relating to all things concerning nutrition. He also can be found in "Shape Up, America," and if his sites weren't so good, and if his pictures were plastered all over them, I'd think he was running for some political office. But his message is serious, and it's for our own good. Be sure to check out "Nutrition for your Condition," "Recipes," and the News section. There's a chat schedule, too, with topics of interest hosted by people in the know.

drkoop.com: **Nutrition During Pregnancy**

www.drkoop.com/wellness/nutrition/healthyliving/index.asp?id=38

At no other time in your life is nutritional health more important than during pregnancy. Fetal growth and development occur rapidly, and changes in your diet -- both positive and negative -- may affect your growing baby's health. Find out if your diet is adequate for two.

drkoop.com: **Nutrition for Healthy Living**
www.drkoop.com/wellness/nutrition/healthyliving

Find out how diet can affect your medical condition -- for better or worse. Click on your condition to learn more about which healthy habits to keep and what unhealthy behaviors to avoid.

drkoop.com: **Nutrition For Infants**
www.drkoop.com/wellness/nutrition/healthyliving/index.asp?id=33

When you think about it, infants really go through some mighty explosive growth cycles. Imagine doubling your weight in 12 weeks! So their nutritional needs are indeed unique. You'll find facts on breastfeeding, formula, soft foods, when to add foods, which foods to avoid, some sample menus. Hmm, no Taco Bell.

drkoop.com: **Nutrition News**
www.drkoop.com/wellness/nutrition/news

Breaking news on the nutritional front can be found at this site. The day I dropped in there were news articles on Vitamin B6 and its role in easing symptoms of PMS, antioxidants and stroke, Vitamin E, and a story saying that the current RDA of Vitamin C should be doubled. Go visit.

drkoop.com: **Spinning**
www.drkoop.com/wellness/fitness/files/spinning.asp

Ever hear of spinning? It has nothing to do with yarn or those old-fashioned spinning wheels. It sounds like it's more like aerobics on wheels. Hop up on a modified stationary bike, listen to some high energy music, and follow you instructor around for an imaginary road trip. This site says that you can lose up to 500 calories in a 45 minute workout. Let's see, 7 workouts a day = 3,500 calories = 1 pound times 7 = 7 pounds a week times 4 = 28-30 pounds a month. Wow! Don't even think about it.

drkoop.com: **Spotting Nutrition Quackery**
www.drkoop.com/wellness/nutrition/healthyliving/index.asp?id=214

Are you looking for instant energy, vitality, and youth? Dr. Koop's site says that quackery lies in the premise, not always the product. Here's seven questions that might send up red flags and make you think twice before donating your money to someone's scam.

drkoop.com: **Stretching**
http://drkoop.com/wellness/fitness/facts/stretching.asp

Is bending down to pick up that pencil you dropped getting harder? Trouble reaching those dishes up in the kitchen cabinet? Getting creaky as you get older? Stretching should be part of any comprehensive exercise program, Dr. Koop says. Check out why you should spend a little bit of time doing this.

 MUST SEE!   VIDEO   AUDIO   SELLS STUFF

 CHAT ROOMS   MAILING LISTS   MESSAGE BOARDS   ADULT CONTENT

 FREE REGISTRATION REQUIRED   MEMBERS ONLY CONTENT   SEARCHABLE

drkoop.com: **Submit Your Nutrition Questions**
www.drkoop.com/wellness/fitness/expert/howard.asp

Submit a question about nutrition, and Sharon Howard, a registered dietician, may answer you via E-mail.

drkoop.com: **Swimming**
http://drkoop.com/wellness/fitness/facts/swimming.asp

Whether you're a beginner or an advanced swimmer, whether you swim laps, or water walk, there seem to be a lot of reasons to take this type of exercise on. Drkoop.com gives you some ideas of what the risks and benefits are.

drkoop.com: **The Food Safety Guide**
www.drkoop.com/wellness/nutrition/healthyliving/index.asp?id=29

Here's a good list of ways to protect yourself from food-borne illnesses, starting with cleaning your kitchen and safe food handling suggestions.

drkoop.com: **Vitamins & Minerals**
www.drkoop.com/wellness/nutrition/vitamins_minerals

Click on a vitamin or a mineral on the list, and you get concise facts on what it is, what is does, where you can get it, and how much is in a typical serving, and how much you should get in your daily diet.

drkoop.com: **Walking**
http://drkoop.com/wellness/fitness/facts/walking.asp

Here's an exercise that doesn't require a personal trainer, a locker full of equipment, or even a drive to the gym. If you can put one foot in front of the other in a repetitive manner, you're halfway there. The secret is that you can burn nearly as many calories per mile as that jogger that passes you by.

drkoop.com: **Women's Nutrition**
www.drkoop.com/wellness/nutrition/healthyliving/index.asp?id=36

Women have special health and nutrition needs that men do not. First of all, they need fewer calories. You'll also find dietary considerations for dealing with PMS and menopause.

Duke University: **The Rice Diet Program** 👁
www.ricediet.com/us/index1.html

The world famous Rice Diet, the original low fat, low salt diet, is a scientific approach to determining what you can eat while maintaining optimal health. This is not a fad diet. The Rice Diet reduces cholesterol, blood pressure, heart size, weight and abnormal blood sugars, thus reducing or eliminating the need for medications. But you don't have to be sick to benefit from the diet. The Diet also prevents the diseases it treats. So belly up to Duke University and see what they have to show you on this extensive web site.

Duke University: **The Rice Diet Program: What Will I Eat?**
www.ricediet.com/us/program/eat.html

Will I have to eat rice? Can I do this at home? Better pack your bags and go to Durham, North Carolina. But read more about the program and contact them to see if this is for you. Oh yes, and what about the cost. Will my health insurance pick up the tab? Just click on that blue button the says "Program Costs."

EarthSave: Healthy People, Healthy Planet

www.earthsave.org

Howard Lyman is the President of EarthSave International. If you followed Oprah Winfrey's trial in Texas, you'll remember him as the "Mad Cowboy" who is now a vegetarian. EarthSave promotes and supports choosing a planet friendly diet. If you lean this way, this web site provides a lot of information on the effects of farm factories on the environment.

Earthy Delights $

http://earthy.com

Looking for a heavenly 30 year Balsamic Vinegar? Truffle Oil? Dried Porcinis? Farro Pasta? Amaranth or Red Himalayan Rice? Black Garbonzo beans? Look no further! This is the place to buy all these and much more.

Easy Ways to Boost Your Activity Level

http://primusweb.com/fitnesspartner/library/activity/activity.htm

Being active is more than going to the gym, or working out. Here's some great suggestions to incorporate more activity into your daily routine. Suggestions include such simple things as "lose the remote!" and "don't look for the closest parking spot!"

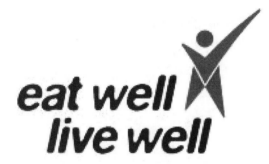

Eat Well, Live Well Research & Information Centre

www.healthyeating.org

Promoting healthy eating to the public down under in Australia is the mission of this organization based at Monash University. This popular site has received over 70,000 hits a week.

Eat Well, Live Well E-mail Newsletter

www.healthyeating.org/submissions

Subscribe to the Eat Well, Live Well e-mail newsletter. It is filled with interesting as well as fun and interactive information.

Eat Well, Live Well Newsletter Archive
www.healthyeating.org/newsletters

I looked up the June, 1999 issue, and played Healthy Food Picnic Panic with my kids. You have 45 seconds to pack a picnic basket with nutritious food. If you have Shockwave, give it a try.

Eat Yourself Slim: The Montignac Method
http://global-m.com/montignac/montignac.htm

This is basically the European version of another low-carb diet in the vein of Atkins and the Hellers. "Think of it as a method of slimming - not a diet." Sure.

Eating Healthy With The Diabetes Food Pyramid As Your Guide
www.diabetes.org/nutrition/article031799.asp

This is a step-by-step guide to getting started with the diabetes food pyramid, and it's packed with useful information. But the best advice suggests you meet with a registered dietician before you try to do it yourself.

EatVeg Menu
www.newveg.av.org/menu.htm

This is a directory that seems to be well-organized. It is organized by subject matter. Sites range from health, animals, fruitarian, to people and transitioning to this lifestyle.

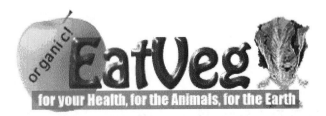

EatVeg.com
www.eatveg.com

Eatveg.com is dedicated to educating people on why an organic plant-based diet is best for personal health, the animals, and the earth. They advocate a cholesterol-free (vegan) diet, emphasizing organic raw foods.

eDiets: Bulletin Boards
www.ediets.com/myediets/quest/webboard.cfm

eDiets has four message boards, each with a distinct area of coverage. There's a Buddy Board where you can find someone to give and get support, a Message Board for discussing eDiet programs with each other, a Motivation Board with techniques and keys to success, and an Administration Board for communicating your ideas and opinions about the program.

eDiets:
Custom Weight Loss Management & Dieting Programs

www.ediets.com

You can become a member of eDiets along with over 640,000 others and get your own personalized diet plan created from your own profile. A free diet newsletter is also available and is delivered right to your Email box.The eDiets Weight Loss Program is a subscription-based information product that uses a proprietary software system to generate professional advice and information that is unique to your needs. The Company operates a central Internet site where you may select an eDiets program for delivery to your PC, receive weekly updates, purchase related items, and attend online motivation meetings.

Emerging Food-Borne Diseases

www.cdc.gov/ncidod/EID/vol3no4/tauxe.htm

Every year, in the United States food-borne infections cause millions of illnesses and thousands of deaths; most infections go undiagnosed and unreported. As the epidemiology of food-borne infections evolves, old scenarios and solutions need to be updated. This article reviews main trends in the evolution of food-borne disease epidemiology and their effect on surveillance and prevention activities.

Encyclopedia of Fruitarianism & Rational Living

www.student.nada.kth.se/~f95-mwi/fun/encyclopedia.html

This encyclopedia contains, basically, two kinds of discussions: ones concerned with what we humans put into our bodies and ones concerned with how we interact with one another and with the other life-forms on this planet. This seems to be quite an extensive list with sources listed from each contributor. But don't look for "brownies" in this encyclopedia.

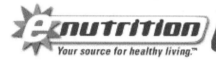

| WEIGHT MANAGEMENT | NATURAL REMEDIES | YOUR HEALTH | SPORTS NUTRITION | VITAMINS & SUPPLEMENTS |

eNutrition $ ♀

www.enutrition.com

Get stuff here: weight loss, vitamin, sports nutrition, and natural remedy stuff. eNutriotion claims to give you unbiased news and information on issues that affect health and wellness, as well as to offer you a selection of products from multiple companies. Their five online magazines: Weight Management, Natural Remedies, Sports Nutrition, Vitamins & Supplements and Your Health, give you the news; this site sells you the stuff. There is an obvious problem with using "unbiased news and information" in the same sentence with "selling stuff." When you choose a product, you have a chance to click onto "relevant articles," which often gives you background info. Product pages do contain ingredients, and directions for use.

 MUST SEE!   VIDEO    AUDIO   SELLS STUFF

 CHAT ROOMS   MAILING LISTS   MESSAGE BOARDS   ADULT CONTENT

 FREE REGISTRATION REQUIRED   MEMBERS ONLY CONTENT   SEARCHABLE

European Vegetarian Union

www.ivu.org/evu

> The European Vegetarian Union is an umbrella organization for most vegetarian groups in Europe. Your choice of 20 different languages. Check out the EVU News for the latest in European vegetarianism.

Exercise Equipment Do's & Don'ts

http://primusweb.com/fitnesspartner/library/equipment/equip01.htm

> Stair climbers, stationary bikes, ski machines, and treadmills all require good technique for a successful ride. Stop leaning on the rails and stand up straight!

Exercise Errors

http://primusweb.com/fitnesspartner/library/activity/errors.htm

> Stretching, warming up, and cooling down are important parts of your exercise program. If you're skipping them, or cutting them short, you may be facing the potential for some costly injuries. Check this site out.

Fad Diet.com

www.faddiet.com

> This web site has compiled a comprehensive list of pretty much well-known fad diets. Find out about the "Russian Air Force Diet," and of course the "Cabbage Soup Diet."

Fad Diet.com: Make Your Own Fad Diet

www.faddiet.com/faddiet/makyourownfa.html

> Want to get rich? Here's some pointers to help you create your own fad diet.

Fake-fat Olestra Sickens Thousands

www.cspinet.org/new/olestra/olestra_12_22_98.htm

> A news release from the Center for Science in the Public Interest dated December 22, 1998 relates that more than 15,000 consumers filed complaints about Olestra, the fat replacer in WOW snacks and Pringles Fat Free chips. Problems ranged from gas, cramps, to bloody stools.

Family Food Zone 👁

www.familyfoodzone.com/fridge.html

> This home page looks like most refrigerators I've seen. The front is cluttered with magnets and notes. Just click open the door, point and click to any of the food items you see, and you'll get information about their nutritional value as well as some serving ideas. What's with the Mom's Food Guide, though? What about us Dads who feed our families? This site is jointly sponsored by the Pacific Science Center and the Washington State Dairy Council.

Family Food Zone: Food Guide Pyramid

www.familyfoodzone.com/pyramid/index.html

> Here's an interactive food pyramid that you can point and click on to learn more detail about each category.

Family Food Zone: Kids Cooking For Healthy Eating
www.familyfoodzone.com/cooking/index.html
> Research shows that children are more open to tasting new foods when they help prepare them. Here's a browsable list of recipes for kids and parents to work on together. I didn't see much in the low-fat area, however.

Family Food Zone: Nutrition Café
www.familyfoodzone.com/game/index.html
> At the Nutrition Café you can play three different games to test your nutritional knowledge. Play a Jeopardy-like game where you must choose the question to a given answer, or you can rate your plate.

Family Food Zone: Pantry Tips for Meals in Minutes
www.familyfoodzone.com/shop/index2.html
> Stock your pantry and fridge with these items and you'll be ready to whip a meal together in minutes.

Family Food Zone: Shopping Tips
www.familyfoodzone.com/shop/index.html
> Here's a few suggestions for quick meals, and some ideas for items to stock in your kitchen for meals in minutes.

Famous Vegetarians
www.chickpages.com/veggiefarm/famousveg
> What do Einstein, Mr. Rogers, Chelsea Clinton, kd Lang, and Doris Day all have in common? They, along with many other people, are on this list of famous vegetarians.

FANSA: Folic Acid:
A Reminder For Women Before & During Pregnancy
http://ift.micronexx.com/sc/sc_h04.html
> The Food and Nutrition Science Alliance provides important information for women. About 2,500 infants are born each year with severe, and sometimes fatal, abnormalities; about half could be prevented if adequate folic acid were consumed. Here you'll learn which foods are good sources, and if you need a supplement.

Farm Catalog: Vegetarian Cookbooks $
www.farmcatalog.com/cgi-bin/Web_store/web_store.cgi?page=cookbooks.html&cart_id=3673722.19484
> There's quite a list here of books that you can order online. You'll find Chinese Vegetarian, Book of Kudzu, Best 125 Meatless Pasta dishes, and more.

 MUST SEE!   VIDEO    AUDIO   SELLS STUFF

 CHAT ROOMS   MAILING LISTS   MESSAGE BOARDS   ADULT CONTENT

 FREE REGISTRATION REQUIRED   MEMBERS ONLY CONTENT   SEARCHABLE

Fast Food Facts - Interactive Food Finder
www.olen.com/food

Here's a nifty, simple to use item. Just enter the fast food restaurant you want to go to and then the item you might order. Then comes the nutritional information. For example, I "went" to McDonald's, typed in "Egg McMuffin," and was shown how many calories and how much fat there was, among other things. It's based on the book, "Fast Food Facts," from the Minnesota Attorney General's Office.

Fasting - Health Promoting Online
www.healthpromoting.com/fast.html

Believing that many of our health problems today are from nutritional excess, the philosophy of conservative therapy espouses fasting as a way to restoration. Here's a good article that could serve as a primer on the subject.

Fatfree: The Low Fat Vegetarian Recipe Archive
www.fatfree.com

This archive has over 2,500 low fat and fat free recipes in a searchable database.

FDA Backgrounder: Olestra & Other Fat Substitutes
http://vm.cfsan.fda.gov/~dms/bgolestr.html

This article was posted in 1995, when P&G wanted to get permission to put Olestra in our potato chips and other salty snacks. The problem's been that toxicology tests had only been done in the lab. Pull up this site to see who the study participants were.

FDA Consumer: Home Cookin' - Consumers' Kitchens Fail Inspections
http://vm.cfsan.fda.gov/~dms/fdcookin.html

"When it comes to food safety, consumers have higher expectations of other food handlers than they do of themselves." This survey conducted in late 1997 revealed that consumers failed to follow food safety guidelines over 99% of the time. And we're worried about eating out?

FDA Guide to Dietary Supplements
http://vm.cfsan.fda.gov/~dms/fdsupp.html

Consumers spent over $6.5 billion on dietary supplements in 1996. Just what are they? Dietary supplements are defined as vitamins; minerals; herbs, botanicals, and other plant-derived substances; and amino acids (the individual building blocks of protein) and concentrates, metabolites, constituents and extracts of these substances. This will help you understand not only what they are, but what they can claim, and how the government is trying to regulate their use. There's also an excellent section on how to recognize fraud.

FDA Kids Home Page
www.fda.gov/oc/opacom/kids

Take the food safety quiz, but first wash your hands with warm soapy water, don't just wipe them on your pants! Check out Yorrick, the bionic skeleton.

FDA's Bad Bug Book: E. coli

http://vm.cfsan.fda.gov/%7Emow/chap15.html

From the FDA and the Center for Food Safety and Applied Nutrition comes this page with a cute picture of this not so cute bug up in the right corner. They seem to love raw hamburger and raw milk. These little guys apparently infested club sandwiches in Ontario in the 1980's and killed 19 people. People shouldn't be allowed to have guns and bugs.

FDA/CFSAN
Dietary Supplement Health & Education Act of 1994

http://vm.cfsan.fda.gov/~dms/dietsupp.html

Signed by President Clinton on October 25, 1994, the DSHEA acknowledges that millions of consumers believe dietary supplements may help to augment daily diets and provide health consumers. The provisions of DSHEA define dietary supplements and dietary ingredients; establish a new framework for assuring safety; outline guidelines for literature displayed where supplements are sold; provide for use of claims and nutritional support statements; require ingredient and nutrition labeling; and grant FDA the authority to establish good manufacturing practice (GMP) regulations.

FDA/CFSAN: Bad Bug Book

http://vm.cfsan.fda.gov/~mow/intro.html

Looking for a particular parasite, bacteria, worm, or toxin? You've come to the right place. This handbook provides basic facts regarding food-borne pathogenic microorganisms and natural toxins. It brings together in one place information from the Food & Drug Administration, the Centers for Disease Control & Prevention, the USDA Food Safety Inspection Service, and the National Institutes of Health. Just scroll down the list of unpronounceable bugs til you think you got what you want and click. Be sure to check out the "typical outbreak" section of each bug, and wash your hands.

FDA/CFSAN: Bad Bug Book: Clostridium Botulinum

http://vm.cfsan.fda.gov/~mow/chap2.html

Botulism is a severe type of food poisoning, with a low incidence; however, it has a high mortality if not treated immediately and properly.

FDA/CFSAN: Bad Bug Book: Salmonella

http://vm.cfsan.fda.gov/~mow/chap1.htmleducation

Somewhere between 2 and 4 million cases occur annually in the U.S. The outbreaks appear to be rising here and in other industrialized nations, with dramatic increases in the northeast US. This page is informative and written in my terms of understanding; a lot of the big words are linked to a glossary to help you understand this stuff. Of particular interest to me is the section titled "typical outbreak," where CDC investigators delved into origins of reported outbreaks. It reads like a Stephen King novel. (We're going to wash our hands and move to Costa Rica.)

MUST SEE!   VIDEO   AUDIO $ SELLS STUFF

CHAT ROOMS   MAILING LISTS   MESSAGE BOARDS   ADULT CONTENT

FREE REGISTRATION REQUIRED   MEMBERS ONLY CONTENT   SEARCHABLE

FDA/CFSAN: Bad Bug Book: **Staphylococcus aureus**
http://vm.cfsan.fda.gov/~mow/chap3.html

Staphylococci exist in air, dust, sewage, water, milk, and food or on food equipment, environmental surfaces, humans, and animals. It's a wonder we can coexist on this planet.

FDA/CFSAN: Can Your Kitchen Pass the Food Safety Test? 👁
http://vm.cfsan.fda.gov/~dms/fdkitchn.html

Food safety concerns revolve around three areas: food storage, food handling, and cooking. This is a multiple choice test of 12 questions, and I flunked the raw cookie dough question because I always have to sample the stuff. Grade your own tests, and read up on the backgrounds of each question. It's a must read.

FDA/CFSAN: Food, Nutrition, & Cosmetics Q&As 🔍
http://vm.cfsan.fda.gov/~dms/qa-top.html

This site contains over 100 food safety, nutrition and cosmetic questions that consumers frequently ask. The answers are from material prepared by the federal public health and regulatory agencies responsible for foods and cosmetics. There are many questions about supplements, additives, food labeling, and food-borne illnesses.

FDA/CFSAN: Policy For Foods Developed By Biotechnology
http://vm.cfsan.fda.gov/~lrd/bioeme.html

Here's a 1995 statement on emerging technologies.

FDA/CFSAN: Seniors & Food Safety 👁
http://vm.cfsan.fda.gov/~dms/seniors.html

As we get older our ability to fight off bacteria becomes weaker. It's a good idea to get up to date on good food handling selection, and storage. The FDA did a nice job on this presentation for seniors.

FDA/CFSAN: Seniors & Food Safety - Preventing Food-Borne Illness
http://vm.cfsan.fda.gov/~dms/seniorse.html

Here's four simple steps to preparing food safely at home.

FDA/CFSAN: Seniors & Food Safety - What's a Senior to Eat?
http://vm.cfsan.fda.gov/~dms/seniorsc.html

Certain foods can pose a significant health hazard for seniors because of the level of bacteria in the product's raw state. Here's a list of things you should probably avoid. Gee, no more oysters on the half shell.

FDA/CFSAN: Seniors & Food Safety - Why Are Seniors at Risk for Food-Borne Illness?
http://vm.cfsan.fda.gov/~dms/seniorsb.html

As we age, the ability of our immune system to function at normal levels decreases. Seems that we just can't fight back like we used to. If you are a senior, or caring for one, this is good stuff to know.

FDA: All About Cooking Thermometers
http://vm.cfsan.fda.gov/~dms/fdtherm.html

One of the critical factors in fighting food-borne illness is temperature. Bacteria grow slowly at low temperatures and multiply rapidly at mid-range temperatures. To be safe, a product must be cooked to an internal temperature high enough to destroy harmful bacteria. Here, you'll learn about the different kinds of thermometers, and once you've got one, where to stick it.

FDA: Center For Food Safety & Applied Nutrition
http://vm.cfsan.fda.gov/~dms/wh-food.html

There's everything you ever wanted to know about food preparation and food-borne illness right here, and there are links to other sites, as well.

Feeding Kids Newsletter
www.nutritionforkids.com/Feeding_Kids.htm

This newsletter is filled with great timely articles on kids and nutrition. This page holds the archives. I read articles like "Nutrient Needs for Active Teen Boys," and "Breakfast as a Science Lesson." It's aimed at parents, teachers, and health professionals. Read back issues or subscribe for free to this bimonthly free E-mail newsletter.

Feeding Kids Newsletter: Subscribe
www.nutritionforkids.com/Subscribe2.htm

Feeding Kids Newsletter comes to your E-mail box every other month. It's uncluttered, easy and fun to read, and informative. It's a useful tool for teachers, health professionals, and parents, too. It's free! Subscribe here.

Feeding the Child With Diabetes - Grade School Through Middle School
www.uchsc.edu/misc/diabetes/nwsntrn1.html

From the Barbara Davis Center for Childhood Diabetes comes this article on food choices. If you're a parent who worries about food that's available at school, read this helpful entry from Markey Swanson, RD, CDE. It contains helpful suggestions for school snacks, lunches, after school, with friends, and emphasizes the importance of exercise and its relationship to carbs.

Fen/Phen Crisis Center: FAQs
www.fenphen.com/faq.html

Frequently asked questions are answered in depth. This drug was removed from the market in 1997, but the site remains. Lawsuits are pending from people who claim to have suffered valvular heart disease from taking this drug.

 MUST SEE!   VIDEO   AUDIO   SELLS STUFF

 CHAT ROOMS   MAILING LISTS   MESSAGE BOARDS   ADULT CONTENT

 FREE REGISTRATION REQUIRED   MEMBERS ONLY CONTENT   SEARCHABLE

Fen/Phen Crisis Center: Home Page
www.fenphen.com

The FEN/PHEN Crisis Center was operated by Dr. Pietr Hitzig, a Harvard-educated, Columbia physician who is widely regarded as the father of the FEN/PHEN protocol. This site now refers you to Phen4.com for the best diet drug ever. He doesn't quit.

Fen/Phen Crisis Center: Treatment Options
www.fenphen.com/top-crisis-treatment.html

Personalized protocols are listed here, emphasizing that with proper dosing and management, the use of this drug can be safe and effective. This web site was posted in 1996, and is obviously out of date, but may be of interest.

Fight BAC! Fighting the Problem of Food-Borne Illness 👁
www.fightbac.org

BAC is an invisible enemy, and you can't smell him or feel him; he's already invaded your kitchen, too. Find out here what the four simple steps are to eradicate this villain. Produced by the Partnership for Food Safety Education.

FitBody 3.0
www.darwin326.com/fitbody

FitBody 3.0 is a complete nutrition, fitness and health tracking system for Apple Macintosh and Microsoft Windows personal computers. By using FitBody, multiple users are able to receive accurate and timely feedback about their nutritional intake, workout progress, and wellness history.

FitenessLink: Pre-Contest Dieting Simplified
www.fitnesslink.com/food/contest.htm

Here's a simple plan for the drug free body builder that takes the mystery out of dieting before a contest.

Fitness Connection $
www.fitness-connection.com

This is the self-proclaimed "one stop supplement shop on the Internet," and they certainly represent many companies. Order your supplements on their secure site.

Fitness Factory Outlet $
www.fitnessfactory.com

This web site offers a full line of free weight machines, treadmills, steppers, exercise bikes, home gyms, commercial machines and accessories. Feel free to browse, order, or even just check in on their fitness tips which they say are changed every other week.

Fitness Find: Cross Training
www.fitnessfind.com/crosstrain.html

Looking for motivation, facts and information, what to look for in equipment before you make your purchase, then how to get started? Check out these links.

Fitness Forum ⚓

http://primusweb.com/fitnesspartner/forum/forum.htm

Do you have a question about exercise equipment? Have you read a particularly inspiring fitness book? Do you need some healthy meal ideas? This is the place to discuss all matters of fitness, nutrition and health.

THE **FITNESS JUMPSITE!**

Your connection to a lifestyle of fitness, nutrition, and health.

Fitness Jumpsite! ⚲ 👁

http://primusweb.com/fitnesspartner/index.html

"Your connection to a lifestyle of fitness, nutrition, and health." If you're struggling with weight loss and trying to get into shape, here's a great place to come to. You'll find places to guide you into a new lifestyle, information on equipment, support, book reviews, and you can join discussions on fitness, nutrition, and health.

Fitness News From the American Heart Association

www.justmove.org/fitnessnews

Here in Fitness News you'll find almost everything you need to know about exercise, fitness, and your health.

Fitness News: Health Facts - Children & the Need for Physical Activity Fact Sheet

www.justmove.org/fitnessnews/healthf.cfm?Target=kidsfacts.html

There's some scary and depressing facts about trends in kids' behavior here. Read this and then kick 'em outdoors!

Fitness News: Health Facts - Exercise & Children

www.justmove.org/fitnessnews/healthf.cfm?Target=exerckids.html

OK kids, here's your guidelines from the AHA for regular physical activity. Put your Playstation away right now, and go outside.

Fitness News: Health Facts - Exercise Tips For Older Americans

www.justmove.org/fitnessnews/healthf.cfm?Target=eldertips.html

Check with your doctor, of course, then check out these brief tips for starting your program.

 MUST SEE!   VIDEO   AUDIO   SELLS STUFF

 CHAT ROOMS   MAILING LISTS   MESSAGE BOARDS   ADULT CONTENT

 FREE REGISTRATION REQUIRED   MEMBERS ONLY CONTENT   SEARCHABLE

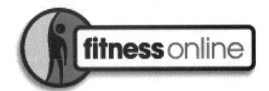

Fitness Online 👁

www.fitnessonline.com/index.asp

> Fitness Online wants to give you all the tools, information, and support you need to help you reach your health and fitness goals. There's lots of quick sites to browse for men and women. Fitness Online is associated with *Shape*, *Men's Fitness*, *Muscle & Fitness*, *Flex*, *Natural Health*, and *Fit Pregnancy* magazines. These are pages from their family of magazines.

Fitness Online: Community ⚓🗣

http://216.33.170.201/community.asp

> Log on to your choice of many chat rooms and message boards. Subjects include getting in shape for men and/or women, nutrition, adding muscle, and fitness.

Fitness Online: Fitness Goals

www.fitnessonline.com/fitnessonline/folCategoryTemplates/category
.asp?Catid=16

> Peruse these articles that previously appeared in *Muscle & Fitness*, *Flex*, and *Shape* magazines.

Fitness Online: Mind & Body

www.fitnessonline.com/fitnessonline/folCategoryTemplates/SuperCat
egory.asp?CatID=6

> Try out a bit of yoga, or other mind/body exercises.

Fitness Online: Personal Profile

www.fitnessonline.com/fitnessonline/folPersonalization/membership
.asp

> Establish your personal profile here and fitness online will be tailored to your personal needs and interests.

Fitness Partner Connection ⚓

http://primusweb.com/fitnesspartner/boards/bb01.htm

> "Jumpsite founders Vicki Pierson and Renee Cloe understand the value of sharing fitness ideas, motivation, and support with a friend. The Fitness Partner Connection Jumpsite was created by these two fitness buddies who met on an Internet discussion group. This is the place to post if you've been searching for a friend who shares your enthusiasm for fitness. Do you need help staying motivated? Are you struggling to maintain a healthy diet? Trying to find someone else with a passion for in-line skating? Are you a fitness professional who wants to meet other instructors?" You can post your own notices here.

Fitness Partner Connection: Bulletin Board: Fitness Equipment ⚓

http://primusweb.com/fitnesspartner/boards/bb03.htm

> Post your message here if you're looking for some exercise equipment, or browse the board for something you want. Buyers and sellers can connect here for free.

Fitness Partner Connection: FAQs

http://primusweb.com/fitnesspartner/library/features/fpcfaq.htm

Here's lots of questions from the Fitness Partners mailbag. Subjects include nutrition, weight loss, and exercise.

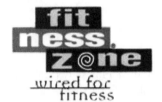

Fitness Zone $

www.fitnesszone.com

FitnessZone is the self-proclaimed premier fitness site on the Internet, featuring an exclusive on-line health and fitness magazine, a nation-wide gym and health-club locator, a fitness library, and a personal fitness profiler -- as well as a comprehensive selection of the highest-quality fitness equipment. FitnessZone is a division of Hot New Products, Inc. of Birmingham, Alabama.

Fitness Zone: Classifieds

www.fitnesszone.com/classifieds

Search for used exercise equipment, or a personal trainer, or for professional equipment.

Fitness Zone: Fitness Profile

www.fitnesszone.com/profiles

Fill in the blanks, and you get a profile of your current fitness level as well as suggestions for improving your workout. It's free, but the site does suggest buying some music to exercise to. Although it's cool to try this profile, make sure you check in with your doctor before doing anything.

Fitness Zone: Fitnesszine

www.fitnesszone.com/features

The online fitness weekly is available here with brief articles on current thought on fitness and nutrition.

Fitness Zone: Fitnesszine: Sports Nutrition Myths

www.fitnesszone.com/features/archives/jul98/3070698.html

Is there any food, drug, or nutrient that can improve speed or performance? Read it and weep if you've already put in your online order for those supplements.

Fitness Zone: Fitnesszine: Staying With the Program

www.fitnesszone.com/features/archives/tips.html

Here's ten tips for staying with a program.

Fitness Zone: Forums ⚓

www.fitnesszone.com/forums

Join in and post messages to various forums like weight training, general fitness, or running. On my last visit I noticed that the forums had not seen any activity since Fall, 1998. Too bad; maybe they're up and running again by now. Seemed like a good idea.

Fitness Zone: Join 📪 ⚓ 🗣

www.fitnesszone.com/join

You can enjoy all of the benefits of FitnessZone membership, including their Fitness Forums, Fitness Classifieds and Personals. And, they'll send you a weekly FitnessZine update if you wish -- all for free!

Fitness Zone: Library ¶

www.fitnesszone.com/library

The FitnessZone library is a searchable repository of the best-known health and fitness FAQs (Frequently Asked Questions), as well as an archive of significant recent contributions to a number of health and fitness newsgroups.

FitnessLink: Choosing Bodybuilding Supplements

www.fitnesslink.com/food/supps.htm

Before you delve into body building supplements learn the basics. What do you need, what's anabolic, thermogenic, or ergogenic? What is creatine? Should you get some dehydroepiandrosterone and how much? Who makes the best? How much should you take? How do you know if it really contains what it says it does?

FitnessLink:
Sports Nutrition Supplements Mislabeled & Misleading

www.fitnesslink.com/food/mislabel.htm

If you're turning to performance enhancing supplements you might want to read this report. In a 1998 lab test, about 50% of supplements chosen at random from retail stores did not contain the amount of ingredients purported on the label. Read the brief summary of the study before you shop.

FitnessMatters: Frequently Asked Fitness Questions

http://lifematters.com/jackfaq.html

Got a question about fitness? There's probably an answer here.

FitnessMatters: Running on Full

http://lifematters.com/rofintro.html

Are you a runner who's pregnant? Or thinking about becoming pregnant? The concept raises lots of questions, and hopefully, your answers can be found here.

Fitting In Fitness

http://primusweb.com/fitnesspartner/library/activity/
fittingfitnessin.htm

Exercise programs always fall victim to the "notenoughtime" syndrome. Here's a worksheet to help you with time management, and to prioritize your activities.

Florida Citrus Land For Kids

www.floridajuice.com/floridacitrus/kids/index.htm

> Let Zippity, the Silly Tangerine, take your kids through a tour of all the benefits of Florida citrus. There are crossword puzzles, word scrambles, and some coloring pages to download for the kids. Go for a tour of how orange juice is made - it isn't just for kids.

Following the DASH Diet

http://dash.bwh.harvard.edu./dashdietservings.html

> Do you want to get started on the DASH diet? Here's basic information on what's included from each of the food groups, and the quantities for a 2,000 calorie diet.

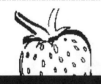 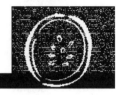 Food & Health Communications, Inc.

Food & Health Communications, Inc. $

www.foodandhealth.com

> Food and Health Communications is a leading publisher of innovative materials for nutrition educators. Subscribe here or shop their catalog.

Food & Nutrition Information Center ♀ ☞

www.nal.usda.gov/fnic

> The Food and Nutrition Information Center (FNIC) is one of several information centers at the National Agricultural Library (NAL), part of the United States Department of Agriculture's (USDA) Agricultural Research Service (ARS). You can access all of FNIC's resource lists and databases, as well as many other food and nutrition related links from this award winning site. Find information on such topics as dietary guidelines, food safety, supplements, report, studies, and links to Internet resources.

Food Allergy Network

www.foodallergy.org

> The Food Allergy Network is a nonprofit organization whose goals are to increase public awareness of food allergies and anaphylaxis, to provide education, and to advance research on behalf of those affected by food allergies. It is a member supported organization. Members receive a bimonthly newsletter, and product alerts. Members range from medical professionals to food manufacturers.

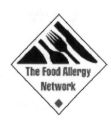

MUST SEE!	VIDEO	AUDIO	SELLS STUFF
CHAT ROOMS	MAILING LISTS	MESSAGE BOARDS	ADULT CONTENT
FREE REGISTRATION REQUIRED	MEMBERS ONLY CONTENT	SEARCHABLE	

Food Allergy Network: Facts & Fiction
www.foodallergy.org/facts_fiction.html
> Who's at increased risk for a food allergy? How long does it take for symptoms to occur? What are the symptoms? Is there a cure? Want to know the answers to these and other questions? Look here for lots of useful information; you'll also find common myths debunked

Food Allergy Network: Food Allergy Research
www.foodallergy.org/research.html
> Here's a list of current research and studies going on. Some are looking for volunteers to participate. You can also sign onto their peanut and tree nut allergy registry, which will help them track reactions and medications that are successfully used.

FOOD Files: Amazing Records
http://library.advanced.org/11960/fun/records.htm
> The longest sausage, the tallest cake, the biggest chocolate, and the biggest donut. Read the facts, and dazzle your dieting buddies with your trivia.

FOOD Files: Fad Diets
http://library.advanced.org/11960/trouble/fad.htm
> Here's a bit of advice regarding fad diets, how they're supposed to work, and of course, the "advice to all" section.

FOOD Files: Kitchen Practices
http://library.advanced.org/11960/handling/kitchen.htm
> Personal hygiene and proper food handling can help you avoid many food-borne diseases. For starters wash your hands, don't sneeze, and leave your nose alone!

FOOD Files: Preparing & Cooking Food
http://library.advanced.org/11960/handling/prepcook.htm
> Want some quick tips on preventing contamination? Go here.

FOOD Files: Storing Food
http://library.advanced.org/11960/handling/storing.htm
> Food spoilage can seriously affect your health. Here are some pointers on storing different kinds of food, including meats, dairy, fruits and vegetables.

Food Finder
www.olen.com/food
> This site is based on the book, "Fast Food Facts," from the Minnesota Attorney General's office. There are over 1,000 items in their database. I typed in "French fries," and I think Burger King won with 20 grams of fat in a medium size order.

Food Fun For Kids
www.nppc.org/foodfun.html

The National Pork Board brings you this kid-oriented site. Come climb the food pyramid, and travel the earth through the magical pantry. Go on the "farmtastic voyage" with Bethany and Michael through their pig farm in Iowa where you'll see baby pigs, how they're fed, and how they are housed. The tour ended before we got to the slaughterhouse. On the left of the page are sections to click on for parents and teachers. (Maybe that's where the slaughterhouse tour is!)

Food Guide Pyramid
www.nal.usda.gov:8001/py/pmap.htm

Click on any section of the food pyramid, and an interactive guide will help you understand things such as what makes up a serving, and even why the food guide is constructed in the shape of a pyramid. I think this may well be the birthplace of the food pyramid; perhaps this web site should be made a shrine. Be sure to make many pilgrimages here.

Food-Borne Bacterial Diseases
www.cdc.gov/ncidod/diseases/bacter/foodborn.htm

Yikes! Did you know that there are over 250 diseases caused by contaminated food and drink? But I'm not worried yet because gin is still safe. This page looks like someone's school report typed up on an old Smith Corona, but be sure to read it. It's downright frightening when you learn that we import over 30 billion tons of food a year, and that there are new and emerging food-borne pathogens. Stir in the increasing immunocompromised population, and we've got trouble, maybe. But fear not, because the CDC says our food supply is the safest it's ever been, in spite of it all. I'm still going to worry.

FoodNet
www.cdc.gov/ncidod/dbmd/foodnet/98surv.htm

The objectives of FoodNet are to determine the frequency and severity of food-borne diseases; determine the proportion of common food-borne diseases that result from eating specific foods; and describe the epidemiology of new and emerging bacterial, parasitic, and viral food-borne pathogens. Read the 1998 report from the CDC on "how we did."

Form YOU 3 International $
www.formyou3.com/products.htm

You can buy all their products here, from complete meals to supplements to cellulite removal systems. The only thing I couldn't find was a home liposuction kit.

Form YOU 3 International Weight Loss Centers
www.formyou3.com/index.htm

There were at least 61 centers in 17 states offering their programs. They take what they call an integrated approach to weight loss, using a food exchange method or a nutrient-rich meal replacement program.

 MUST SEE!   VIDEO   AUDIO   SELLS STUFF

 CHAT ROOMS   MAILING LISTS   MESSAGE BOARDS   ADULT CONTENT

 FREE REGISTRATION REQUIRED   MEMBERS ONLY CONTENT   SEARCHABLE

Foundation for the Macrobiotic Way
www.enjoy-life.com/health

The Foundation for the Macrobiotic Way is a non-profit organization that was formed in New Orleans, Louisiana in 1987 by macrobiotic students who were interested in providing education about healthy ways of living. The Foundation has been dedicated to offering educational programs, teachers, and resources to help those interested in maintaining their mental, physical and spiritual well-being.

Foundation for the Macrobiotic Way: A Marcobiotic Diet
www.enjoy-life.com/health/corepages/macrodiet.html

What is it they chew? There's a pie chart here that clearly depicts the diet of a macrobiotic. I did not see any brownies.

Four Food Groups
www.vegsource.com/food_groups.htm

This is an excerpt from the "Vegetarian Starter Kit," from the Physicians Committee for Responsible Medicine.

Frequently Asked Questions About Vegetarianism
www.veg.org/veg/FAQ/rec.food.veg.html

This is actually a Usenet site, and is loaded with common questions

Fresh Network
http://easyweb.easynet.co.uk/karenk/top.html

The Fresh Network exists to bring together those who have an interest in a 100% or high percentage raw food diet. A Network to exchange vital education information, ideas and person experiences so that individuals can change their diet and lifestyle with help and support from others, to suit their own personal set of ever changing needs and circumstances.

Fruitarian Foundation
www.fruitarian.com/ar/AboutFruitarianFoundation.htm

"We at The Fruitarian Foundation share a vision of a world that is enhanced through a better community of healthy human beings which promote the highest values of the human race: Intellectual, Artistic, and Spiritual. We are convinced that only a nutrition system of Raw Food, can liberate the human mind and spirit and offer the biological support for a superior health, necessary condition for the complete unfold of all the creative powers of human beings and their harmonic relationship to the earth and the Universe."--The Vision Statement of the Fruitarian Foundation.

Fruitarian Network
http://spot.acorn.net/fruitarian

From the Akron Community Resource Network comes this Fruitarian web site, you will find an extensive definition of what a fruitarian is and the benefits of being one; you'll also find poems to fruit trees and their parents.

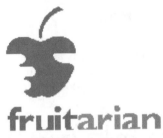

Fruitarian Site

www.fruitarian.com

This is the international meeting place for people who love to eat fruit. Fruitarians are vegetarians (kind of) who subsist on fruit only. Here you can learn about fruitarian nutrition.

Fruitarian Universal Network

www.student.nada.kth.se/~f95-mwi/fun

Fruitarians eat raw fruit primarily. The FUN says, "All you need for cooking as a fruitarian is a knife, a spoon, and a plate." We're thinking of selling the pots, pans, and stove. This sounds good.

Fruitarian Universal Network: FAQs

www.student.nada.kth.se/~f95-mwi/fun/faq.html

How do you get enough protein, and what about the essential fatty acids? Can you get that in a wholly fruit diet?? Look here for the answers.

Fruitarian Universal Network: How to Become a Fruitarian

www.student.nada.kth.se/~f95-mwi/fun/howTo.html

Warning! If you want to become a fruitarian don't change overnight. Your body might react in a negative way.

Fruitarian Universal Network: Nutrition Calculator

www.student.nada.kth.se/~f95-mwi/fun/calc.html

Here's an interesting tool to help you calculate the energy in a fruit or fruit meal. You can then compare to Recommended Daily Intake Table for which there is a link. The RDI table is from the Swedish National Board for Health and Welfare, and I suspect it is outdated because it recommends 100g of fat a day for a man, or 78g for a woman. They must all be a bit chunky over there!

Fruitarian Universal Network: What Do Fruitarians Eat?

www.student.nada.kth.se/~f95-mwi/fun/whatEat.html

There's a decent chart here describing the 6 "energy levels" according to fruitarianism, and there's some recipes which give you an idea of what and how they eat.

 MUST SEE!   VIDEO   AUDIO   SELLS STUFF

 CHAT ROOMS   MAILING LISTS   MESSAGE BOARDS   ADULT CONTENT

 FREE REGISTRATION REQUIRED   MEMBERS ONLY CONTENT   SEARCHABLE

Fruitarian Universal Network: What is a Fruitarian?

www.student.nada.kth.se/~f95-mwi/fun/whatIs.html

"A fruitarian is a person who eats fruit and only fruit. What we in FUN mean by fruit is all the sweet fruits such as mangos, bananas, melons, oranges, etc., all kinds of berries, and the vegetable fruits such as tomato, cucumber, olives, etc." - from the Fruitarian Universal Network. Here's a good description of your basic fruitarian.

Fruitarian Universal Network: Why Become a Fruitarian?

www.student.nada.kth.se/~f95-mwi/fun/why.html

"The 'less-killing principle' or the 'non-killing principle' is an important part of fruitarianism. The less violence, the more love. Violence and killing in all forms should be rejected to make room for love." - from the Fruitarian Universal Network. If you like simplicity in your food, you might be interested in fruitarianism.

Frutiarian Network Around the World

http://www3.islandnet.com/~arton/fruitnet.html

"The Fruitarian Network News provides the means by which aspiring fruitarians/raw fooders/people in transition to a healthy and radiant well-being can communicate with like-minded people. It publishes general information, articles and letters relating to the fruitarian/raw food diet, provides mental and spiritual support, discusses problems and experiences arising therefrom."- from the Fruitarian Network Around the World Web Site. There is a nice section with frequently asked questions about the movement.

Genetically Modified Foods

www.healthyeating.org/general/gmf.htm

From Eat Well, Live Well comes this article on genetically altered foods. In May, 1999, new standards for food labeling came into force in Australia and New Zealand. Labeling such foods is still under debate here in the USA.

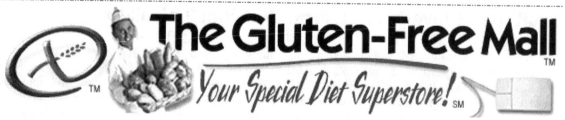

Gluten-Free Mall $👁

www.glutenfreemall.com

This is your one-stop shop for special dietary foods. Order online, and have it delivered to your door.

Go Ask Alice Home Page 👁

www.goaskalice.columbia.edu

This is a highly informative and entertaining way to deliver sound advice from Columbia University. Point and click to any area of health concerns, and you're on your way.

Go Ask Alice: Fitness & Nutrition 👁

www.goaskalice.columbia.edu/Cat3.html

If you remember the Jefferson Airplane, you know how Columbia University got this name. What's more amazing is that we boomers who were part of that culture can remember anything! But this site has a great list of questions that were E-mailed to "Alice" at Columbia. Just skim the list and there's sure to be some questions of interest that you will want to pursue. I particularly liked "Ice cream for breakfast?" and "How to eat your veggies, even if you don't like them."

Going Vegetarian: Part I

http://vegetarian.about.com/library/weekly/aa022398.htm?pid=2757&cob=home

So you've been thinking of moving toward a vegetarian diet and/or lifestyle, but you're not sure how to get it started? This article, by Tiffany Refior, your vegetarian guide in "About.com," is a good place to start.

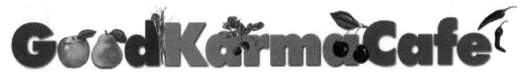

Good Karma Café 🔍 👁

www.goodkarmacafe.com

Here's a nice place to look for, exchange, or send vegetarian recipes. Check out their city guides to vegetarian eating, and send a veggie greeting card to someone. There's book reviews with a direct link to Amazon.com for buying them.

Good Karma Café - Our Karma, Our Bodies

www.goodkarmacafe.com/body/karma.shtml

Find some good help here on vegetarian weight loss, nutrition, and health here. There are also links to other sites.

Good Karma Café - Vegetarian Recipe Exchange ⬇

http://freshpages.com/Vegetarian_Recipes/Vegetarian_Recipes.html

Ask for, or post, veggie recipes on this message board. If you ask for help, you most likely will get it.

Good Karma Café - Welcome to Recipe Central ⬇

www.goodkarmacafe.com/recipes/recipes.shtml

There's a recipe exchange board here, and a recipe "re-do," where meat recipes are transformed into veggie fare.

 MUST SEE!   VIDEO   AUDIO $ SELLS STUFF

 CHAT ROOMS   MAILING LISTS   MESSAGE BOARDS   ADULT CONTENT

 FREE REGISTRATION REQUIRED   MEMBERS ONLY CONTENT   SEARCHABLE

Good Nutrition - A Look at Vegetarian Basics

http://mars.superlink.com/user/dupre/navs/nutri.html

If you're thinking about taking on a vegetarian lifestyle and have concerns if you'll get adequate protein, carbs, vitamins, and minerals, read this article.

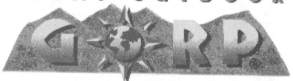

GORP: Great Outdoor Recreation Pages ⚓👁

www.gorp.com/default.htm

Interested in doing something outdoors? GORP has ideas and suggestions for you, whether it's walking, biking, paddling, climbing, skiing, or bird watching. Be sure to check out the forums where you can post messages on nearly everything outdoors. You can find lots of links to further your knowledge on any outdoor subject, and get lost somewhere in cyberspace. Be sure to leave a trail of gorp so you can find your way home.

GORP: Great Outdoor Recreation Pages: Biking 👁

www.gorp.com/gorp/activity/biking.htm

Here's a good resource for you if you think you might be interested in bicycling for fitness and fun.

Grab A Grape

http://exhibits.pacsci.org/nutrition/grape/grape.html

If you like to play Jeopardy, this nutrition game's for you. Pick four categories out of seven relating to nutrition, and then play it just like Jeopardy. Categories include Food and Sports, Weight Control, Fast Foods, and several others. Give it a try.

Grass Roots Veganism with Joanne Stepaniak

www.vegsource.org/joanne

Joanne Stepaniak, MSEd, is a writer, counselor, educator, and recipe innovator who has been involved with vegetarian- and vegan-related issues for over three decades. Joanne is the author of The Vegan Sourcebook, a comprehensive guide to compassionate vegan living encompassing the history, ethics, and philosophy of the vegan movement, as well as environmental, sociological, psychological, and nutritional perspectives. She must be Mother Nature! Really though, her web site is easy to navigate, not cluttered with dancing elephants, and very informative for any vegetarian or aspiring vegetarian.

Griffin's Weightlifting Page: Weighty Matters 👁

http://weber.u.washington.edu/~griffin/weights.html

Wow, this is huge. Weighty Matters is a selective archive of weightlifting and bodybuilding posts from the old misc.fitness and the newer misc.fitness.weights and other newsgroups, plus bits and pieces from the "weights," "strength" and "weights-plus" mailing lists. There are links galore, and if you can't find it here, it doesn't exist.

Harvard School of Public Health: The Olestra Project

www.hsph.harvard.edu/Academics/nutr/olestra/olestra.html

This site holds the proceedings of a workshop held in January, 1996, on The Potential Effects of Reducing Carotenoid Levels on Human Health. This is, of course, the basis for the Olestra controversy.

Health Implications of Obesity

http://text.nlm.nih.gov/nih/cdc/www/49txt.html

From the National Institutes of Health Consensus Conference in 1985 comes this statement showing the adverse effects of obesity on longevity, and the clear association with hypertension, diabetes, and cancer. This should help you with any lifestyle change you may have been thinking about.

Health Specialists: Malibu Beach Two Day Diet $

www.thehealthspecialists.com/product.html

Do you want to lose 10 pounds in 2 days? And 2 inches per thigh in just 2 weeks? And if you have MPEG video/audio files you can see and hear testimonials of how people lost as much as 17 pounds in 2 days! Just $62 gets you this magic potion. Want to buy some ocean front property in Kansas?

Health Steps

www.ghc.org/health_info/self/fitness/hlthstep.html

Group Health Cooperative of Puget Sound presents this site that will help you plan and begin your own personal walking program.. A regular walking program can reduce your risk of heart disease, help you lose weight and lower body fat, tone flabby muscles, keep bones strong, improve your energy level, and help you manage stress. Go for it!

HealthWeb: Nutrition

www.libraries.psu.edu/crsweb/hw/nutr

If you're looking for some in-depth information, HealthWeb along with the University of Pennsylvania, can help you find electronic journals, research centers, and other publications to help you find what you're looking for.

Healthy Athlete

http://bewell.com/healthy/athlete/index.asp

Healthy Athlete E-zine comes to us weekly from Healthgate, a leading provider of biomedical information on the Web. This is a crisp production filled with helpful news on such things as sports injuries, equipment reviews, sports nutrition, and up-to-date articles on fitness. You can access Medline, or search Healthgate's large database from here. Look for your ailment on the browsable list of sports injuries. There's even a medical dictionary to help you with the big words.

 MUST SEE!   VIDEO   AUDIO   SELLS STUFF

 CHAT ROOMS   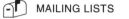 MAILING LISTS   MESSAGE BOARDS   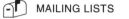 ADULT CONTENT

 FREE REGISTRATION REQUIRED   MEMBERS ONLY CONTENT   SEARCHABLE

Healthy Athlete: Energy Bars & Gels 👁

http://bewell.com/healthy/athlete/1999/barsgels/index.asp

Are those bars and gels worth the price? Do they really work? What do they do? Could I just get my fuel from a banana and save the difference? Here's a good, in-depth article on these high carb boosters. There are even pop quizzes along the way to see if you're alert while reading.

Healthy Eating 🔍 👁

http://bewell.com/healthy/eating/index.asp

Healthy Eating brings you timely articles on good food and nutrition. Open up this magazine to such articles as food in the news, vitamins and health, and nutrition during pregnancy. There's a browsable database of herbs and vitamins, and you can search Medline, or use the medical dictionary. Visit here for useful nutrition information in a pleasant format.

Healthy Heart Handbook for Women 👁

www.nih.gov/health/chip/nhlbi/heart

The National Institutes of Health brings you this online booklet about women and heart disease. It starts out with definitions of cardiovascular disease, discusses major risk factors for women, prevention strategies, and tells us about research on heart disease with focus on women.

Healthy Heart Handbook for Women: The Healthy Heart

www.nih.gov/health/chip/nhlbi/heart/aheart.htm

Every year 245,000 women die of heart disease, and another 90,000 women die of stroke. Over 10 million women have heart disease. Just what is coronary heart disease? Who gets it? Here's an easy reading primer on the number one killer of women.

Healthy Weight Network

www.healthyweightnetwork.com

Healthy Weight Network brings you the latest information on eating and weight, and helps you apply it in your life. It comes from the editorial offices of Healthy Weight Journal, and is most helpful on bridging the gap between research and practical application.

Healthy Weight--Healthy Steps

www.4meridia.com/consumer/archive/steps/fitness.cfm

A target heart rate calculator is on this page. Just enter your age and you get your target.

Healthy Weight--Healthy Steps Calorie Burning Guide

www.4meridia.com/consumer/archive/steps/cal.cfm

Here are lists of calorie values for ten minute periods of regular activities based on various weights.

Healthy Weight--Healthy Steps--Walking Test

www.4meridia.com/consumer/archive/steps/walkingtest.cfm

A walking test to measure your fitness level, this page will tell you what shape you're in and give suggestions for improving your fitness level.

Heart & Stroke Foundation of Canada
www.hsf.ca/main_e.htm
> The equivalent of the American Heart Association, the Heart and Stroke Foundation of Canada offers a more inviting web site for the general public. It just looks user friendly, and it is. There are well-presented sections for women and heart disease, stats and news, kids, and food. Go to "Test Your Knowledge" to take the "Ticker Test" to determine your risk for stroke or heart disease.

Heart Information Network:
DASH Diet Lowers Blood Pressure
www.heartinfo.com/news97/dash61797.htm
> High blood pressure affects one in four Americans, and there seems to be few dietary guidelines to control its effects. However, in a study funded by the National Heart, Lung, and Blood Institute, a diet low in fat and high in fruits and vegetables appears to lower blood pressure. Find out what participants ate, and how it worked.

Heart Smart
www.siestasoftware.com/hsmart.htm
> Heart Smart is designed to help you plan and maintain a healthy diet. Set up your diet according to your health needs. You can download a trial version for free, or buy one if you like it.

Heart Watch Newsletter
www.betterhealth.com/heartwatch/jul99
> From the publishers of The New England Journal of Medicine, this newsletter is full of up-to-date information. You can search the archives or simply peruse previous issues online. You can also subscribe and have it mailed monthly for $29/year.

Heart Watch Newsletter:
Can Vitamin E Pills Protect the Heart?
www.betterhealth.com/seniors/alternative/nejm/0,4802,1958_124100,00.html
> According to the authors, it is known that antioxidants contained in fruits and vegetables can lower the risk of coronary heart disease, but studies of antioxidant supplements have less clear results. The bottom line? Eat plenty of fruits and vegetables to get your antioxidants, and of course, always consult your doctor.

Heart Watch: Fiber Lowers Heart Disease Risk in Women
www.betterhealth.com/nejm/0,4802,7016_127321,00.html
> Heart Watch Newsletter is published by The New England Journal of Medicine. Read this article which describes how by eating a bowl of cold fiber containing cereal (about 5 grams), women were able to lower their risk of heart disease by 37%.

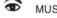 MUST SEE!   VIDEO   AUDIO   SELLS STUFF
 CHAT ROOMS   MAILING LISTS   MESSAGE BOARDS   ADULT CONTENT
 FREE REGISTRATION REQUIRED   MEMBERS ONLY CONTENT   SEARCHABLE

Heartsmart Family Fun Pack 👁

www.hsf.ca/En/funpack/index.html

Here's an interactive site from the Heart and Stroke Foundation of Canada that seeks to educate kids in a fun way about adopting a lifestyle that can lead to a longer, healthier life. Try going to TV Talkback, then click on the remote control as you learn how TV commercials lead you to your kitchen for junk food. It can stimulate good conversation in the family room, after Dad hides his chips and beer behind his recliner.

Help for Carbohydrate Addicts - Books by Drs. Richard & Rachael Heller

www.carbohydrateaddicts.com/cabooks.html

The books provide a choice of programs that include step-by-step plans and jump-start plans. Some focus on health issues, some on weight loss, some on both. Some plans are more appropriate for kids, some for those over 40, and some are appropriate for adults of all ages.

Herbalife $

www.herbalifediet.com

Herbalife's secure online shopping center for weight loss programs and products. The true miracle product we've been looking for must be in here somewhere.

Hinduism Online: Discussing Vegetarianism With a Meateater

www.hinduismtoday.kauai.hi.us/ashram/Resources/Ahimsa/WinMeatEaterArgument.html

From "Hinduism Today," this is a discussion of vegetarianism, its basis in scripture, and statements from the Physicians Committee for Responsible Medicine.

Home Enterprises - Beer Blok $

www.homent.demon.co.uk/beerblok.htm

Stop worrying about developing a "beer belly" when you supplement your beer with this!

Home Enterprises - Diet & Health $

www.homent.demon.co.uk/main.htm

From the UK, you can order fat burners and fat binders.

Hopkins Technology Health CD-ROMs 🔽

www.hoptechno.com/healthp.htm

Hopkins Technology has been developing software since the early 80's. Order their CD-ROMs on topics ranging from nutrition analysis to diet, exercise, and weight control.

HotJ-Heavyweights on the Journey
http://recovery.hiwaay.net/hotj/index.html

The HotJ loop focuses on compulsions and addictions relating to food. Many of its members weigh or weighed over 400 pounds, and may be members of Overeaters Anonymous, a twelve step program. These twelve steps are the guidelines which this support group focuses on. The subject is treated with great sensitivity and compassion. However, OA does not support, endorse, or recommend any one Internet chat or support site.

How to Read a Food Label 👁
www.4meridia.com/consumer/archive/label.cfm

A sample nutrition fact chart is shown and is interactive. Choose any item on the nutrition label and a description of its importance and an interpretation of what it actually means pops up.

IAEA/ICGFI: Facts About Food Irradiation
www.iaea.or.at/worldatom/inforesource/other/food/index.html

The safety and benefits of foods processed by ionizing radiation are well documented. In an effort to provide governments, especially those of developing countries, with scientifically accurate information on issues of general interest to the public, the International Consultative Group on Food Irradiation (ICGFI), which was established under the aegis of the Food and Agriculture Organization of the United Nations (FAO), the World Health Organization (WHO), and the IAEA, decided at its 7th Annual Meeting in Rome, Italy, in October 1990, to issue a series of "Fact Sheets" on the subject.

Idaho Potato
www.idahopotato.com/index.html

If the dairy people and the citrus people and the fruit people get to be listed, so do the potato people. Why not join the "Spuddy Buddy Fan Club?" or learn to make a mashed potato snowman?

Identifying Weight Loss Fraud & Quackery
www.healthyweightnetwork.com/fraud.htm

This is a good article from Healthy Weight Network on how to identify fraud, questionable weight loss products, and how to report it.

IFIC Food Insight: Calcium for All Ages & Genders
http://ificinfo.health.org/insight/janfeb99/calcium.htm

Did you know that less than half of adults are consuming adequate amounts of calcium, although they think they are? And it's not just for bones? And that if you don't take in enough calcium you're body will leach it from your bones? There are dietary sources other than dairy that give you calcium as well. Got broccoli?

 MUST SEE!   VIDEO   AUDIO   SELLS STUFF

 CHAT ROOMS   MAILING LISTS   MESSAGE BOARDS   ADULT CONTENT

 FREE REGISTRATION REQUIRED   MEMBERS ONLY CONTENT   SEARCHABLE

IFIC Foundation: Search
http://ificinfo.health.org/search.htm

The International Food Information Council has provided this search site so you can search their vast library. For example, I typed "diabetes," and got back 43 abstracts from past articles.

IFIC Insight: Antioxidants: Working Toward A Definition
http://ificinfo.health.org/insight/NovDec98/antioxidants.htm

Antioxidants seem to be the rage, so to speak. We're all taking them because we know they can reduce the risk of cancer and cardiovascular disease by preventing free radicals from attacking cells and damaging DNA. And I thought we were done with radicals after the '70's.

IFIC Insight: Extreme Eating - Are Teens Compromising Their Health?
http://ificinfo.health.org/insight/NovDec98/extremeeat.htm

Many teens aren't getting the nutrients they need due to their eating behaviors. Some eat too much fat, some are dieting in dangerous ways, and many don't get enough fruits and vegetables, and vegetarianism among this group is increasing in prevalence. Balance, variety, and moderation: How do you make that cool?

IFIC Insight: Recommended Dietary Allowances
http://ificinfo.health.org/insight/septoct98/rdas.htm

RDAs are becoming RD's right before our very eyes. What's this all mean? This article from IFICs Insight takes us ehind the scenes through the evolution of this revision. Find out what RDIs, EARs, AIs, and ULs are.

IFIC Insight: The High Protein Myth
http://ificinfo.health.org/insight/septoct98/proteinmyth.htm

From Sept/Oct 1998, comes more fuel for the fiery debate over those high protein diets. Read this before you go visit Dr. Atkins and the others.

IFIC Review: Caffeine & Health: Clarifying the Controversies
http://ificinfo.health.org/review/ir-caffh.htm

After reading this review of the current literature, you just might want to go out and get yourself a cappuccino or even an espresso. Supposedly caffeine is cool, and don't worry about a moderate intake even if you're a kid, or pregnant, or have a heart arrhythmia, or you're hypertensive. Caffeine addiction? No such thing. Coffee growers must have funded this one!

IFIC Review: Intense Sweeteners: Effect on Appetite & Weight Management
http://ificinfo.health.org/review/ir-intsw.htm

Read about sweeteners and their effect on appetite, their role in weight loss and weight management from this in-depth review of research literature from the International Food Information Council.

IFIC Review: **Sorting Out the Facts About Fat**

http://ificinfo.health.org/review/ir-fat.htm

Fat is the good guy. Fat is the bad guy. If this were a Western, I'd be totally confused. But once I read the article, I was able to follow the characters a lot better.

IFIC Review:
Uses & Nutritional Impact of Fat Reduction Ingredients

http://ificinfo.health.org/review/fatr.htm

This review will give you a really good foundation of fat knowledge in a nutshell. Quick, how much fat's in a walnut? What kind of fat? Good or bad? Are there good nuts around? This site really isn't about nuts, but you can call a dietician (900-CALL-AN-RD will put you in touch with a registered dietician for $1.95 for the first minute, and $.95 for each additional minute.).

IFIC: **A Fountain of Youth**

http://ificinfo.health.org/insight/janfeb98/fountain.htm

Read this interesting abstract on the effects of strength training on bone density. Forty women participated in this Tufts study, and you may be convinced to pick it up a notch.

IFIC: **Backgrounder - Food Labeling**

http://ificinfo.health.org/backgrnd/bkgr5.htm

All food labels are required to include a statement of identity or product name, net contents, name and address of manufacturer, ingredient labeling and nutrition labeling (the "Nutrition Facts" panel). Read the background to find out why things go on to a label, and who dictates what should go there.

IFIC: **Backgrounder on Sugars & Sweeteners**

http://ificinfo.health.org/backgrnd/bkgr8.htm

Did you know that aspartame is 200 times sweeter than sugar and has a whopping 4 calories per gram? But because it's so sweet, hardly any is needed to sweeten foods, and thus barely any calories are added to foods. You too will be able to sprout some cool trivia about sweeteners after you read this brief and informative primer brought to you from the International Food Information Council.

IFIC: **Backgrounder: Fat & Fat Replacers**

http://ificinfo.health.org/backgrnd/bkgr7.htm

Do you think you know all about fats and their role in your diet? OK, then tell me about fatty acids, trans fats, hydrogenation, fat soluble vitamins, and cholesterol. All I really knew was that I wanted to keep my fat intake to under 30% of caloric intake each day, whatever that meant. This is highly informative, and written for we who are not nutritionists.

  MUST SEE!   VIDEO   AUDIO   SELLS STUFF

  CHAT ROOMS   MAILING LISTS   MESSAGE BOARDS    ADULT CONTENT

  FREE REGISTRATION REQUIRED   MEMBERS ONLY CONTENT   SEARCHABLE

IFIC: Brittle Bones:
Osteoporosis Education for Asian Americans
http://ificinfo.health.org/insight/brittlebones.htm

According to the National Osteoporosis Foundation, the disease is responsible for 1.5 million fractures annually; hip, spine, wrist and ribs are the most common sites. And women are four times more likely to experience this than men . More here.

IFIC: Diet & Environment in Cancer Risk
http://ificinfo.health.org/insight/dietenv.htm

In this 1995 interview with the American Cancer Society's Clark W. Heath, Jr., M.D., you'll find out how diet, environment, and exercise affect your risk. It is still a timely interview. You'll learn that researchers estimate that if we apply everything currently known about cancer prevention, roughly two thirds of all cancers would not occur. See the list here.

IFIC: Everything You Need About the Function of Fats in Foods
http://ificinfo.health.org/brochure/functfat.htm

Do you know how dietary fats affect cholesterol? Do we really need fats? Read this interesting site from the IFIC written in collaboration with the American Dietetic Association. If you don't have time to read the whole thing, read the "bottom line," which is really the common thread running through any credible weight loss program: Balance, Variety, and Moderation.

IFIC: Everything You Need to Know About
Acesulfame Potassium
http://ificinfo.health.org/brochure/aceK.htm

Say what? Well, most likely we've eaten it because it's used in over 4,000 products around the world. In fact, you've probably put it in your coffee. So read these Q&As, and next time you're milling about the coffee station at work you can dazzle your co-workers with tidbits of trivia. You'll be able to tell them if it promotes tooth decay, if it is or is not a carcinogen, and if it's OK for pregnant women.

IFIC: Everything You Need to Know About Aspartame
http://ificinfo.health.org/brochure/aspartam.htm

Can aspartame cause weight gain? Should children with ADD (attention deficit disorder) touch this stuff? What about diabetics? These questions, and more, are answered here in an informative Q&A format.

IFIC: Everything You Need to Know About Sucralose
http://ificinfo.health.org/brochure/sucralose.htm

Some scientists were playing with a sugar molecule one day in 1976, and substituted three chlorine atoms for three hydrogen oxygen groups. From this came a sweetener that's 600 times sweeter than ordinary sugar, and it has no calories! So is it safe? What about putting those chlorine atoms I'm eating now in my nonfat food? Here's an article with questions and answers that's easy to read and to digest.

IFIC: Experts Agree on Key Advice to Reduce Cancer Risk
http://ificinfo.health.org/insight/novdec97/cancerrisk.htm

From the American Institute for Cancer Research and the World Cancer Fund comes this report, issued in late 1997 that between three and four million cases of cancer worldwide could be prevented annually through dietary changes. Read why a predominantly plant-based diet comprised of vegetables, fruits, and grains is recommended. I'm going vegetarian tomorrow.

IFIC: **Fats & Fat Replacers**
http://ificinfo.health.org/press/fatmyths.htm

> From a brochure published in early 1998, separate fact from fiction regarding an aspect of diets and nutrition that can be very difficult to digest. Does low-fat mean low-calorie? Are all calories created equal? Look it up right here.

IFIC: **Food Additives**
http://ificinfo.health.org/backgrnd/bkgr9.htm

> Find out what additives are, how they're defined, regulated and used. Who determines their safety? What about color additives? Is there any relationship between additives and hyperactivity?

IFIC: **Food Biotechnology**
http://ificinfo.health.org/backgrnd/bkgr14.htm

> Here's an overview of what biotechnology is, and how it's used in farming today. This science is responsible for helping farmers get higher crop yields, improving disease and insect resistance, and even getting firmer tomatoes to your market. Read this primer, but you won't find much criticism of the process if you have concerns.

IFIC: **Food Insight: Food Biotechnology: Benefits for Developing Countries**
http://ificinfo.health.org/insight/janfeb99/foodbiotechnology.htm

> From the Jan/Feb 1999 issue of the IFIC's Food Insight comes this piece on what's up in the biotechnology arena for the third world. The focus currently is on biogenetically improving crop yields, implanting vaccines in some foods, and on transferring resistance genes to combat plant diseases.

IFIC: **Glossary of Food-Related Terms**
http://ificinfo.health.org/glossary.htm

> Want to know what bovine spongiform encephalopathy is? What about xenobiotics? Anything related to food is defined here.

IFIC:
International Food Information Council Foundation
http://ificinfo.health.org

> Consumers today are more aware of the relationship between diet and health than ever. They genuinely desire information about food safety and nutrition so they can make informed decisions about the foods they eat. Founded in 1985, the International Food Information Council (IFIC) is a non-profit organization whose mission is to communicate science-based information on food safety and nutrition to health and nutrition professionals, educators, government officials, journalists and others providing information to consumers. It is funded by the food, beverage, and agriculture industry in case you're wondering who's behind this organization.

 MUST SEE!   VIDEO   AUDIO $ SELLS STUFF

 CHAT ROOMS   MAILING LISTS   MESSAGE BOARDS   ADULT CONTENT

 FREE REGISTRATION REQUIRED   MEMBERS ONLY CONTENT   SEARCHABLE

IFIC: Ordering Information $

http://ificinfo.health.org/order.htm

Order brochures, IFIC reviews, and other publications here. There's an extensive list. Most are free, but if you order quantities, you pay.

IFIC: Organizations, Agencies, & Associations

http://ificinfo.health.org/resource/orgs.htm

This is a listing of government agencies, professional organizations, health and medical organizations, and food industry groups. Look here to find how to get in touch with them.

IFIC: Questions & Answers About Cancer, Diet, & Fats

http://ificinfo.health.org/qanda/diet_cancer.htm

The relationship of diet to cancer is a subject that continues to evolve, and there are few definitive answers regarding its cause. What we have learned is that several dietary factors affect the risk of cancer. Read what the most important dietary step you can take to reduce the risk of cancer is.

IFIC: Questions & Answers About Food Irradiation

http://ificinfo.health.org/qanda/qairradi.htm

Food irradiation is the process of exposing food products to ionizing energy for a specified length of time. The amount of exposure is controlled to produce various preservation effects, such as retarding spoilage or killing any harmful bacteria. So if you wonder if your food is radioactive, this is suggested reading.

IFIC: Questions & Answers About Trans Fats

http://ificinfo.health.org/qanda/transqa.htm

When it comes to reducing risk for heart disease, what should people pay more attention to: total fats, saturated fats or trans fats? What does that mean when it comes to choosing among the many different types of foods available today? Here's a timely site to aid you in your quest for knowledge.

IFIC: Sweet Facts About Sugars & Health

http://ificinfo.health.org/review/swtfact.htm

Sugars rank as one of the most misunderstood components of our food supply, and many people wonder about their effect on their health. Read this in-depth report from the IFIC and learn about sugar's impact on behavior, weight, coronary heart disease, and teeth.

IFIC: The Benefits of Balance: Managing Fat in Your Diet

http://ificinfo.health.org/brochure/balance.htm

"Fats are necessary to good health... Dietary fats provide energy, vital hormone-like substances and essential fatty acids for healthy skin. They also carry and help the body absorb the fat-soluble vitamins A, D, E and K."- from the Benefits of Balance brochure. Read this excellent online brochure which separates fact from myth

IFIC: What The Experts Say About Food Biotechnology

http://ificinfo.health.org/foodbiotech/whatexpertssay.htm

This is a list of brief quotations from scientists and organizations on the safety and benefits of agricultural biotechnology, genetic manipulation, and recombinant DNA technology.

IFIC: What You Should Know About Sugars

http://ificinfo.health.org/brochure/sugar.htm

> Although this Q&A is from 1994, not much has changed about this molecule my sweet tooth yearns for. Get up to speed on fructose, glucose, corn sweeteners, and sucrose in this Q&A from the International Food Information Council.

IFIC: U.S. Consumer Attitudes Toward Food Biotechnology

http://ificinfo.health.org/press/quest.htm

> Here's the actual questions, along with the tabulated responses to the survey about genetically altered foods. I was surprised about how little we knew, or for that matter, cared. The most controversial aspect seemed to be questions regarding food labeling of genetically altered products.

Incredible Internet Guide Series

www.brbpub.com/iig

> This is the home page for the Incredible Internet Guide Series. Find out what other titles are available in the series, get free e-mail addresses, and use our message boards.

Index of Food & Nutrition Internet Resources ♀

www.nal.usda.gov/fnic/etext/fnic.html

> Here's a comprehensive list of food and nutrition resources available on the Internet. It is compiled and maintained by the Food and Nutrition Information Center, part of the United States Department of Agriculture.

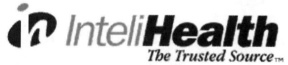

InteliHealth: Home to John Hopkins Health Information: Feeding Your Baby

www.intelihealth.com/IH/ihtIH?t=3481&p=~br,IHW|~st,7165|~r,WSIHW0
00|~b,*|&st=3324

> John Hopkins gives you some help on breastfeeding, maternal nutrition, and bottle feeding basics as well.

InteliHealth: Home to John Hopkins Health Information: Fitness & Sports Medicine 👁

www.intelihealth.com/IH/ihtIH?t=7165&p=~br,IHW|~st,7165|~r,WSIHW0
00|~b,*|

> Interested in starting a fitness program? What do you want to know about sports nutrition? John Hopkins Health Information will provide you with virtually all you need to know. The rest will be up to you!

 MUST SEE!   VIDEO   AUDIO   SELLS STUFF

 CHAT ROOMS   MAILING LISTS   MESSAGE BOARDS   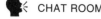 ADULT CONTENT

 FREE REGISTRATION REQUIRED   MEMBERS ONLY CONTENT   SEARCHABLE

InteliHealth: Home to John Hopkins Health Information: Fitness & the Elderly

www.intelihealth.com/IH/ihtIH?t=8923&p=~br,IHW|~st,7165|~r,WSIHW0
00|~b,*|&

Walking, gardening, and housecleaning are just a few of the ways that seniors can enhance their quality of life. Studies are showing the importance of strength conditioning and its positive effect on muscles and bones. Start here to get with the program. Soon our health clubs may not just be for the twentysomethings anymore.

InteliHealth: Home to John Hopkins Health Information: Fitness Quiz

www.intelihealth.com/IH/ihtIH?t=2415&c=81&p=~br,IHW|~st,334|~r,WS
IHW000|~b,*|&d=dmtQuiz

Here's a 12 question test on fitness. Go ahead, it's easy, but if you miss any get on the floor and give me 20 pushups.

InteliHealth: Home to John Hopkins Health Information: Five Tips For Planning & Losing Weight 👁

www.intelihealth.com/IH/ihtIH?t=20704&c=224700&p=~br,IHW|~st,1422
0|~r,WSIHW000|~b,*|&d=dmtContent

Losing weight or maintaining a healthful weight brings the promise of feeling great, looking good and decreasing the negative impact that being overweight has on your health. Here's a rundown of the factors that most weight-loss experts agree will help you succeed.

InteliHealth: Home to John Hopkins Health Information: Fundamentals of Fitness 👁

www.intelihealth.com/IH/ihtIH?t=8901&p=~br,IHW|~st,7165|~r,WSIHW0
00|~b,*|

Fundamentals of Fitness puts it all together, walking you through such topics as how your muscles, ligaments, tendons, heart, and lung work together when you work out, the risks of exercise, and setting up your own fitness, aerobic, strength training, or flexibility programs. It's presented in a neat progression.

InteliHealth: Home to John Hopkins Health Information: Gadgets & Quizzes

www.intelihealth.com/IH/ihtIH?t=20705&c=225043&p=~br,IHW|~st,1422
0|~r,WSIHW000|~b,*|&d=dmtContent

Test your knowledge about food, calories, diet, and fitness with these interactive quizzes.

InteliHealth: Home to John Hopkins Health Information: Index of Medication for Weight Control

www.intelihealth.com/IH/ihtIH?t=20705&c=225105&p=~br,IHW|~st,1422
0|~r,WSIHW000|~b,*|&d=dmtContent

Here's a nifty chart of weight loss drugs, both prescription and nonprescription, that are currently available. Don't look for advice, or safety or efficacy here. Just the facts, ma'am.

InteliHealth: Home to John Hopkins Health Information: Nutrition for Mom

www.intelihealth.com/IH/ihtIH?t=4461&p=~br,IHW|~st,3324|~r,WSIHW0
00|~b,*|&

> If you are breastfeeding, you need to check up on your dietary intake. This site will give you insight into your recommended caloric intake and what to eat to ensure your baby's nutrition.

InteliHealth: Home to John Hopkins Health Information: Nutrition Headlines

www.intelihealth.com/IH/ihtIH?t=8015&p=~br,IHW|~st,9103|~r,WSIHW0
00|~b,*|

> John Hopkins University hosts this highly informative site with breaking news on nutrition related topics.

InteliHealth: Home to John Hopkins Health Information: Sports Nutrition

www.intelihealth.com/IH/ihtIH?t=8933&p=~br,IHW|~st,7165|~r,WSIHW0
00|~b,*|

> Want to know the latest reports on creatine, aminos, anabolics, caffeine, and other purported performance enhancers? What's the role of fluid and hydration in exercise? What to eat for a precompetition meal? Read this info before you buy. It may prove that an educated consumer ends up with more money in his pocket.

InteliHealth: Home to John Hopkins Health Information: Starting a Fitness Program

www.intelihealth.com/IH/ihtIH?t=8916&p=~br,IHW|~st,7165|~r,WSIHW0
00|~b,*|

> If you're just thinking of getting started on a fitness program, this is the place to start. Here's an informative "how to," presented in a logical order of progression. You'll start with the issue of medical evaluation, as in will this help me or hurt me? Then you'll go to confronting obstacles, maintaining motivation, and more. Work out at home or go to a gym? Get a trainer?

InteliHealth: Home to John Hopkins Health Information: The Aging Adult

www.intelihealth.com/IH/ihtIH?c=34061&t=8923&p=~br,IHW|~st,7165|~
r,WSIHW000|~b,*|&d=dmtJHE

> Successful aging vs. usual aging: the choice may be yours. Check in here for the dietary requirements and changes you may need to make. If you've made lifestyle changes for good health, the changes may be minimal.

 MUST SEE!   VIDEO   AUDIO $ SELLS STUFF

 CHAT ROOMS   MAILING LISTS   MESSAGE BOARDS   ADULT CONTENT

 FREE REGISTRATION REQUIRED   MEMBERS ONLY CONTENT   SEARCHABLE

InteliHealth: Home to John Hopkins Health Information: Vitamin & Nutrition Resource Center ♀ ☜

www.intelihealth.com/IH/ihtIH?t=325&p=~br,IHW|~st,325|~r,WSIHW000|~b,*|

This web site is jam-packed with vitamin, nutrition, and weight loss information from a most reliable source. Click to interactive meals where you can break Mom's rules and play with your food, ask a question of their nutrition experts, and sign up for their free Nutrition E-Mail. Can't find something? Search their nutrition database.

InteliHealth: Home to John Hopkins Health Information: Weight Management News Headlines ☜

www.intelihealth.com/IH/ihtIH?t=20833&p=~br,IHW|~st,9103|~r,WSIHW000|~b,*|

"Fat-free Chocolate Worth Screaming For!" was among the headlines in John Hopkins' weight management news. Updated daily, you can read the latest on news stories such as the class action lawsuit being brought up by users of "fen-phen."

InteliHealth: Home to John Hopkins Health Information: Weight Management Timeline ☜

www.intelihealth.com/IH/ihtIH?t=14285&p=~br,IHW|~st,14220|~r,WSIHW000|~b,*|

If you think that weight problems are a 20th century phenomenon, check out this historical timeline dating way back, where Doctor Hippocrates noted that overweight people seemed to pass on before the thin ones. Proceed to the 18th century where you'll learn that the chemist who figured out how to count calories gets beheaded in the French Revolution. We are not alone in this fight against fat, nor are we pioneers.

InteliHealth: Home to John Hopkins Health Information: Weight Management Zone ♀ ☜

www.intelihealth.com/IH/ihtIH?t=14220&p=~br,IHW|~st,14220|~r,WSIHW000|~b,*|

Need to know more about food, obesity, exercise, weight and youth? Give this nicely done page a try. Check out "Weight Loss for Life," or their "Guide to Behavior Change." There's lots of no nonsense information you can use if you're serious about losing weight. You can also search their weight management database if you can't find what you're looking for.

International Food Information Council: Ten Tips To Healthy Eating

http://ificinfo.health.org/brochure/adult10.htm

In cooperation with the American Dietetic Association, the International Food Information Council has listed 10 tips to making sense of your daily food intake. Again, it boils down to three words: Variety, Balance, and Moderation. Perhaps these tips should be posted on everyone's refrigerator along with the school pictures of the kids and the Christmas picture of the dog in front of the tree wearing a red bow.

International Laparoscipic Obesity Surgery Team

www.obesitylapbandsurgery.com/teammain.htm

Here's a surgical group doing Lap-Band surgery in Europe and in Mexico. Read about this minimally invasive surgery and how it works.

International Vegetarian Union

www.ivu.org/evu

The major aim of IVU is to further vegetarianism worldwide by promoting knowledge of vegetarianism as a means of advancing the spiritual, moral, mental, physical and economic well-being of mankind.

International Vegetarian Union: Recipes Around the World ♀

www.ivu.org/recipes

Search for recipes by ingredient, or search by region. So far, there were over 1,600 recipes on file. You can even submit your favorite to be included in their database.

Internet Scambusters

www.scambusters.com

Keep up to date with the latest Internet scams, viruses, and report fraudulent sites you may have visited. Subscribe to their "Internet Scambusters" E-mail newsletter. They promise that they won't invade your electronic privacy by sharing your address.

Iowa State University: Food Safety Project 👁

www.exnet.iastate.edu/Pages/families/fs

Study up on the food safety lessons, and take a test after each section. Do it! There's lots more on this page, too. You can bone up on common food-borne pathogens and learn the ten steps to a safe kitchen.

Iowa State University: Food Safety Project: Irradiation

www.extension.iastate.edu/foodsafety/rad/irradhome.html

Everything you always wanted to know about food irradiation, and more. You can even virtually visit Iowa State University's Linear Accelerator, and see what it does to a chicken, for example.

Irradiation: A Safe Measure For Safer Food

www.fda.gov/fdac/features/1998/398_rad.html

In December, 1997, the FDA approved treating red meat with a measured dose of radiation to combat E. coli 0157:H7, which has been known to cause over 20,000 illnesses and 500 deaths a year. Here's some good information on the process, the whys, whens, and whats. It touches a bit on the controversy surrounding radiation and on the question of consumer acceptance.

 MUST SEE!   VIDEO   AUDIO $ SELLS STUFF

 CHAT ROOMS   MAILING LISTS    MESSAGE BOARDS   ADULT CONTENT

 FREE REGISTRATION REQUIRED   MEMBERS ONLY CONTENT   SEARCHABLE

Jean Frermont's Food & Nutrition on the Web 👁

www.sfu.ca/~jfremont

Jean Fremont, RD, who hails from Simon Fraser University's School of Kinesiology in British Columbia, has compiled a remarkable list of links with commentaries on food, nutrition, exercise, and education. Many sites are for us laypeople who still can't determine if a tomato is a fruit or a vegetable, or if corn is a starch or a junk food item.

Jennie's Vegetarian Info Page

www.frognet.net/~jsg22/VEGINFO.html

Find information here in nontechnical terms on vegetarianism. If you're considering this as a new lifestyle, or newly into it, you'll find answers and support. The different kinds of vegetarians are defined.

Jenny Craig 👁

www.jennycraig.com

This is your opportunity to utilize Jenny's tools that are available in her weight loss programs, go shopping, or find tips for success. Her web site is still in the development phase, apparently, but shows promise of growing. The program is one of only a few that encourages more than supplemental feeding, or counting; it is based more on lifestyle changes, one at a time. It's about building balance and is worth looking into.

Jenny Craig Store $

www.jennycraig.com/store/index.html

Buy your Jenny Craig supplements and cookbooks here. You can also get exercise machines, videos, and audio tapes.

Jenny Craig: Guide to Feeling Fit

www.jennycraig.com/guide/index.html

Just click on any of the topics on the left side of your screen, and you'll pull up brief discussions for support and motivation. Jenny promises that her online site will be growing and blossoming into something better soon.

Jewish Holiday Fare

http://vegetarian.about.com/msubholjewish.htm?pid=2757&cob=home

Vegetarian cooking ideas are here for the Jewish Holidays.

Jewish Vegetarians of North America

www.orbyss.com/jvna.htm

The purpose of Jewish Vegetarians of North America is to promote the practice of vegetarianism within the Judaic tradition, and explore the relationship between Judaism, dietary laws, and vegetarianism.

JHS Natural Products: Coriolus $

www.jhsnp.com/about_coriolus.html

JHS Natrual Products is "committed to bringing you the world's finest all-natural products for immune health." Commonly known as the "turkey tail" in North America, Coriolus versicolor (also known as Trametes versicolor), is unique among the medicinal mushrooms, with extensive use in both traditional medicine and modern clinical practice. JHS has in depth information about coriolus, what it is and how it works. You can also order online.

JHS Natural Products: PSK Mushrooms $

www.jhsnp.com/index2.html

The immuno-stimulating compounds extracted from the mushroom Coriolus versicolor generate sales of several hundred million dollars a year in Japan, making them the top selling all-natural nutritional product used by cancer patients in that country. Read all about it, and order online. The goal of JHS Natural Products is to bring you the finest all-natural products for immune health, the information you need to choose the highest quality product and an easy to use shopping environment.

Joanne Stepaniak - Recipes

www.vegsource.org/joanne/recipes.htm

Recipes from Joanne Stepaniak are changed weekly, so keep checking in.

Joslin Diabetes Center ☜

www.joslin.org

Joslin Diabetes Center is an International leader in diabetes treatment, research, and education. Established in 1898, and affiliated with Harvard Medical School, Joslin leads the field in both basic and clinical research, and is devoted to educating both patients and professionals. This is their home page, and it will open many doors to a wealth of information.

Joslin Diabetes Center: Carbohydrate Counting

www.joslin.org/education/library/wcarbsug.html

Diabetics need to maintain their blood sugar to as close to normal as possible. Carbohydrate counting is one of the methods used because carbs tend to have the greatest affect on your blood sugar. Learn how to count 'em here.

Joslin Diabetes Center: Eating For Life: Discussion ⬇

www.joslin.org/managing/eating.html

This is an active discussion group for people with diabetes, and their families, to learn more about nutrition and diabetes. Topics have covered carbohydrate counting, snacking, and dining out. Log on and join in.

 MUST SEE!   VIDEO   AUDIO $ SELLS STUFF

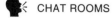 CHAT ROOMS   MAILING LISTS   MESSAGE BOARDS   ADULT CONTENT

 FREE REGISTRATION REQUIRED   MEMBERS ONLY CONTENT   SEARCHABLE

Joslin Diabetes Center: Fitting Alcohol Into Your Meal Plan
www.joslin.org/education/library/walohol.html

Beginning with a strong suggestion to consult with your medical team, this page gives suggestions about fitting alcohol into your meal plan - in moderation, of course. There's a chart of alcoholic beverages which shows their caloric and carbohydrate content. 105 calories in a shot of gin? Is there Gin Lite? There are lots of tips and guidelines to responsibly include alcohol in your plan.

Joslin Diabetes Center: Fitting Sugar Into Your Meal Plan
www.joslin.org/education/library/wcarbsug.html

I always thought diabetics had to avoid sugar. Find out how to fit sugar into your plan responsibly. And once you've learned how to fit sugar, count carbs, and control portions, try putting a meal plan together, just for practice on this site. And please see you dietician!

Joslin Diabetes Center: Portion Control
www.joslin.org/education/library/wcarbsug.html

Calories, carbs, and portions. I don't like to count, and I like to binge eat while standing at the refrigerator. I would make a lousy diabetic. But the fact is the amount you eat is closely related to blood sugar control, and here's some good ideas to help you watch your portions.

Joslin Diabetes Center:
There's No Such Thing As A Diabetic Diet
www.joslin.org/education/library/nodiet2.html

"It's not about avoiding sugar!" and "How does carbohydrate counting work?" are two of the areas of diabetes and nutrition covered in this informative article from the library of the Joslin Diabetes Center. But you'd be foolish to go this alone, it emphasizes, and strongly urges you to work closely with a dietician and your health care provider.

Joslin Diabetes Center:
Recommended Cookbooks & Resource Books
www.joslin.org/education/library/wcbook.html

They're not selling books here, but offering a comprehensive list of books to help you manage your diet. Most are available in your bookstore, or ordering instructions are given.

JPFS Workouts
www.jeanpaul.com/workouts.html

Jean-Paul Fitness Specialists is a contract association of personal trainers founded by Jean-Paul Francoeur. "Committed to your individual wellness," is the company motto. This site enables you to choose a strength program, with routines to follow, and pictures of the right way to lift your weights. However, he counsels that you must stretch and warm-up before and after lifting, and suggests that you have an experienced spotter or trainer when doing these exercises.

Jupiter Rising: Online Vegetarian Resource
http://members.aol.com/khlisson/vegetarian.html

Although the "Jupiter Rising" newsletter is apparently closed, there are some good articles on choosing vegetarianism from the still open archives. There's some great stuff for beginners.

Just Move! ⚲ 👁

www.justmove.org/home.cfm

The American Heart Association hosts this Fitness Center, and throughout their home page, you can see how you measure up to their national data base, keep track of your progress online, and have your own personal trainer. There are also E-cards to send, Cyberteams to join, and a listing of events. Try it out!

Just Move: AHA Events Calendar

www.justmove.org/events/August.html

See if there's anything going on in your area.

Just Move: Body Composition

www.justmove.org/myfitness/actarticles/acframes.cfm?Target=bodycomp.html

Figure out your body mass index to see where you're classified; then do your waist/hip ratio. Eat one last huge dish of ice cream, and straighten up.

Just Move: Cyberteams 👇 👁

www.justmove.org/cyberteams

Are you interested in walking, running, cycling, rock climbing, or other activities? Connect with other like-minded people in these health fitness forums. Ask questions, share stories, respond to other postings or hear what others have to say.

Just Move: Exercise & Your Heart - A Guide to Physical Activity

www.justmove.org/myfitness/actarticles/acframes.cfm?Target=ex_yrhart.html

Everything you need to know to get started is here. Should you see a doctor? What are the risks of exercising? What if you get a heart attack? Your questions answered plus you'll find some sample exercise programs for the beginner. If you can walk 5 minutes, you're in. Get started, kid.

Just Move: Exercise Diary 👁

www.justmove.org/diary/login.cfm?CFID=22458&CFTOKEN=30300

Track your progress towards chosen fitness goals using their online exercise diary. Just record your daily, weekly or monthly exercise regimen, and they'll give you feedback reports and statistical summaries. For extra motivation, your own personal trainer will e-mail you encouragement and suggestions to ensure that you're working towards your goals. It's easy to register, and once you're in your personal trainer will E-mail you with encouragement and suggestions to help you reach your goals.

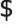 MUST SEE!   VIDEO   AUDIO   SELLS STUFF

 CHAT ROOMS   MAILING LISTS   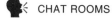 MESSAGE BOARDS   ADULT CONTENT

 FREE REGISTRATION REQUIRED   MEMBERS ONLY CONTENT   SEARCHABLE

Just Move: Healthy Heart Workout Quiz
www.justmove.org/myfitness/lowarticles/lowframes.cfm?Target=www.j
ustmove.org/myfitness/workoutquiz.cfm

Time for a pop quiz, but don't stress, it won't count toward your final grade.

Just Move: Measure Up
www.justmove.org/measureup

How does your fitness level compare with that of other Americans?

Just Move: My Fitness
www.justmove.org/myfitness

Just click on the level of activity that describes you, and you'll get lots of helpful ways to take it up a notch.

Just Move: Physical Activity
www.justmove.org/myfitness/actarticles/acframes.cfm?Target=exerci
se.html

"Physical inactivity has been established as a major risk factor for the development of coronary artery disease. It also contributes to other risk factors including obesity, high blood pressure and a low level of HDL cholesterol. Even modest levels of physical activity are beneficial." This is from the American Heart Association's Scientific Position on Physical Activity. Read more on their recommendations and the benefits. Don't just sit there, move!

Just Move: Physical Activity Calorie Use Chart
www.justmove.org/myfitness/actarticles/acframes.cfm?Target=calori
echart.html

Find out how many calories you're burning per hour with your chosen exercise.

Just Move: Target Heart Rates
www.justmove.org/myfitness/actarticles/acframes.cfm?Target=hartra
tes.html

How do you figure out your own target heart rate? Why? What's it for? It's easy to do, and it's good for measuring your progress. Try it out here.

Just Move: The Benefits of Daily Physical Activity
www.justmove.org/myfitness/actarticles/acframes.cfm?Target=dailyb
ene.html

Do you want to manage stress better, boost your energy level, release tension, sleep better, get stronger, and live longer? Guess what - it's free, and you don't have to use a secure line to order this.

Keeping Your Food Safe 👁
www.cdc.gov/ncidod/dbmd/foodspot.htm

Millions of people become sick every year from food-borne infections. The CDC posted this easy-to-read, non-scientific site to help us prevent these bad bugs from ruining your party.

Keto Perfect

http://lonestar.texas.net/~jsaravia/epilepsy.html

Keto Perfect is a Windows program that helps to establish a ketogenic diet for those who need it for seizure control. Download it and give it a try. There's also a good history of the ketogenic diet and its use in controlling seizures.

Ketogenic Diet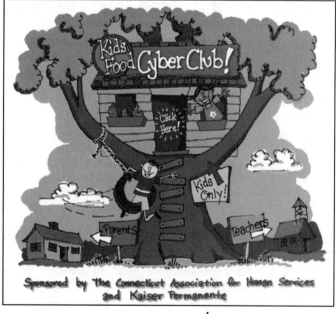

www.ketogenic.org

A good site for resources, menus, and links.

Ketogenic Diet Programs

www.stanford.edu/group/ketodiet/ketocenters.html

Here's a growing list of places in the U.S. and abroad that offer the Ketogenic Diet.

Ketogenic Diet Software

www.infinet.com/~ophir/keto

The program was written by Robert Stump, Jr., whose sister was struggling with all the calculations for her son. Her gives you instructions for downloading. Good Luck.

Ketogenic Option, The

http://member.aol.com/ketooption

The purpose of this site is to create an international forum for the promotion, access, and exchange of information for this diet.

Kids Food CyberClub

www.kidsfood.org

This CyberClub was created by the Connecticut Association for Human Services and Kaiser Permanente. There's sections for kids only, for teachers, and for parents. It's an interactive site to teach kids about good food choices.

 MUST SEE!   VIDEO   AUDIO $ SELLS STUFF

 CHAT ROOMS   MAILING LISTS   MESSAGE BOARDS   ADULT CONTENT

 FREE REGISTRATION REQUIRED   MEMBERS ONLY CONTENT   SEARCHABLE

Kids Food CyberClub: Cyber Food Shopper

www.kidsfood.org/choices/shopper.html

The Cyber Food Shopper has $5.00 and is going to buy snacks for you, but four of them have to be low in fat and come from four of the five food groups. If you're thrifty you can buy junk food with any leftover money after the above criteria have been met.

Kids Food CyberClub: Food Guide Pyramid

www.kidsfood.org/f_pyramid/pyramid.html

Test your knowledge about the food groups and build your food pyramid.

Kids Food CyberClub: Nutrition Sleuths

www.kidsfood.org/sleuths/sleuths.html

Here's a cool game for kids. It's a kind of scavenger hunt they play on the Internet. It's a cool tool to teach nutrition and at the same time how to use search engines.

Kids Food CyberClub: Rate Your Plate

www.kidsfood.org/rate_plate/rate.html

Test your knowledge of the food pyramid, and find out not only what goes where, but just what makes up a "serving."

Kids Food CyberClub: Winning Choices

www.kidsfood.org/choices/winning/winning.html

Help your friends make smart choices and get points.

Kidshealth.org: Food Guide Pyramid

http://kidshealth.org/kid/food/pyramid.html

Here's the ubiquitous pyramid, except this time it's animated and written in kids' terms.

Kushi Institute

www.macrobiotics.org/ki.html

The Kushi Institute was founded in 1978 by Michio and Aveline Kushi to provide education for leadership toward the creation of a healthy and peaceful global community based on sound dietary, physiological and common sense practices of macrobiotic principles. For 20 years people from around the globe have come to the Kushi Institute for the ultimate experience in learning the macrobiotic lifestyle and diet. The Kushi Institute is located in Becket, Massachusetts, in the heart of the beautiful Berkshire Mountains.

La Leche League International ⚓ 🗣 ↑ 👁

www.lalecheleague.org

La Leche League International is an international, nonprofit, nonsectarian organization dedicated to providing education, information, support, and encouragement to women who want to breastfeed. You'll find lots of good information, resources, and links.

La Leche League International: Breastfeeding Chats 🗣

www.lalecheleague.org/Chat/chat.html

This is the Chat schedule, how to use it, and what times they're talking. Feel free to join an online conference.

La Leche League International: FAQs About Breastfeeding
www.lalecheleague.org/FAQ/FAQMain.html

There's a long list of questions pertaining to breastfeeding, along with concise answers.

La Leche League International: Useful Links
www.lalecheleague.org/links.html

Interested in further information on breastfeeding and infant nutrition? Browse these links.

LEARN Education Center $
www.learneducation.com

LEARN stands for Lifestyle, Exercise, Attitude, Relationships, Nutrition. Order the LEARN Program, as well as other weight loss books and cassettes.

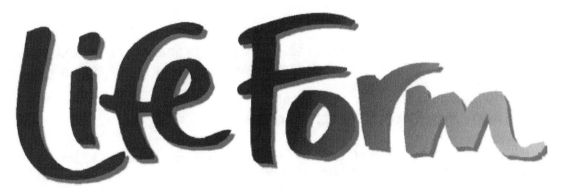

Life Form
www.fitnesoft.com

This software allows you to track everything about your health. You can keep track of the foods you eat, your measurements, log your exercise, and track your chemistry from lab reports. An information page keeps track of your medical history as well as all the health care professionals you are involved with. Download a version for free, or buy the software for about $49.

Light Living
www.lightliving.com

Light Living formerly was known as Light Cooking. It is not just about changing your diet, it's about changing your life. A healthy lifestyle includes: healthy cooking, good nutrition, exercise and a healthy home life. Light living is about moderation, not sacrifice. From here you can go into Kids Cooking Corner, FAQs, Tip of the Day, Recipe of the Week, and more.

Lipoinfo.com
www.lipoinfo.com

Here is the most comprehensive liposuction information site on the Internet. Up-to-date and comprehensive, it is sponsored by Dr. Paul Weber, out of Fort Lauderdale, Florida.

 MUST SEE!   VIDEO   AUDIO $ SELLS STUFF

 CHAT ROOMS   MAILING LISTS   MESSAGE BOARDS   ADULT CONTENT

 FREE REGISTRATION REQUIRED   MEMBERS ONLY CONTENT   SEARCHABLE

Lipoplasty Society
www.lipoplasty.com

Many of your questions answered, and you can see some before and after pictures. The Society is an association of over 1,000 Board Certified plastic surgeons.

LipoSite-Liposuction Online Chat 🗣
www.liposite.com/chat

If you have a browser that supports JAVA, you can chat.

LipoSite: Frequently Asked Questions
www.liposite.com/faq

Your questions are answered here, from what is it to how do I choose a surgeon to recovery to techniques.

Liposuction
www.geocities.com/HotSprings/5142/liposuction/liposuctions.html

Your questions answered here. It is important to emphasize that liposuction is a method of spot reduction, but not weight loss.

Liposuction Before & After Photos
www.liposite.com/photos

View before and after photos of face, neck, arms, trunk, and legs of people who have undergone liposuction. There were 67 sets of photos at this viewing.

Liposuction Interactive Information Resource-LipoSite
www.liposite.com

LipoSite is an interactive liposuction information resource web site. From here you can find information and advice, and read about others' experiences with this procedure. The site is sponsored by Board Certified Plastic Surgeons.

Liposuction True Life Journals
www.liposite.com/journals

Here's an opportunity to read in diary format the journey through liposuction both from the patient and the surgeon's eyes. They share their observations all the way through recovery.

LipoSymposium
www.liposymposium.com

This informative web site provides lots of information about the procedures as well as links to qualified Board Certified Plastic Surgeons.

Listeriosis
www.cdc.gov/ncidod/diseases/foodborn/lister.htm

Now we have to be concerned about soft cheeses, hot dogs, and deli meats. What is it? How does it get into food? How do you know if you have it? How is it treated? If you're pregnant, have a newborn, or are immunocompromised, put this on your required reading list.

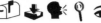

LIVING AND RAW FOODS
THE LARGEST COMMUNITY ON THE INTERNET
DEDICATED TO EDUCATING THE WORLD ABOUT
THE POWER OF LIVING AND RAW FOODS

Living & Raw Foods
www.rawfoods.com/index.shtml

This is a helpful site dedicated to educating the world about the power of living and raw foods. Here you can find resources, links, recipes, and support. This web site is neatly laid out, easy to navigate, and will lead you to a wealth of information.

Living & Raw Foods: Articles & Information
www.living-foods.com/articles

There's a wealth of information on this site for anyone who is, or is interested, in a living and raw food diet. Read about the health benefits of this lifestyle. You'll also find book and literature reviews, info on juicing, sprouting, and dehydrating.

Living & Raw Foods: Chat
www.living-foods.com/chat

Want to talk about it? Enter here for live chat about raw food, and the lifestyle.

Living & Raw Foods: City Guide
www.living-foods.com/cityguide/index.cgi?db=default&uid=

OK, so you want to go down the raw living road. Where do you buy the stuff you'll need? Click here and search this city guide to find a natural foods store in your area. You'll find a listing of farmers' markets, natural and organic food stores, farms, and support groups. This is a great resource if you are new to an area, or if you plan to travel.

Living & Raw Foods: FAQ
www.living-foods.com/faq.html

Just what is living and raw food? Where's the protein? What are enzymes? Isn't this just a fad? Get your answers to these and more here.

Living & Raw Foods: How to Become a Fruitarian
www.living-foods.com/articles/fruitarian.html

Here's an in-depth article about fruitarianism, the logic behind it, the whys, and a synopsis of a typical food day in a fruitarian's life.

Living & Raw Foods: In the News
www.living-foods.com/news

This page features articles and media clips about living and raw foods. Read what others are saying about this lifestyle.

 MUST SEE!   VIDEO   AUDIO $ SELLS STUFF

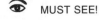 CHAT ROOMS   MAILING LISTS   MESSAGE BOARDS   ADULT CONTENT

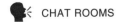 FREE REGISTRATION REQUIRED   MEMBERS ONLY CONTENT   SEARCHABLE

Living & Raw Foods: Marketplace $
http://www.living-foods.com/marketplace
> Do you want to buy a juicer, a dehydrator, or a sprouter? This looks like the right place with its secure, online ordering feature.

Living & Raw Foods: Recipes
www.living-foods.com/recipes
> Are you looking for a good recipe for Energy Soup? Sea Veggie Pizza? Mango salsa? You will not find even a bad recipe for beef stew here.

Living & Raw Foods: Register for Membership
www.living-foods.com/register.html
> Once you become a member, you will automatically be added to the living and raw foods mailing list and will receive e-mail when there are new happenings at the web site as well as stay in touch with the living and raw food community online by receiving e-mails from people who are subscribed to the list. You will also have special access to the members area of the web site.

Living & Raw Foods: The Personals
www.living-foods.com/personals
> Want to find a vegetarian for a date? Or are you looking for someone who is raw? Here's where you should start.

Low Carb Connoisseur $
www.low-carb.com/low-carb/index.html
> The Low Carb Connoisseur is dedicated to helping the low carb, sugar-free dieter obtain the highest quality and best selection of products available. Get stuff for the Atkins Diet, the Sugar Busters Diet, and other low carb, or sugar free programs.

Macrobiotic Questions & Answers
www.macrobiotic.org/letters1.html
> Fred Pulver answers your questions about macrobiotics from the Carbondale Center. The questions come from E-mails received and replies sent

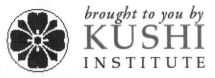

Macrobiotics Online ☞
www.macrobiotics.org
> Macrobiotics Online contains a wealth of information including articles, recipes, case histories, and an online catalog of organic foods, cookware, and books. You can view and sample recipes from books that are for sale. Read about the Kushi Institute's "Way to Health" program, along with some fabulous recovery stories.

Macrobiotics Today

www.natural-connection.com/resource/macro.html

> Macrobiotics Today is the leading voice of modern macrobiotics with informative articles, interviews, and reports representing diverse views in the macrobiotic community. Macrobiotics Today presents issues, information, and activities on diet, health, and environmental consciousness from a macrobiotic perspective that combine traditional macrobiotic views on physical, emotional, and spiritual health with contemporary thinking and scientific knowledge. Macrobiotics Today has been published continuously since 1960. You can subscribe or read articles online from back issues.

MacroNews: Cooklets $

www.macronews.com/cooklet.htm

> Christina Pirello appears on PBS in this whole foods cooking show. She is a whole foods cooking teacher, gives seminars and workshops, and is based in the Philadelphia area. Buy her videos here.

Magic of Believing-A Weight Loss Support Group

www.swlink.net/~colonel

> "We understand the pain and the torment of being heavy. On our e-mail support list we discuss diets, dieting, losing weight, obesity, medical advances in relation to weight loss, fitness, and nutrition. Sometimes we just share the everyday difficulties of life. We 'talk" about how hard it is, we listen and sometimes even cry together." Get information on how to join the group here. They warn you that you will get deluged with support mail, however. I guess they figure the more time you spend reading your E-mail, the less time you'll have to eat.

Make Fitness Fun For Kids

http://primusweb.com/fitnesspartner/library/activity/funkids.htm

> It's time to get the kids away from the TV, the computer games, and the couch. See here how the epidemic of inactivity can do great harm to our kids.

Making Time For Strength Training

http://primusweb.com/fitnesspartner/library/activity/traintime.htm

> Most fitness experts agree that even devoting 30 minutes to strength training two or three times a week is sufficient for strength and muscle development. Here's some help for you to be more efficient with your limited time.

Man's Life: Fitness

www.manslife.com/fitness/bigsweat

> "Here's your body. What's your problem?" That's what it says, then you just point to a place on the body shown, click, and they'll fix you up with some exercises.

 MUST SEE!　　 VIDEO　　 AUDIO　　$ SELLS STUFF

 CHAT ROOMS　　 MAILING LISTS　　 MESSAGE BOARDS　　 ADULT CONTENT

 FREE REGISTRATION REQUIRED　　 MEMBERS ONLY CONTENT　　 SEARCHABLE

Man's Life: Fitness Forum
www.manslife.com/stickit/display/ml_fitness?TOPID=u9Myaxw3

Yak it up here on the message board. When I visited there were postings on love handles, creatine, diets, abs, and more abs, creatine, andro, and, oh yeah, abs. I guess we think about our stomachs a lot, both what's inside and outside.

Man's Life: Psycho Trainer
www.manslife.com/fitness/trainer

"Imagine the kind of fitness program you'd have if you handed over your towels and locker keys to the boys from the Hamas. You'd have pain so good it hurts real bad." Now you have an idea of where this site will take you, if you want to get fit fast.

Marcus' Vegetarian Page
http://marcussharpe.com/veg1.htm

It doesn't look very active, but the links are good, and the guestbook is frequently visited.

Mass Attack ☞
www.geocities.com/HotSprings/Spa/9598/home.html

Pick up the "remote control," and click any part of the body to see some great animation to help you learn how to properly do some exercises. I clicked on "upper body," then went to abdominals, and watched the animation on how to execute the proper crunch. The description of the movement is alongside.

Mayo Clinic - Subscribe to Nutrition Update
www.mayohealth.org/cgi-bin/apps/list_mailer2?list=nutrition

This free E-mail bulletin keeps you up-to-date with what's new in the Mayo Clinic's Nutrition Center.

Mayo Clinic Diet Center: Weight Loss ☞
www.mayohealth.org/mayo/common/htm/dietpage.htm

This is the renowned Mayo Clinic's informative diet and nutrition magazine of the Internet. There's lots of useful info. Search recipe files, ask questions to a dietician, and sign up for nutrition updates to be sent to your Email. Bookmark this user friendly site; it's kept updated, it's science-based, and they won't sell you any quick fixes.

Mayo Clinic Health Oasis: Antioxidants
www.mayohealth.org/mayo/9308/htm/antioxid.htm

Although written in 1993, this article will help you understand just what antioxidants are, and how they keep you healthy. This is an excellent primer for us laypeople who should learn a bit about free radicals and toxic molecules. Now only if I can remember what I've read.

Mayo Clinic Health Oasis: Buyer Beware
www.mayohealth.org/mayo/9707/htm/me_5sb.htm

In 1994, Congress passed and President Clinton signed the Dietary Supplement Health and Education Act. Sounds good, right? But now the FDA doesn't need to regulate the safety of your supplements before they go to market; now it intervenes only if people get sick, injured, or die. Then they have to prove that the product is harmful before issuing warnings. It sounds like we're the laboratory animals, and the FDA observes us as we pop our supplements each day. Read on.

Mayo Clinic Health Oasis:
Cancer - What You Eat Can Affect Your Risk
www.mayohealth.org/mayo/9509/htm/cancer.htm

> Here's a good, easy to read article on what to eat more of, and what to eat less of, to help reduce your risk of cancer.

Mayo Clinic Health Oasis:
Carbohydrates: Their Role in Your Diet
www.mayohealth.org/mayo/9903/htm/carbohyd.htm

> Your brain uses carbs as a source of energy. Learn to eat the right kind of carbohydrates.

Mayo Clinic Health Oasis: Childhood Obesity
www.mayohealth.org/mayo/9705/htm/overweig.htm

> One in five kids between the ages of 6 and 17 are classified as obese. There are several reasons for this, but the sad news is that most will grow up to be obese adults. Along with this will go the numerous health risks. Find out what to do about it.

Mayo Clinic Health Oasis: DHEA - Hype or Health
www.mayohealth.org/mayo/9612/htm/dhea.htm

> Do you want to slow down the aging process, build muscle mass, burn fat, strengthen your immune system, avoid cancer, heart disease, and diabetes? So do I. Is DHEA the answer? What is it? Should you take it? How much? Does it even work? Once again, the Mayo Clinic sorts out fact from fiction and updates us on where research is going. There's also good links to further info on hormone supplements.

Mayo Clinic Health Oasis:
Diet & Exercise Guidelines For Overweight Children
www.mayohealth.org/mayo/9705/htm/over_2sb.htm

> Overweight kids need a diet for weight loss somewhat different from adults. Read up on what to do.

Mayo Clinic Health Oasis:
E coli Bacteria - Protecting Yourself From Food-Borne Illness
www.mayohealth.org/mayo/9511/htm/ecoli.htm

> There's more to healthy eating than just choosing the right foods. Wash your hands, clean and cook your food properly, and watch for the symptoms you'll read about on this page from the Mayo Clinic.

Mayo Clinic Health Oasis: Energy Gels
www.mayohealth.org/mayo/9510/htm/energyge.htm

> "Carbo goo," does it work? Find out if it's for you.

 MUST SEE!   VIDEO   AUDIO $ SELLS STUFF

 CHAT ROOMS   MAILING LISTS   MESSAGE BOARDS   ADULT CONTENT

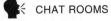 FREE REGISTRATION REQUIRED   MEMBERS ONLY CONTENT   SEARCHABLE

Mayo Clinic Health Oasis:
Food Allergies - Widely Misunderstood
www.mayohealth.org/mayo/9908/htm/foodal.htm?ref=nutrition

Only 1 percent of Americans actually have food allergies, yet 20 percent believe they do. Separate fact from fiction, allergies from intolerances, here at the Mayo Clinic Health Oasis.

Mayo Clinic Health Oasis:
Food Irradiation: The Answer to E. coli?
www.mayohealth.org/mayo/9709/htm/food_irr.htm

Gamma rays in your hamburger? I prefer ketchup, pickles, lettuce, tomatoes, etc. But the bottom line is that your food is not radioactive, just somewhat cleaner. Read all about it in this article from Mayo.

Mayo Clinic Health Oasis:
Food Storage - Knowing When to Toss or Keep Shelf Goods
www.mayohealth.org/mayo/9610/htm/storage.htm

What is that green thing in the back of your cupboard? What? You never put it there? Here's some helpful hints to ensure that your foods remain fresh and don't lose important nutrients.

Mayo Clinic Health Oasis: Guide to Food Storage
www.mayohealth.org/mayo/9610/htm/stor_sb.htm

I hate throwing things away, but in some cases it just makes sense.

Mayo Clinic Health Oasis: Health Quiz
www.mayohealth.org/cgi-bin/apps/quiz.cgi/mayo/expert/htm/9603quiz.txt?/mayo/common/htm/top.txt,/mayo/common/htm/bottom.txt

Here's a pop quiz for you. Take it if you think you know it all. Then check your answers. It's only ten questions, and it won't affect your grade point average.

Mayo Clinic Health Oasis: Listeria - A Deadly Bacteria
www.mayohealth.org/mayo/9902/htm/listeria.htm

I thought Listeria was a kind of flower in our garden until I read this. It's a food-borne bacteria that resists heat, acidity, and refrigeration; you can't taste it or smell it either. And wait til you read where it can be found. You'll be scrubbing your produce and ordering your steaks and burgers well-done after you read this.

Mayo Clinic Health Oasis: Managing Childhood Obesity
www.mayohealth.org/mayo/9705/htm/over_1sb.htm

Some helpful hints are on this web site from Mayo Clinic's Health Oasis.

Mayo Clinic Health Oasis: Mediterranean Diet
www.mayohealth.org/mayo/9906/htm/mediet.htm

Studies have shown that people with heart disease who follow this diet style may have a reduced risk of a second heart attack by as much as 70%. And Greek men have a 90% lower premature death rate from heart attack than American men. But read on to find out what kinds of foods they eat over there. While you're reading, I'm packing my bags and moving to the Mediterranean.

Mayo Clinic Health Oasis:
Muscle-Building: Do Andro & Creatine Work?
www.mayohealth.org/mayo/9811/htm/muscle.htm

People have spent billions of dollars on stuff to lose fat, build muscle, and improve performance. But can you really find the answer in a bottle of pills? Read this superb article that explains it all in a manner even I can understand. What I really like is that Health Oasis links you to more information if you want to go deeper into creatine and androstenedione.

Mayo Clinic Health Oasis: Pregnancy & Nutrition Update
www.mayohealth.org/mayo/9601/htm/pregvit.htm

Read up on the importance of folic acid and vitamin A in pregnancy.

Mayo Clinic Health Oasis: Quizzes From the Nutrition Center
www.mayohealth.org/mayo/common/htm/dietquiz.htm

Here are nine quizzes ranging from diet, fast food, alcohol, to fat. They're quick and they're informative.

Mayo Clinic Health Oasis:
The "Bug" That Made Milwaukee Famous
www.mayohealth.org/mayo/9606/htm/cryptosp.htm

It was a tiny parasite that sickened over 400,000 people and killed over 100. It was found in their drinking water. Check this page out while sipping some tap water. You'll find that it resists treatment with chlorine, and is so small that municipal water plants can't even filter it out. But the good news is that if you're not immunosuppressed, it's self-limiting; that is, your diarrhea will pass, so to speak.

Mayo Clinic Health Oasis: The DASH Diet
www.mayohealth.org/mayo/9805/htm/dash_sb.htm

This site contains a chart that shows number of servings from each food group that are recommended when following the DASH diet.

Mayo Clinic Health Oasis:
The DASH Diet - It May Benefit Your Blood Pressure
www.mayohealth.org/mayo/9805/htm/dash.htm

A new eating guide called the DASH diet may help you prevent or lower high blood pressure. And, the diet may have other health benefits.

Mayo Clinic Health Oasis: There Is No "Mayo Clinic Diet"
www.mayohealth.org/mayo/9806/htm/mayodiet.htm

The Mayo Foundation Web Site receives about 2,000 hits daily looking for this nonexistent miracle diet. It just isn't there. But you can read about its origins in the 1940's and how the myth has prevailed. Then you'll read about what you should be doing to lose weight.

 MUST SEE!   VIDEO    AUDIO   SELLS STUFF

 CHAT ROOMS   MAILING LISTS   MESSAGE BOARDS   ADULT CONTENT

 FREE REGISTRATION REQUIRED   MEMBERS ONLY CONTENT   SEARCHABLE

Mayo Clinic Health Oasis:
Vitamin & Nutritional Supplements 👁

www.mayohealth.org/mayo/9707/htm/me_jun97.htm

> A wealth of information is contained in the Mayo Clinic's Health Oasis, and if you get as confused as I do when you look at the vitamin section, your best bet is to take a couple of minutes and read this page. It's easy to read, and the vocabulary is within my level of understanding. Thank you, Mayo.

Mayo Clinic Health Oasis:
Weight Control: What Works & Why

www.mayohealth.org/mayo/9406/htm/main.htm

> Over 97 million American adults are considered to be overweight or obese and we spend over $33 billion on weight loss products and services. Find where you fit and what you need to do.

Mayo Clinic Health Oasis:
Weight Self-Assessment: Should You Shed Pounds?

www.mayohealth.org/mayo/9707/htm/weight.htm

> Calculate your BMI, answer a few questions, and find out what health risks you may have. Then you'll get the answer.

Mayo Clinic Health Oasis: Weight Control

www.mayohealth.org/mayo/9903/htm/weig_sb4.htm

> Here's some sound advice on how to lose weight safely and how to keep it off. If you want to join a weight management program, look for the five criteria listed on this site.

Mayo Clinic Health Oasis: Weight Training

www.mayohealth.org/mayo/9905/htm/weight.htm

> The American College of Sports Medicine has fitness guidelines that recommend weight training for people over 50 in addition to aerobics and stretching. Read how muscle shrinks and bones deteriorate as we age, and how weight training can help ward off that feeling of not being able to get out of our recliners. Hmmm, maybe they should make our TV remotes in five and ten pound models.

Mayo Clinic:
Diet & Nutrition Resource Center - Library References

www.mayohealth.org/mayo/common/htm/dietpg2.htm

> Search their archives of previous articles and chances are you'll find information on anything you might be looking for. From weight management to nutrition for children, it's all here.

Mayo Clinic: Virtual Cookbook 👁

www.mayohealth.org/mayo/recipe/htm/maintoc.htm

> The Mayo Clinic's Nutrition Center has an entire cookbook here. Recipes are shown in their original form and in their modified form. A nutritional analysis is shown for both. Modified forms obviously reflect lower fat, lower calorie, lower sodium, etc. There's a wealth of good and smart recipes here.

McDougall Newsletter:
The Great Debate: High vs. Low Protein Diets
www.drmcdougall.com/debate.html

> This is another newsletter bebunking the myth of "The Zone," as well as the other high-protein, low carb diets. It's very convincing.

McDougall Online Wellness Center
www.drmcdougall.com

> Dr. McDougall is the founder of the McDougall Plan for Healthy Living, and he's been writing about the effects of nutrition on disease for over 20 years.

Meat.org
www.meat.org

> Stay away if you are easily grossed out because this site doesn't come from the Beef Council or the Cattlemen's Association. But if you are curious you can go visit a slaughterhouse and see it from a rather militant vegetarian's eyes.

Meet Benny Goodsport & the Goodsport Gang
www.bennygoodsport.com

> Here's a very interactive site for kids, but be careful, they just might drag you out of your couch for a game of kickball.

Men's Fitness
www.mensfitness.com/mensfitness/index.asp?catid=184

> This is the online version of *Men's Fitness*. Sections include fitness and training, nutrition, sports and adventure, of course, sex and behavior.

Men's Fitness: Chat
http://216.33.170.200:4080/chat/world/html/login.html?uri=/*index

> Just enter your username and password, and start chatting.

Men's Fitness: Discussion
http://216.33.170.201/magcommunity/threads.asp?topicID={84F6F35B-281F-11D3-9691-0090277C0BFE}

> Looks like you can post just about anything on this message board.

 MUST SEE!   VIDEO   AUDIO $ SELLS STUFF

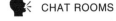 CHAT ROOMS   MAILING LISTS   MESSAGE BOARDS   ADULT CONTENT

 FREE REGISTRATION REQUIRED   MEMBERS ONLY CONTENT   SEARCHABLE

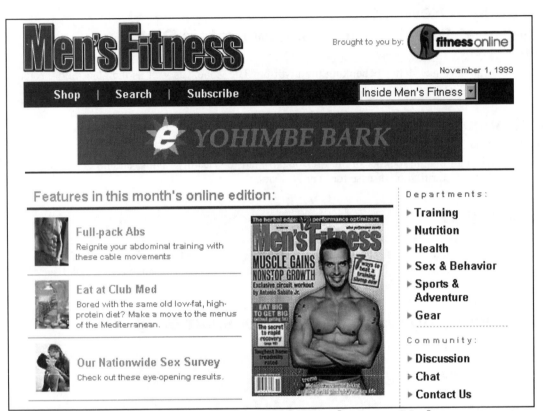

Men's Fitness: Ten Gym Mistakes Beginners Make

www.mensfitness.com/magazines/magViewer/FitnMagArt.asp?Catid=234&
Objid={49EC4C5A-2382-11D3-ACE5-
00A0244A08DA}&curpage=1&curCatID=184

   Going to a gym for the first time can be awkward, and it feels like you're being watched. A list of ten
   common mistakes to avoid can be found here.

Men's Health

www.menshealth.com

   Men's Health Magazine has a bit of everything for men. There's even a searchable section on nutrition
   which allows you to search their archives.

Men's Health: Caloric Calculator

www.menshealth.com/features/eat_this/sports/index.html

   Type in your bodyweight and activity level and *Men's Health* will calculate your required calorie
   intake. Not only that, it will tell you how many calories you should get from carbs, from fat, and from
   protein.

Men's Health: Eat This

www.menshealth.com/features/eat_this/quick/index.html

   From *Men's Health Magazine* comes this handy browsable site for recipes. Just scroll down one of
   three choices: Recipes by ingredient, or on the side, or by situation. Then your choices pop up.

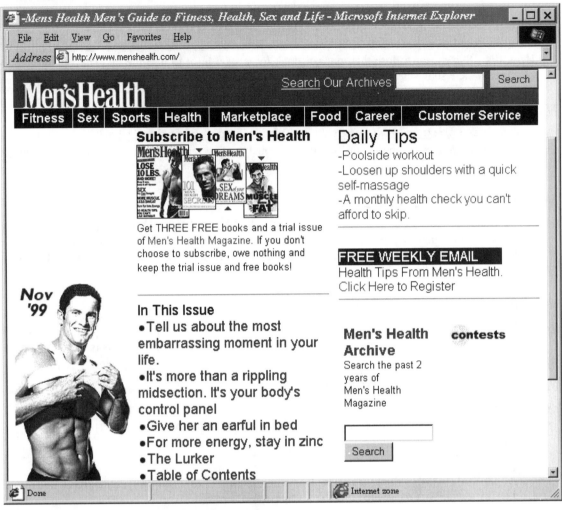

Men's Health: Personal Trainer

www.menshealth.com/personaltrainer/index.html

> Do you want a bulletproof chest, legs like oak, iron arms, or to go from scrawny to brawny? Then start here, point and click. But pointing and clicking is not the exercise; wait 'til you see what you have to do.

Men's Health: Personal Trainer - Scrawny to Brawny

www.menshealth.com/personaltrainer/t2_routines/original_index.html

> This is the recommended workout to get brawny. And I thought this was a web site to get a brownie.

 MUST SEE!   VIDEO   AUDIO   SELLS STUFF

 CHAT ROOMS   MAILING LISTS   MESSAGE BOARDS   ADULT CONTENT

 FREE REGISTRATION REQUIRED   MEMBERS ONLY CONTENT   SEARCHABLE

Men's Health: Personal Trainer - Unbelievable Abs

www.menshealth.com/personaltrainer/t4_routines/original_index.html

Here it is: 8 exercises to lose that gut, but don't forget you have to lose the fat. The rippled look is underneath there somewhere.

Men's Health: Sports Nutrition

www.menshealth.com/features/eat_this/sports/index.html

This is a good primer on sports nutrition if you're just starting out. You can focus on strength and/or endurance.

Men's Nutrition: Quiz

http://primusweb.com/fitnesspartner/library/nutrition/mensquiz.htm

Do men usually gain weight around their stomachs? Do light beers have less fat? Do protein supplements really work? Test your knowledge about men's nutrition, but relax, it won't take your grade point average down.

Meridia

www.4meridia.com

Meridia is a prescription medication used for medical management of obesity. This is their home page.

Metabolife International $

www.metabolife.com

There are over 50,000 distributors and 1,000 retail outlets waiting to sell you this stuff or to sign you up as a distributor.

Metabolism Diet

www.dietnutrition.com/metabolism.html

Psst! Do you want to lose 14 pounds in 7 days?

Migraines and MSG

www.magicnet.net/~btnature

You may be sensitive to Monosodium Glutamate (MSG) in your food and drink -- and this may be the source of your pain and misery. Read more about it here.

Milk - It's On Everybody's Lips

www.whymilk.com

It's a great site even if you don't like milk! Click on "famous faces" for a list of all who have appeared with the mustache, then click on the picture for an enlargement. My favorites? Donna Shalala and Dennis Rodman. Too bad they didn't appear in the same photo. Or go to the Milk Mustache Mobile and play The Milk Mustache Game.

Minnesota Obesity Center

http://www1.umn.edu/mnoc

The Minnesota Obesity Center is a Obesity Nutrition Research Center. Their goal is to find ways to prevent weight gain, obesity, and its complications.

Miracle Exclusives Online
www.miracleexclusives.com

Extractors, juicers, blenders, dehydrators, flakers, graters, grinders, mills, everything but the kitchen sink is right here. After you find what you're looking for, go to retailers and find a dealer near you. You can't order online unless you're a retailer and are registered.

Momentum AIDS Project: Nutrition News
www.aidsinfonyc.org/momentum/nutrition/bignut.html

Because malnutrition is a leading cause of death among AIDS victims, the subject of diet and nutrition is extremely important. This site helps you understand why good nutrition is important and takes on such areas as food safety, poor appetite, nausea, and problems with swallowing or chewing.

Motivation to Move
http://primusweb.com/fitnesspartner/library/activity/motomove.htm

It could be that as much as 40% of Americans are completely sedentary, and probably 80% don't get enough exercise. Not only that, but of those who start an exercise program, roughly 50% drop out after only 6 months. If you can get off the couch, read why and what to do. Let's get started!

MSNBC Calorie Calculator
www.msnbc.com/modules/quizzes/caloriecalc.asp

All you have to do is enter the number of minutes you spend doing any of the activities in this pretty long list, and you'll find out how many calories you've burned in a day.

MSO Surgery Information
www.drrossfox.com/surgery.html

The types of surgery for weight loss are discussed here. Candidate criteria, what to expect, and follow up care are also included. You can also get a tummy tuck there, not online.

MSO-Weight Loss Surgery for the Treatment of Obesity
www.drrossfox.com/home.html

The Medical Services Organization specializes in the surgical treatment of obesity. It's a practice located in the Pacific Northwest Area.

My Experience with Phen-fen
www.syspac.com/~hahn/phenfen.html

You can read Anita Hahn's journey through weight loss while using Phen-fen. Although this drug combination's use was halted in 1997, her diary can be used as a tool for support and motivation for many.

 MUST SEE!   VIDEO   AUDIO   SELLS STUFF

 CHAT ROOMS   MAILING LISTS   MESSAGE BOARDS   ADULT CONTENT

 FREE REGISTRATION REQUIRED   MEMBERS ONLY CONTENT   SEARCHABLE

My Personal Weight Loss Story $

http://www1.mhv.net/~donn/prime.html

This is a lengthy story about Donn Jasura's diet odyssey. It finally leads us to PrimeQuest Products, where you can order all the shakes you want. It explains "adaptogens," and how Russian Olympic teams won all kinds of gold medals while using this. This must be the true miracle we've been searching for. His web site is really pretty good for finding links and support, motivation and diets. If you visit all his links, you'll be too smart to fall for this stuff.

National Association to Advance Fat Acceptance

http://naafa.org

NAAFA is a non-profit human rights organization dedicated to improving the quality of life for fat people. NAAFA has been working since 1969 to eliminate discrimination based on body size and provide fat people with the tools for self-empowerment through public education, advocacy, and member support. This is the home page of this organization.

National Cancer Institute:
Information For People With Cancer

http://rex.nci.nih.gov/PATIENTS/INFO_PEOPL_DOC.html

From the National Cancer Institute comes these articles about current or recent studies using various supplement such as beta-carotene, selenium, and vitamin E. You can read how the studies were done, and if the outcomes were successful in reducing the incidence of certain types of cancer.

National Council Against Health Fraud ♀

www.ncahf.org

The National Council for Reliable Health Information maintains this web site. The NCAHF is a non-profit, tax-exempt voluntary health agency that focuses its attention upon health fraud, misinformation and quackery as public health problems. It is private, nonpolitical and nonsectarian. The organization is comprised of health professionals, educators, researchers, attorneys and concerned citizens. Its officers and board members serve without compensation. It derives 75% of its financial support from dues paid by members.

National Food Safety Database ♀

www.foodsafety.org/index.htm

The goal of the National Food Safety Database project is to develop an efficient management system of US food safety databases that are used by the Cooperative Extension Service (CES), consumers, industry, and other public health organizations. The end result of such a management program is a highly informative, efficient and accurate web site which will provide one-stop shopping for food safety information. It is supported by the USDA and the Food Research Institute.

National Food Safety Database: Bacteria on Cutting Boards

www.foodsafety.org/il/il114.htm

Do you only have one cutting board in your kitchen? Fix your chicken on it? Cut up your vegetables on it? Cut up an apple and give it to your kids? Go directly to jail, do not pass go.

National Food Safety Database:
Beware the Unknown Brew: Herbal Teas & Toxicity
www.foodsafety.org/sf/sf184.htm

Herbal teas have been enjoyed for centuries throughout the world. But they have been the subject of controversy in the United States since their introduction into the mainstream marketplace two decades ago. I just learned that chamomile is in the same family as ragweed, and that anaphylactic cases have been reported about people who consumed the tea, but were allergic to ragweed. Rare, but it's happened.

National Food Safety Database:
Consumer's Guide to Natural Toxicants in Food
www.foodsafety.org/fs/fs044.htm

Naturally occurring chemical components of fruits and vegetables may be toxic to your health. Be sure to check out the "Holiday Menu."

National Food Safety Database:
Critical Issues in Food Safety
www.foodsafety.org/hothome.htm

Bookmark this page if you want to be kept up to snuff on latest food safety news. When I peeked here one day, I found news on allergy alerts (presence of undeclared peanuts in a product), latest E. coli outbreaks, and much more. It's kept up-to-date and there's more here than you'll ever find in your local newspaper or on TV.

National Food Safety Database:
Germs, Chemicals, & Other Hazards
www.foodsafety.org/conthome.htm

From here, you can jump to biological or chemical or physical contaminants pages. This is a highly informative and thorough database.

National Food Safety Database: Test Your Food Safety IQ
www.foodsafety.org/register.htm

Register here, then take the Quiz. It's a ten question test that really does count, because if you don't get it, you could get really sick. This is a required course.

National Food Safety Database: The Bugs Within Us
www.foodsafety.org/sf/sf033.htm

"A microscopic zoo inhabits our armpits and groins, our eyes and ears, the entrances to our respiratory tracts, and the exits from our urinary tracts. Our digestive systems are continuous tubes along which bacteria congregate. Our urine, sterile as it collects from our kidneys, picks up bacteria as it leaves our bodies. The contents of our colons harbor 10 billion microbes per gram." Ricky Lewis, Ph.D., wrote this piece and will both fascinate you and gross you out. It's great bedtime reading.

MUST SEE!	VIDEO	AUDIO	SELLS STUFF
CHAT ROOMS	MAILING LISTS	MESSAGE BOARDS	ADULT CONTENT
FREE REGISTRATION REQUIRED	MEMBERS ONLY CONTENT	SEARCHABLE	

National Institutes of Health:
Headache: Hope Through Research

www.ninds.nih.gov/patients/disorder/headache/head2.htm

Get up to speed on migraine headaches here. There is a discussion about food triggers and how they work.

National Institutes of Health: The DASH Diet

www.nih.gov/news/pr/apr97/Dash.htm

"Dietary Approaches to Stop Hypertension" (DASH) is a way to decrease or prevent high blood pressure. The eating plan is published here by the NIH; it is a combination diet that is rich in fruits and vegetables and low fat dairy foods, and low in saturated and total fat. It was also high in dietary fiber, calcium, magnesium, and potassium. Check out the sample menu based on a 2,000 calorie diet.

The Natural Child Project™
All children behave as well as they are treated.

Natural Child Project

www.naturalchild.com/home

On the table of contents page, click on "breastfeeding," and you'll be led to some articles on the subject.

Natural Home & Travel Guide ♀

www.naturalusa.com/index.html

This self-proclaimed "America's Favorite" online natural consumer guide receives over 160,000 hits a month. Here you can find thousands of resources in over 34 sections. Find food co-ops, health food stores, vegan, vegetarian, macrobiotic, and live food resources. Search by city, state, company, or even category. Or you can browse categories if you choose. Lots of links

---

Natural Land - Award Winning Natural Living Supersite ⬇ 👁

www.naturalland.com

Read the latest news in the organic, cooking, healing, fitness, and nutrition realms. And that's not all; there's a recipe search, health quizzes, and a weekly poll you can participate in.

Natural Land: Chat Room 🗣

www.naturalland.com/chat.htm

Chat rooms are open from 10:00 AM - 12:00 PM. Scheduled topics are posted here. Jump right in!

Natural Land: Cooking Village

www.naturalland.com/cv.htm

Enter the "Cooking Village" of Natural Land, the publisher of Veggie Life. You'll find "Meals in Minutes," to "Preventing and Healing Foods."

Natural Land: eNaturalMall $

www.naturalland.com/shop.htm

Go to Natural Land's Natural Mall where you can shop in stores for aromatherapy, home & garden, fitness aids, and books. It's quite extensive, and your shopping cart is allowed in the mall!

Natural Land:
Free E-mail Newsletter & Free Magazine Trial Subscription
www.naturalland.com/sub.htm

Subscribe here for a free E-mail newsletter from Natural Land. You can also sign up for a free trial subscription to one of their magazines.

Natural Land: Nutrition Village
www.naturalland.com/nv.htm

Which has higher nutritional value: cooked or raw veggies? How much Vitamin C is really required in your diet? And learn about antioxidants and phytonutrients, among many other articles.

Natural Land: Support Platform Discussion
www.naturalland.com/disc/support.htm

Join any of Natural Land's 18 support groups and seek help, ask questions, or even give advice on subjects ranging from asthma and AIDS to family issues, cancer, and PMS.

Natural Land: Weight Loss Village
www.naturalland.com/nv.htm

Finally, some weight loss help for the vegetarian. Peruse a list of healthful, helpful topics to help with your battle.

Natural Land: Community Platform Discussion
www.naturalland.com/disc/community.htm

Join ongoing discussion groups on dieting, gardening, nutrition, cooking, healing, organic living, and fitness, and others on Natural Land's Community Platform.

NCI/CDC 5 A Day Online Tracking Chart
http://5aday.nci.nih.gov

The National Cancer Institute and the Centers For Disease Control and Prevention have produced a little test to help you see how you stack up on your fruit and vegetable intake.

NetSweat.com: The Internet's Fitness Resource
www.netsweat.com

This is one of the largest directories of fitness, sport and nutrition sites on the Internet! Get lost here in tons of links and lists, but chances are you'll find what you want if you've got the time.

Never Say Diet: Putting It On
www.betterhealth.com/neversaydiet/0,4787,1205,00.html

This area of the Never Say Diet Center is devoted entirely to the physical and emotional needs of those who want to gain weight healthfully. There's not a whole lot of depth, but you might find something to get you started.

 MUST SEE!   VIDEO   AUDIO $ SELLS STUFF

 CHAT ROOMS   MAILING LISTS   MESSAGE BOARDS   ADULT CONTENT

 FREE REGISTRATION REQUIRED   MEMBERS ONLY CONTENT   SEARCHABLE

New Century Nutrition 👁

www.newcenturynutrition.com

This is the site for "Living on the Planet Continuum, " they proclaim. This is a nicely done web zine with a virtual kitchen, newsletter archives, and message boards. There's a section on nutrition research findings from the China Project.

New Runner

www.newrunner.com

The editors of Runner's World bring you this remarkably helpful site for the beginner who wants to give running a go for fitness, and maybe on to more serious stuff. Register to use the training log where you can track your progress, and they'll send you notes of encouragement. It's easy to use.

New Runner: Step by Step 👁

www.newrunner.com/step

Physical exams, choosing shoes, breathing, first steps, aches and pains; it doesn't get any more basic (but helpful) than this.

New York Times on the Web:
Women's Health: Diet & Exercise 🔍 👁

www.nytimes.com/specials/women/whome/diet_exercise.html

There's lots of news for women interested in diet and exercise to peruse from the *New York Times*. What's great is that you can link right to the source of the news item. You can also search their archives.

Newest Weight Loss Gimmicks

www.weight.com/gimmick.html

Read the latest on "fat binders," ear patches, and even slimming soaps right here as Dr. Myers explains how their proponents say they work. He debunks the myths one by one. I guess we just have to keep waiting for that magic bullet!

NIH Office of Dietary Supplements 🔍

http://odp.od.nih.gov/ods/databases/ibids.html

The International Bibliographic Information on Dietary Supplements (IBIDS) is a database of published, international, scientific literature on dietary supplements, including vitamins, minerals, and botanicals. IBIDS is produced by the Office of Dietary Supplements (ODS) at the National Institutes of Health to assist the public, health care providers, and researchers in locating credible, scientific literature on dietary supplements. There's over 300,000 citations and abstracts here. Gotta do a science project? A term paper?

NIH Technology Assessment-Voluntary Weight Loss
http://text.nlm.nih.gov/nih/ta/www/10.html

One quarter to one third of Americans are overweight; many have tried a variety of methods to lose weight, with limited success in retaining weight loss. In controlled settings, diets, behavior modification, exercise, and drugs produce short-term weight losses with reasonable safety. Unfortunately, most people who achieve weight loss with any of these programs regain weight. For many overweight persons, achieving and maintaining a healthy weight is a lifelong challenge. Various methods are reviewed here by the National Institutes of Health, concluding with benefits and risks associated with each strategy. Future directions for weight loss management and research are discussed.

North American Vegetarian Society
www.cyberveg.org/navs

NAVS is a nonprofit educational organization dedicated to the promotion of vegetarianism. They work in a variety of ways to promote the nutritional, health, environmental, and compassionate benefits of a meatless diet.

Nutri/System Center Locations
www.nutrisystem.com/centers.html

Find a diet center near you. They are located in 47 states with over 500 centers.

Nutrient Data Laboratory
www.nal.usda.gov/fnic/foodcomp

From the United States Department of Agriculture, the Agricultural Research Service brings you nutrient data of the stuff you eat. You'll find no flashy graphics, dancing elephants, or talking vegetables here. But the information, along with links, are all here on a searchable database.

NutriGenie Diabetes Meal Planner
http://users.aol.com/nutrigenie/ngdmp44.html

This is a dietary management system that claims to be good for those who count carbohydrates, or fat grams, or use the ADA food exchange system. Download evaluation software for free, and try out this meal planner.

NutriGenie: Managing Diabetes Version 3.6 For Windows
http://users.aol.com/nutrigenie/nsmd36.html

This software utilizes ADA guidelines and is a companion to ADA publications. It can also keep track of blood glucose, blood pressure, has a weight log, and can maintain a diet history. Try the trial version for free.

Nutripeak.com: Sports Nutrition For the Serious Athlete $
www.nutripeak.com

Lose fat, gain muscle, endurance and energy, and get a free T-shirt.

MUST SEE!	VIDEO	AUDIO	$ SELLS STUFF
CHAT ROOMS	MAILING LISTS	MESSAGE BOARDS	ADULT CONTENT
FREE REGISTRATION REQUIRED	MEMBERS ONLY CONTENT	SEARCHABLE	

Nutrition Action Healthletter: Healing Broken Hearts
www.cspinet.org/nah/6_99/heart.htm

Dean Ornish, M.D., is director of the nonprofit Preventive Medicine Research Institute, and author of five best-selling books. His philosophy is that heart disease can be reversed or prevented by intensive diet and lifestyle changes. This is an interview with him, and although his methods were highly controversial, studies are showing that his system works.

Nutrition Action Healthletter: Index
www.cspinet.org/nah/index.htm

Read highlights of past issues. Entertaining and informative is the section called "Right Stuff vs. Food Porn," where you'll see just what's in a Coolatta, and find out which foods get a thumbs up or thumbs down.

Nutrition Action Healthletter: Subscribe
https://vs.cais.com/cspi/join4.html

Become a member of the Center for Science in the Public Interest, and for your $24, you'll receive 10 issues of their Nutrition Action Healthletter. This organization was founded in the 1970's by a group of scientists associated with Ralph Nader's Center for the Study of Responsive Law. Since then it has grown to over 1,000,000 members. This is the group who saved us from the death strangle of movie theater popcorn and caused them to lighten it up with air popping or canola oil instead of hydrogenated shortening.

Nutrition Action Healthletter: Trans Fat
www.cspinet.org/nah/6_99/transfat3.html

The Nutrition Action Healthletter comes from the Center for Science in the Public Interest. This June, 1999, article is an excellent source of information, especially if you eat out at fast food places, cafeterias, stores, and snack bars. Trans fats, simply stated, raises your blood cholesterol and thus, your risk of heart disease. Here's a look at how to avoid them when eating out. Read about those blooming onions that are the rage, and those Burger King fries that are supposed to be better than McDonalds. The bottom line? Cut the fat, whatever it is.

Nutrition Action:
Carbo-Phobia-Zoning Out on the New Diet Books
www.cspinet.org/nah/zone.html

From the Center for Science in the Public Interest comes this newsletter joining the debate over the Zone, Protein Power, and Healthy for Life.

Nutrition for Kids: Recommended Links
www.nutritionforkids.com/Links.htm

This is a list of links for kids, parents, teachers, and health professionals.

Nutrition Sleuth
http://exhibits.pacsci.org/nutrition/sleuth/sleuth.html

You will be Inspector Snarfengood, and your victims are missing important nutrients. You will find them. It's a lot like Hangman, but you only get three tries.

Nutritional Analysis Tool
www.ag.uiuc.edu/~food-lab/nat/mainnat.html

From the University of Illinois comes this handy calculator. Enter a food item, the number of servings, how it will be cooked, and it will give you an analysis. It takes a little time, but if you're interested, or counting something, it can be handy.

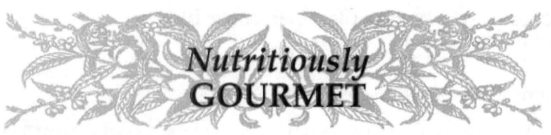

Nutritiously Gourmet
www.nutritiouslygourmet.com

Do you want to eat a well-balanced diet that gives you the food pyramid without the monotony of eating the same old thing? Look at these monthly menu ideas that bring you good food that's good for you.

Obesity & Weight Control from Michael D. Myers. M.D. Inc.
www.weight.com

The purpose of this site is to provide objective medical information on obesity, eating disorders, and associated medical conditions in a non-commercial environment where any editorial comment is appropriately noted. It is maintained by Dr. Michael D. Myers, a practicing physician and lecturer, who has treated obesity and eating disorders for over 17 years. You'll find current topics on obesity to obesity related medical conditions to information on eating disorders.

Obesity Complications from Michael D. Myers M.D. Inc.
www.weight.com/complications.html

Obesity can lead to many medical complications, from hypertension to sleep disorders The bottom line is that obesity can lead to premature death..

Obesity.com 👁
www.obesity.com

Obesity.com provides the latest information about weight loss and obesity. It is published by Mathew Naythons, MD, and the staff of NetHealth.

 MUST SEE!   VIDEO   AUDIO   SELLS STUFF

 CHAT ROOMS   MAILING LISTS   MESSAGE BOARDS   ADULT CONTENT

 FREE REGISTRATION REQUIRED   MEMBERS ONLY CONTENT   SEARCHABLE

Obesity.com--Community Board & Support ⚓

http://WeightLoss2000.com/support/support_00_intro.htm

If you want to get tips or support from other people who are going through the trials and tribulations associated with weight loss, this page allows you to use a personal mailbox for added privacy. You can post messages, queries, or respond to others' questions.

Obesity: The World's Oldest Metabolic Disease

www.quantumhcp.com/obesity.htm

Dr. Michael Blumenkrantz discusses obesity and its implications on mortality and morbidity.

Official Mad Cow Disease Home Page

http://mad-cow.org

Want to learn a bit about Mad Cow Disease? How does over 5,100 articles sound for starters? This is an excellent place to start, and it's up-to-date.

Olwen's Links on Obesity Surgery

http://homepages.ihug.co.nz/~olwen/ocwlnkws.htm

Here's a list of web sites devoted to the education and business of weight reduction surgery. Some are surgical groups and some are university or hospital based. Always remember to do your homework before you jump into this! There's also a good link list of E-mail support groups, and finally, there's the Obesity Law Center if you need help there.

On Safari Through the Vitamin Jungle

http://primusweb.com/fitnesspartner/library/nutrition/vitamins.htm

Millions of people take vitamins, say the Dieticians of Canada, for the wrong reasons. Check this site out to see reasons why people say they need them, then read on to see who should be taking vitamins. You'll aslo learn how to choose them.

OncoLink: Nutrition During Cancer Treatment: FAQs

www.oncolink.upenn.edu/support/nutrition/faq

Here are many good questions people have asked about nutrition during cancer treatment. There's questions about vitamin supplements, herbal therapies, the Gerson Diet, and many others. It's a good place to look if you're new to this.

OncoLink: Onco Tip: Macrobiotic Diet

www.oncolink.upenn.edu/support/tips/tip24.html

The macrobiotic diet has often been promoted for both the prevention and treatment of cancer, and there are numerous testimonials testifying to its effectiveness. However, the medical community feels there haven't been any controlled studies to verify the accolades. OncoLink issues several cautions for you to consider.

OncoLink: Onco Tip: Megadose Vitamin C

www.oncolink.upenn.edu/support/tips/tip25.html

Megadosing of vitamin C is not recommended for prevention or treatment of cancer at this time due to the current scientific literature. Read the details in this "Onco Tip."

OncoLink: NCI/PDQ Physician Statement: Nutrition
www.oncolink.upenn.edu/pdq_html/3/engl/304467.html

OncoLink is one of the premier oncology sites on the web. Sponsored by the University of Pennsylvania Cancer Center, it holds a wealth of information. Although this particular statement is intended for use by doctors and health care professionals, it can be very helpful for anyone who needs to understand the nutritional needs of an oncology patient. If you need help, you can call their toll free number and speak to an information specialist.

One Peaceful World
www.macrobiotics.org/OPW.html

As a non-profit educational foundation with international headquarters in Becket, Massachusetts, One Peaceful World is engaged in a variety of activities. They have published over 30 books on diet, health, and the evnironment. They have organized airlifts of macrobiotic food to Russia, and frequently donate food, seeds, clothing, and supplies to other organizations around the world who are subjected to disease, poverty, or war.

Optifast
www.optifast.com

Another weight management program offering treatment protocols using a dietary supplement, all under the watch of health professionals. You can find out if there is someone near you offering this program.

Oregon Dairy Council
www.oregondairycouncil.org

A nice web site from the Oregon Dairy Council, with recipes, links, and more information. Guess what's in the recipes. Hint: it isn't soy milk.

Original Fruitarian Guidebook:
How to Become a Fruitarian
www.islandnet.com/~arton/fruitext.html

This is the best primer on Fruitarianism I ran across, explaining in good detail why one would choose a fruit diet, and how one lives the life.

Original Hollywood Celebrity Diet $
www.celebritydiet.com

Do you want to be cleansed, detoxified, and rejuvenated in just two days? Me too. Do you want to drop a dress size in two days? Me too. Order the juice, order the pills, and order the sculpting crème, but you might want to ask for the scientific studies first.

 MUST SEE!   VIDEO    AUDIO $ SELLS STUFF

 CHAT ROOMS   MAILING LISTS   MESSAGE BOARDS   ADULT CONTENT

 FREE REGISTRATION REQUIRED   MEMBERS ONLY CONTENT   SEARCHABLE

Orlistat for Obesity Treatment from Michael Myers M.D. Inc
www.weight.com/orlistat.html

Approved by the FDA in April, 1999, Xenical is used to aid in weight reduction by interfering with fat absorption. Read Dr. Myers article about how it works, as well as potential side effects you might experience. He stresses that it should be used only as a part of a comprehensive treatment plan in the management of obesity.

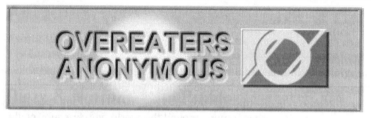

Overeaters Anonymous 👁
www.overeatersanonymous.org

Overeaters Anonymous is a Fellowship of individuals who, through shared experience, strength and hope, are recovering from compulsive overeating via a twelve step program. They welcome everyone who wants to stop eating compulsively. You'll find instructions on how to locate meetings in your area.

Overeaters Anonymous: Online Catalog $
https://www.overeatersanonymous.org/catalog.htm

Order pamphlets, books, cassettes, workbooks on a secure site.

Oxford University Libraries Automation Service
www.lib.ox.ac.uk/internet/news/faq/archive/dieting-faq.part1.html

This is an extensive and exhausting list of frequently asked questions on weightloss and dieting. It's very informative but grueling to get through. Chances are if you have a question, you'll find the answer here with perhaps a link or suggestion where to go for more information. Want a good description of the Atkins diet, the Zone diet, or how Jenny Craig diets work, look here. You'll find a factual description with no hype, just the facts. There's lots of links to be found here and send you on your way.

Pacific Bariatric Surgical Medical Group
www.pbsmg.com

This is a San Diego based surgical group, specializing in surgery for obesity. They also offer informative seminars and monthly support groups.

Parent's Place: Blood Sugar Control During Pregnancy
http://www4.parentsplace.com/pregnancy/nutrition/qa/0,3105,11195,00.html

Blood sugar control and gestational diabetes are discussed here.

Parent's Place: Preparing For Pregnancy: A Nutritional Guide
http://www4.parentsplace.com/pregnancy/nutrition/qa/0,3105,11763,00.html

What are the correct amounts of vitamins and minerals to take during pregnancy? Any diet changes necessary? Read this brief primer on nutrition and pregnancy.

Parent's Place: Veganism & Pregnancy

http://www4.parentsplace.com/pregnancy/nutrition/qa/0,3105,5161,00.html

Can a vegan diet be safe during pregnancy? What adjustments are needed, if any? Which nutrients do I need to be especially aware of ?

Parents Place: Pregnancy: Nutrition 👁

http://www4.parentsplace.com/pregnancy/nutrition

This web site has a list of topics relating to pregnancy. If you have questions on supplements, exercise during pregnancy, iron, protein, calcium, or nursing nutrition, look here for concise answers.

Partnership For Healthy Weight Management

www.consumer.gov/weightloss

The Partnership for Healthy Weight Management is a coalition of representatives from science, academia, the health care profession, government, commercial enterprises and organizations whose mission is to promote sound guidance on strategies for achieving and maintaining a healthy weight. Together they have agreed on "Voluntary Weight Loss Guidelines." These voluntary guidelines were developed by the Partnership to give consumers who are seriously and conscientiously trying to lose and maintain weight loss the information they need when comparing products and services. Imagine, Slim-Fast and the American Dietetic Association on the same page.

Past Carrots - Nutrition for Kids

www.nutritionforkids.com/Carrots/All_Carrots.htm

On this site are the archives of past "Weekly Carrots" which are short tidbits of information you can use for kids' nutrition. For example, one weekly carrot said that only one in five kids eats the minimum of three vegetable servings, and of those veggies nearly 60% come from potatoes and tomatoes. French fries and ketchup, it suspects.

People Against Cancer Home Page

http://main.dodgenet.com/nocancer/index.html

People Against Cancer is a grassroots, non-profit, public benefit organization dedicated to "new directions in the war on cancer." They distribute a wide range of educational materials about non-toxic innovative forms of cancer prevention, diagnosis and therapy, publish "Options: Revolutionary Ideas in the War on Cancer," and administer the Alternative Therapy Program for people seeking treatment options.

PHYS - The Place for Health, Fitness, Nutrition, Wellness, Weight Loss Exercise, Diet, & More 👁

www.phys.com

This is a kind of online magazine from CondeNet, the people who publish Glamour, Vogue, Self, Allure, and others. There's lots of information and self assessment quizzes. It's loaded with graphics. Although many articles are brief, you can often choose links to other sites for in depth information.

 MUST SEE!   VIDEO   AUDIO $ SELLS STUFF

 CHAT ROOMS   MAILING LISTS   MESSAGE BOARDS   ADULT CONTENT

 FREE REGISTRATION REQUIRED   MEMBERS ONLY CONTENT   SEARCHABLE

PHYS: Aerobics
www.phys.com/f_fitness/03encyclopedia/02database/aerobics.html

Basically, the purpose of aerobics it to get your heart rate up by doing a mixture of dance and calisthenics. But now don't be surprised if there's a few boxing and martial arts techniques thrown in. This site will walk you through the benefits, advantages, the warm-ups, the stretching, the gear, and finally, will link you to other resources. But don't start linking now, get up!

PHYS: Are You Fit or Fat?
www.phys.com/b_nutrition/01self_analysis/04fitorfat/fitorfat.cgi

Just fill out this calculator, and you'll instantly get back results about your BMI, body fat percentage, health risk assessment, and your ideal weight.

PHYS: Bicycling
www.phys.com/f_fitness/03encyclopedia/02database/bicycling.html

This is one of the fastest ways to achieve cardiovascular fitness, and to burn calories. It also boosts muscle strength, and is relatively easy on your joints. What do you mean, you don't know how to ride a bike? Try a stationary one. Don't forget to try out the calorie calculator where it says "go figure."

PHYS: Calculators 👁
www.phys.com/c_tools/calculators2/01home/calculators.htm

"When it comes to your health, everything does add up." This is a page of interactive calculators which may or may not be fun, depending on the outcomes. Regardless of results, it is true that everything does add up. Punch in a few numbers, and you'll not only get your BMI, but also your caloric, fat, carb, and protein needs.

PHYS: Chat ⚓ 🗣
www.phys.com/c_tools/chat/chat.htm

"Whether you're trying to find the nutritional value of sticky buns, tighten your own buns or get a bun in the oven, you'll find someone here who's been there and done that and has advice to share."

PHYS: Exercise Guide
www.phys.com/f_fitness/03encyclopedia/01home/exercise.html

This exercise guide looks like just the thing for the person who wants to start working out but doesn't know where to begin. You can start with a risk assessment, and go from there. There's plenty of motivational help because at times we all get bored or disillusioned.

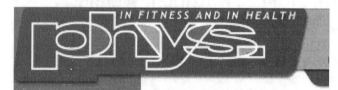

PHYS: Fitness Main Page ⚓ 👁
www.phys.com/f_fitness/00home/home.htm

Phys is produced by the editors of Vogue, Glamour, Mademoiselle, SELF, Allure, and Women's Sports & Fitness. This is a site to bookmark because it's both fun and it's a valuable resource. It's packed with tools, calculators, articles, and advice for all. You could easily spend too much time here instead of exercising. Make this a favorite so you can keep coming back to this dynamic web site.

PHYS: Forums ⚓ ⚲
www.phys.com/d_forums/allforums.html

Come over here to discuss such matters as fitness, weight loss, exchange recipes, and so much more that there is a search feature to help you find any boards that might be what you're looking for.

PHYS: Portion Finder 👁
www.phys.com/b_nutrition/02solutions/05portion/game.htm

Here's an interactive game called "Wheel of Portion," which uses Shockwave to help you learn just what a portion of food is. The food pyramid always uses "portion," and this game will help you understand the terminology. Actually, it's fun, and informative.

PHYS: Self Analysis
www.phys.com/b_nutrition/01self_analysis/01home/self.htm

Here you can do a self evaluation with various scales and get your calorie, fat, protein, and carb needs. You can also do a health risk assessment, find out your BMI, body fat percentage, as well as ideal weight. PHYS comes to us from CondeNet; they publish Vogue, Glamour, Self, and Women's Sport and Fitness, among others.

PHYS: Sitewide Search ⚲
www.phys.com/e_search/search.htm

Enter any word regarding diet or fitness, and PHYS will search it's past issues. I entered "cabbage soup," and got a brief review of the diet philosophy, how it is supposed to work, along with a critique of its philosophy

PHYS: Snack Bandit
www.phys.com/c_tools/gadgets/snackbandit/snackbandit.html

This looks like a Las Vegas style slot machine. All you have to do is browse the fairly extensive list of snacks, how many, and what you want to do to exercise those calories off. I had just eaten 6 Oreos so that's what I entered. I chose walking as my punishment and it said I should have to walk the dog only two minutes! I Think I'll have some more Oreos, then take a longer walk.

PHYS: Spinning
www.phys.com/f_fitness/03encyclopedia/02database/spinning.html

Spinning has nothing to do with wool or yarn these days. Today it's studio cycling, and can be extremely demanding. So be sure you're ready for it. Because so much is put into it, the benefits can be enormous. Check it out if you're game. Be sure to click on "go figure."

PHYS: Sports Activity Data Base
www.phys.com/f_fitness/03encyclopedia/01home/activity.html

Pick a sport, form aerobic boxing to snowboarding to yoga, and anything in between. PHYS will help you with ideal training routines to the equipment you'll need to get started. Just click on something that interests you, read it, and get up and outside.

 MUST SEE!   VIDEO   AUDIO   SELLS STUFF

 CHAT ROOMS   MAILING LISTS   MESSAGE BOARDS   ADULT CONTENT

 FREE REGISTRATION REQUIRED   MEMBERS ONLY CONTENT   SEARCHABLE

PHYS: The Personal Nutritionist

http://www4.phys.com/b_nutrition/01self_analysis/06pyramid/pyramid.html

Fill in a simple questionnaire and you'll get your ideal diet, or it can analyze your current diet.

PHYS: Trigger Food Quiz

www.phys.com/b_nutrition/01self_analysis/03trigger/trigger.html

Everyone has at least one trigger food: A sinful, satisfying treat whose taste sets off an almost insatiable desire for more, such as chocolate or potato chips.You may already know which foods get you going, but have you ever wondered why? With this quiz, PHYS will uncover why you find certain foods irresistible, and show you how to enjoy them without becoming enslaved. I answered the five questions and was told that my love of salty snacks was based on some Neanderthal yearnings for salt. It's nice to know my roots.

PHYS: Walking

www.phys.com/f_fitness/03encyclopedia/02database/walking.html

"Walking is the oldest mode of transportation - after all, humans have been doing it for more than 1.5 million years. It's also the cheapest, easiest form of aerobic exercise: All you have to do is open your front door, step outside and get moving." PHYS said it all in that intro. You'll also read about the benefits, advantages, and what equipment you need.

PHYS: Weight Training

www.phys.com/f_fitness/03encyclopedia/02database/weights.html

Studies show that weight-bearing exercises (like weight lifting) can help make your bones stronger, lowering your osteoporosis risk and leaving you less vulnerable to fractures in the future. In addition to an aerobic type exercise, weight training should be part of your regimen.

Physical Activity & Health: A Report of the Surgeon General

www.cdc.gov/nccdphp/sgr/sgr.htm

This is the report in its entirety, which is quoted in part everywhere on fitness sites on the World Wide Web. The bad news is that about 60% of Americans are not regularly active, and 25% are totally sedentary. Read it and weep, or read it and go for a walk.

Physician & Sports Medicine: Exercising When You're Overweight

www.physsportsmed.com/issues/oct_96/weight.htm

If you are like many overweight people, you have tried dieting and exercising with varied success. Problems such as barriers, phasing in fitness, and goal setting are discussed in this short page. Getting motivated, and staying on the program are addressed.

Physicians Committee for Responsible Medicine: Calcium & Strong Bones

www.strongbones.org

From the PCRM comes this convincing article about your bones and calcium. You'll learn that calcium doesn't just come from dairy products, but from leafy green vegetables and legumes. You'll learn that in a 12 year Harvard study, women who got their calcium from dairy actually broke more bones than women who rarely drank milk. Got greens?

Physicians Committee for Responsible Medicine:
Vegetarian Starter Kit 👁

www.pcrm.org/health/VSK/starterkit.html

There's a wealth of information about vegetarianism presented in a logical, factual, easy-to-read manner. You'll get tips on how to get started, vegetarianism for children, and answer to your nutritional concerns.

Physicians WEIGHT LOSS Centers $

www.pwlc.com

Over 90 products are related to weight loss are available via online shopping. They also have franchise locations across the country, specializing in counseling and support.

Plastic Surgery FAQs-Liposuction

www.plasticsurgery.org/faq/lipo.htm

Six questions answered, emphasizing that liposuction is not to be considered as an effective method of weight loss.

Porridge People

www.geocities.com/HotSprings/Sauna/7015

This is a page of vegan recipes, from breads, soups, and stews, to main dishes and desserts.

PowerBar Online $👁

www.powerbar.com

The PowerBar web site doesn't just sell stuff here; they have lots of articles on training and performance. It's interactive and fun to use.

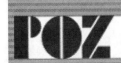

POZ Magazine 👁

www.poz.com

Since their first issue in 1994, POZ has become a lifeline for thousands of people living with HIV. Each month the magazine reports on the impact that AIDS has on life, politics, culture and society. It profiles people living with the virus and delivers important health information. It's diet and nutrition section is well done. You can subscribe online, and it's free if you are HIV positive.

 MUST SEE!   VIDEO   AUDIO $ SELLS STUFF

 CHAT ROOMS   MAILING LISTS   MESSAGE BOARDS   ADULT CONTENT

 FREE REGISTRATION REQUIRED   MEMBERS ONLY CONTENT   SEARCHABLE

POZ Partner: Grandma's Recipe
www.thebody.com/poz/survival/7_99/diet.html

This site has some simple down to earth suggestions for choosing the right foods and is especially helpful for those with limited resources who can't shell out for vitamins and minerals. The basic rule is to eat what your ancestors did; if they didn't eat it, you shouldn't either. Foods are categorized into energy, constructive, and protective groups.

POZ: All You Can Eat
www.thebody.com/poz/survival/4_99/diet.html

If you're losing weight or ill you need to consume 19 or 20 calories per pound per day, according to this article in POZ. The bottom line: Eat well and eat more often.

Pregnancy Today Online:
ACOG Guidelines for Exercise in Pregnancy
www.pregnancytoday.com

These are the official recommendations for exercise in pregnancy from the American College of Obstetricians and Gynecologists

Prevention of Major Medical Problems With Diet
www.neat-schoolhouse.org/diet-prev.html

Rosemary C. Fisher searched over 200 medical studies to find how diet affects health and well-being as one ages. Check out what she's learned about food and its relationship to various diseases.

Prosource $
www.psperformance.com

Anti-catabolics, protein powders, meal replacements, testosterone boosters, fat burners, prohormones, success stories, and more! Step right up, folks.

Pure-food.com
www.pure-food.com/food.htm

"The intent of this web site is to educate and raise awareness of the issues of food safety and the degradation of our food supply, including: Food irradiation and pesticides, and the public relations ploys designed to hide the truth." - from the Purefood.com web site. Here's a non-governmental point of view on irradiation, and uses of pesticides and herbicides.

Pure-food.com: Alerts - What Can I Do?
www.pure-food.com/alerts.htm

Feeling frustrated and powerless about food irradiation, pesticides, and herbicides? Well, here's a list of things to do, people to call, and let them know how you feel.

Pure-food.com: Facts About Herbicides & Pesticides
www.pure-food.com/pesticid.htm

Here's some questions and answers about America's use of pesticides and herbicides. Ever consider going organic?

Quack Watch: Appropriate Use of Supplements

www.quackwatch.com/03HealthPromotion/supplements.html

> Who should take supplements? How much should you take? Why take them? Here's a few obviously basic questions to ask yourself before you go down to your local vitamin store.

Quack Watch: DHEA: Ignore the Hype

www.quackwatch.com/01QuackeryRelatedTopics/dhea.html

> Superhormone? The mother of all hormones? Fountain of youth? After you read this, you might find these hormones a tough pill to swallow.

Quack Watch: Don't Buy Phony Ergogenic Aids

www.quackwatch.com/01QuackeryRelatedTopics/ergo.html

> If you're considering using performance enhancing aids such as vitamins, minerals, amino acids, or other supplements to build muscles or tweak your performance, do your best to get informed. Here's one place to go.

Quackwatch

www.quackwatch.com

> Quackwatch is your guide to health fraud, quackery, and intelligent decisions. This web site is maintained by Stephen Barrett, M.D., and should be bookmarked as a guide to help you make informed decisions. There are links to take you to alternative cancer treatment scams, to questionable multi-level marketing organizations, and you'll find sources of reliable information.

Redux & "Phen/fen" Medical Problems from Michael Myers.M.D. Inc.

www.weight.com/medprob.html

> You can refer to articles referring to residual problems related to these drugs.

Rosanna's Marcobiotic Kitchen

www.rosanna.com

> "Our mission is health, yours and ours. Through our letter, you will have the expert guidance to assure proper and balanced nutrition for anyone in the temperate climate zones." Rosanna Martella and James McCaig live the macrobiotic life. Rosanna is the Master Chef/Counselor and James is Editor/Publisher of the letter. Subscribe to their free newsletter and receive recipes and insightful comments about the effects of certain foods on our bodies.

Runner's World Online 👁

www.runnersworld.com

> The home page of Runner's World Online, this is the place to start. Catch up on the daily running news, sign up to receive Runner's World Extr@, their free weekly E-mail newsletter, and read the tip of the day.

 MUST SEE!   VIDEO   AUDIO $ SELLS STUFF

 CHAT ROOMS   MAILING LISTS   MESSAGE BOARDS    ADULT CONTENT

 FREE REGISTRATION REQUIRED   🔒 MEMBERS ONLY CONTENT   SEARCHABLE

Runner's World: Claim Check

www.runnersworld.com/nutrition/nu4supps.html

Nutritional supplements are the hottest rage, and we are spending tons of money on them. Liz Applegate, Ph.D., is nutrition editor for Runner's World, and a member of the National Triathlon Training Camp Elite Team. She gets us up to speed on four popular supplements: ginseng, sodium bicarbonate, creatine, and branched-chain amino acids. This is worth reading before you load your shopping cart.

Runner's World: Energy To Go

www.runnersworld.com/nutrition/gels.html

For the past few years, many endurane athletes have been using energy gels and research is showing that they do have some benefit. This brief article gives good advice on how to use them.

Runner's World: For Sweet Teeth Only

www.runnersworld.com/nutrition/nusweets.html

Oh no, a sugar/cancer link. I knew it was coming. My fingers are crossed that this goes the way of saccharin.

Runner's World: Mother Nature's Super Foods

www.runnersworld.com/nutrition/nusuperfood.html

What do Asian Fish Sauce, Oysters, Garlic, and Tofu have in common? Would you eat them all in the same meal? (Ginny Lewis is the only person I know who would do that.) Anti-oxidants, phytochemicals, beta-carotene, and fiber: some of these things just can't be put into a pill. But read what's so powerful about these "superfoods" in this Runner's World article.

Runner's World: Performance Pick-Me-Ups

www.runnersworld.com/nutrition/nuperform.html

Water, sports drinks, energy bars, or energy gels: which should your choose? Liz Applegate, Ph.D., is nutrition editor of Runner's World, and she gives us the scoop on the strengths and weaknesses of each.

Runner's World: Taking the Bar

www.runnersworld.com/nutrition/nuenergybar2.html

What's in those energy bars, and when is their use appropriate or recommended? There's also a chart comparing some of the best sellers. The good news is that there's one that tastes and looks just like a brownie. My search may be over.

Runner's World: You Can Take It With You

www.runnersworld.com/nutrition/nuenergybar.html

From Runner's World, here's a good primer on energy bars, what's in them, and how to choose one. But no matter how good they may be for you while exercising, the bottom line will be how they taste. I wonder how they stack up against a simple brownie.

Salmonellosis ☞

www.cdc.gov/ncidod/diseases/foodborn/salmon.htm

An American scientist name Salmon discovered this tiny bug, and decided that it could not be tamed, or used as a house pet. We probably all have contracted this little fella at some time, and I suspect it was no laughing matter. Put this in your shopping cart of required reading.

Salton - The Industry Leader in Home Products $

www.salton-maxim.com

> Just click on the Juiceman here on this page, and you'll get to the guy with the eyebrows you may have seen on those late-night infomercials. There are a few pages that discuss the benefits of juicing, and a brief bio of Jay Kordich, the Juiceman. Go ahead and buy the juicers here, too.

Sante (For Good Health)

www.hoptechno.com/santeall.htm

> Sante is an all-in-one weight control, cookbook, exercise, and nutrition program. Just enter your personal details and Sante does the rest. I wonder if it exercises for me.

Sante 7000 Search Form ⚲

http://209.98.30.12/sante7000/sante7000_search.cfm

> Search this database of over 7,000 foods and you'll get a list of at least 29 nutrients contained within. I typed in "brownie," and found a lot of stuff in one. That's why they comprise the foundation of my own food pyramid.

Search the USDA Nutrient Database ⚲

www.nal.usda.gov/fnic/cgi-bin/nut_search.pl

> I wanted to know the nutritional value of a brownie. I just typed in "brownie," and got a a list of choices of brownies. Eventually, I learned that there's a lot of potassium in a brownie. Therefore, I consider them an essential building block for good health.

Shape Up America 👁

www.shapeup.org

> C. Everett Koop, MD, is the founder of this organization, which is a high profile national initiative to promote healthy weight and increased physical activity in America, Their web site is designed to provide you with the latest information about safe weight management, healthy eating, and physical fitness.

Shape Up America! Support Center

www.shapeup.org/support/index.htm

> Shape Up America's Support Center is designed to help you learn more about some of the barriers that stand between you and successful weight management. Here you'll find solutions and strategies for success.

Shape Up America! Survey on Physical Activity in the U.S.

www.shapeup.org/surveys/physical.htm

> About 40% of American adults are found to be completely sedentary. Activity levels for children are decreasing as well, especially among teens. What's going on here? Here's a summary of the survey's findings.

Shape Up America: Cyberkitchen ✐
www.shapeup.org/kitchen/frameset1.htm

Shape Up America's Cyberkitchen is designed to "show you how to balance the food you eat with physical activity so that you can achieve and maintain a healthy weight." The program involves seven steps. You must provide personal information, and the program includes healthy recipes.

Shape Up America! Fitness Center 👁
www.shapeup.org/fitness/index.htm

Shape Up America believes that fitness means different things to different people, so they devised this center to help you no matter what level of fitness you are. They can develop an activity program that is just right for you. Go ahead, give it a try. This web site is big, and very interactive, but you just may find that it's just what you need to get started. On your mark, get set, go!

Shape Up America! Fitness Center - Assessment 👁
www.shapeup.org/fitness/assess/fset2.htm

There are five tests for you to take here, with the results giving you an idea about the shape you're in. The information is also used in other parts of the fitness center; for instance, it will help determine your calorie level when you enter the nutrition center, and it will help to calculate calories burned when you exercise. Pretty nifty, don't you think? Then click onto the information center for a quiz on how much you think you know about physical activity.

Shape Up America! Fitness Center - Improvement 👁
www.shapeup.org/fitness/improve/fset4.htm

Once you've taken all the assessment tests, you're ready to enter the improvement section. Here you will choose a focus area where you think you fit, depending on your level of daily activity. So if you are at a computer all day, or watch TV a heck of a lot, you'll be sent to the appropriate focus area. Then you'll be given a tracking form. Before you know it, you've ditched the remote and you're in the Boston Marathon! Well, not quite, but you will be moving.

Shape Up America! Fitness Center - Nutrition 👁
www.shapeup.org/fitness/nutrition/fset3.htm

The Nutrition Center is designed to help you better understand the nutrition requirements of active people. If you have taken the tests in the Assessment Center, then you can check out your daily calorie goals in line with the food guide pyramid. There's also vast amounts of information in the supplements section, ranging from antioxidants to hormones to sports drinks.

Shape Up America! The X-Factor Survey
www.shapeup.org/surveys/x-factor.htm

32 million women and 26 million men in America are classified as being either overweight or obese. 78% of these people are currently NOT dieting. This is an interesting survey completed by Louis Harris on the factors contributing to this troublesome trend in what is becoming an American lifestyle.

Sibutramine from Michael Myers. M.D. Inc.
www.weight.com/sibutramine.html

Here's a discussion of Meridia, which was approved in 1997 for use in weight management. Dr. Myers explains in laymen's terms just what it is and how it works. He stresses that it's use must be in combination with a low-calorie diet, exercise, and behavior modification.

Slim-Fast Online
www.slimfast.com

Slim-Fast has been around for over 20 years, and here is where you can learn about the program. Nothing is sold here.

Slowing the Aging Clock
http://primusweb.com/fitnesspartner/library/activity/agingclock.htm

If you think you have no control over the aging process, read this brief, but interesting, site.

Small Household Vegetarian Recipes
www.boutell.com/vegetarian/index.html

Are you cooking for just two or a small family? Check out these recipes.

Sports Nutrition Connection
http://rampages.onramp.net/~msam/home.html

"Providing accurate, scientifically-based sports nutrition information to help the competitive and recreational athlete reach their maximum potential." This is the mission of the sports nutrition connection, and its authors seem serious about providing accurate, science-based information in sports nutrition. If you are an endurance athlete, a body builder, or even a weekend jogger, check out this site. These authors are not trying to sell you anything but good advice.

Sports Nutrition Connection: An Overview of Ketogenic Diets
http://rampages.onramp.net/~msam/index.html

What are ketogenic diets, and how do they work? Read about complications, effects, and risks. At least you don't have to buy anything. Jeff Edmunds, RD, just sells you some sound facts.

Sports Nutrition Connection: Basic Nutritional Considerations For the Endurance Athlete
http://rampages.onramp.net/~msam/enduranc/basicE.html

Calories, carbs, protein, and fat; yes, even fat is an essential nutrient for every cell in our body. This article by Matt Samuels, RD, will get you headed into the right direction.

Sports Nutrition Connection: Basic Nutritional Considerations for the Strength Athlete/Bodybuilder
http://rampages.onramp.net/~msam/strength/basicS.html

This article by Matt Samuels, RD, focuses on kcal and macro nutrient intakes. It will tell you how to calculate your kcalorie needs, as well as your carb and fat requirements.

 MUST SEE!   VIDEO   AUDIO   SELLS STUFF

 CHAT ROOMS   MAILING LISTS   MESSAGE BOARDS   ADULT CONTENT

 FREE REGISTRATION REQUIRED   MEMBERS ONLY CONTENT   SEARCHABLE

Sports Nutrition Connection:
Dietary Intake & Supplementation: Effects On Testosterone
http://rampages.onramp.net/~msam/misc/testoste.html

Zinc, boron, DHEA, and androstenedione; they sound like extraterrestrial elements from Star Trek. But people are spending millions of dollars for supplementation. Jeff Edmunds, RD, brings us back to earth with this in-depth article.

Sports Nutrition Connection: How to Get Lean & Ripped
http://rampages.onramp.net/~msam/strength/ripped.html

Mike Darnley, RD, leads us through the maze of diet, exercise, and genetics to reach that goal of being "lean and ripped." I guess being able to control two out of three isn't so bad.

Sports Nutrition Connection:
Nutrition For Gaining Muscle Mass
http://rampages.onramp.net/~msam/strength/weightga.html

If you're looking for a miracle potion, you've come to the wrong place. But if you need sound nutritional advice, this article by Jeff Edmunds, RD, set you straight.

Sports Nutrition Connection: Questions & Answers
http://rampages.onramp.net/~msam/qa.html

The guys who write the articles for the Sports Nutrition Connection answer your questions.

Sports Nutrition Connection: The Beneficial Effects of Fat
http://rampages.onramp.net/~msam/enduranc/fat.html

Here's a primer on fat and its role in performance for the endurance athlete. Maybe there's some truth that "it ain't over 'til the fat lady sings." Read Matt Samuels, RD, well-footnoted, well-researched article on the necessity of fat in your diet.

Sports Nutrition Connection:
Why Water Is The Most Important Nutrient
http://rampages.onramp.net/~msam/enduranc/water.html

Mike Darnley, RD, presents this page with a focus on the role of water in athletic performance. Read the astounding facts on how much water we can lose just through our skin, and learn of water's importance in hydration. The author has degrees in Nutrition and a Masters in Exercise and Sports Nutrition.

Stanford Medical Center: FAQs About the Ketogenic Diet
www.stanford.edu/group/ketodiet/FAQ.html

Questions most often asked by parents are answered here. There's also a section of questions that health care providers have asked the Stanford team.

Stanford Medical Center: Ketogenic Diet Program 👁
www.stanford.edu/group/ketodiet

The ketogenic diet is a special method of treating epilepsy (seizure disorders). This Web Site was created by the Pediatric Neurology Division at Stanford University School of Medicine to facilitate communication between health care providers who are using the ketogenic diet to treat epilepsy. Here's a good resource for information and communication.

Starting An Exercise Program

http://primusweb.com/fitnesspartner/library/activity/startexercise.htm

> So you want to start exercising and you're not even sure what to exercise, how to do it, and when. This page is a great place to start your new lifestyle.

Strength Training Basics

http://primusweb.com/fitnesspartner/library/activity/trainbasics.htm

> Major muscle groups, sequence, speed, sets, reps, resistance, range, progression, and frequency: if you're just thinking about strength training, there's a lot of vocabulary you might want to become familiar with to eliminate any fear and ignorance. Read this to enable you to have a safe and successful workout.

Stretching & Flexibility

http://galway.informatik.uni-kl.de/staff/weidmann/pages/stretch/stretching_toc.html

> Everything you ever wanted to know about stretching and flexibility, plus more.

Structure House:
Unique Center for Weight Loss & Lifestyle Change

www.structurehouse.com/shouse/about.htm

> People from 50 states and 35 countries have come to Structure House to learn how to break eating cycles and change self-defeating patterns into a healthy way of life. It's located in Durham, NC.

Stupid Things Vegetarians Hear

www.boutell.com/vegetarian/stupid.html

> Here's a list of a few things you may have heard from non vegetarians. Pretty funny.

Sugar Busters

www.sugarbusters.com/sbfiles/home.html

> Sugar Busters is a diet plan which operates on the premise that low-fat, high carbohydrate diets are a flop, that people usually end up putting their weight back on, and then some. Well, according to them, the culprit isn't fat or carbs; it's sugar! Sugar causes the production of insulin which keeps you from losing weight no matter how much you diet or exercise. Now what? So if you're in a rut with your fad diet, buy this book online, and follow this 14 day meal plan. What's so cool about this program? You can't eat carrots or corn, but you can have red wine! Visit with the authors, Drs. Andrews, Balart, Bethea, and Mr. Steward, a geologist; part with some money, and deny yourself the pleasures of sugar. Me? I'll stick with my brownies and take walks.

 MUST SEE!   VIDEO   AUDIO   SELLS STUFF

 CHAT ROOMS   MAILING LISTS   MESSAGE BOARDS   ADULT CONTENT

 FREE REGISTRATION REQUIRED   MEMBERS ONLY CONTENT   SEARCHABLE

Sugar Busters Comments & Experiences
www.sugarbusters.com/sbfiles/questions/comments.html

People who have been on the diet relate their experiences with bloating and flatulence, headaches and energy, bowel movements and pregnancy.

Sugar Busters Glossary
www.sugarbusters.com/sbfiles/questions/glossary.html

What are atheroma, glucagon, and amylase? Are bioflavonoids coming to take us away? Sugar Busters supplies you with definitions of terms to help you better understand the thinking behind the program.

Sugar Busters Interview Form
www.sugarbusters.com/sbfiles/communicate/interview.html

Help out the authors of "Sugar Busters" by relating your experiences with this diet plan in this interview form.

Sugar Busters: Kitchen Form
www.sugarbusters.com/sbfiles/communicate/kitchen.html

Submit your favorite recipe that follows the sugar busters guidelines, and they'll review it for possible posting to their web site or include it in a cookbook.

Surgical Treatment of Obesity
www.weight.com/obesitysurgery.html

Various kinds of surgical are discussed, along with who may be regarded as a candidate for these procedures. Benefits and risks are an important part of the discussion.

Surgilite
http://surgilite.hypermart.net

This bariatric practice is located in Hollywood, CA. Many questions about surgical obesity are answered here. Even if you don't live near here, this site proves to be very informative if you are considering surgery.

Susan Powter
www.susanpowter.com

Susan Powter's home page is a jumping off point to find products, advice, support, and ideas for successful weight management.

Symmetry International $
www.go-symmetry.com

Symmetry International is a multi-level organization selling a product line of dietary supplements; they seem to have a focus on herbs and vitamins. They don't like to use the term "multi-level," but rather, "cellular marketing." Go ahead, give it a try, get filthy rich, and make your own infomercials with bikinis, boats, and bimbos in the background.

Take The Food Pyramid Challenge
www.bennygoodsport.com/food.htm

This is fun. Check off the foods you want as you plan your menu for the day. There's more than one answer, so choose foods you like. Then Benny Goodsport will help you tally your results, comparing them with the food pyramid.

Talk With The Experts: Ask the Mayo Dietician
www.mayohealth.org/mayo/expert/htm/ask2.htm

Your questions regarding nutrition can be answered here; in fact, it may have been asked before. Just scroll through the archives before you send one off. This is a very informative site, and there is no selling, no hype - only informed news.

Tarla Dalal
www.tarladalal.com

Tarla Dalal is India's best-selling author of cookbooks, with over 20 titles to her credit. Her first book, The Pleasures of Vegetarian Cooking, is in its 25th printing. Her recipes are known for their ease and simplicity. This online cookbook is really easy to for finding recipes, or for trying out new ones. You can also use a shopping cart to add ingredients; then you can print out your shopping list.

Taste of Heaven & Earth
www.amacord.com/taste

Try some sample recipes from Bettina Vitell's book. She was once the head chef of a Zen monastery.

The Body: Alternative & Complementary Treatments, Including Natural & Herbal Remedies
www.thebody.com/treat/herbal.html

Milk thistle, glutamine, and Chinese herbs? Read up on these alternative treatments from a list of links to articles compiled by The Body, and AIDS and HIV information resource.

The Body: An AIDS & HIV Information Resource
www.thebody.com/index.shtml

This web site is an incredible resource for anyone. It holds a wealth of information from basics of HIV, to treatment and prevention, to listing conferences. You can be updated on drug trials and newest therapies, or even enroll in clinical trials. There are chat rooms, bulletin boards, and insight from experts. It's easily navigable, uncluttered, and presented in understandable language. Register for updates in HIV news, too. Their diet, nutrition, and exercise sections are useful and current. This site should be bookmarked!

 MUST SEE!   VIDEO   AUDIO   SELLS STUFF

 CHAT ROOMS   MAILING LISTS   MESSAGE BOARDS   ADULT CONTENT

 FREE REGISTRATION REQUIRED   MEMBERS ONLY CONTENT   SEARCHABLE

The Body: Diet & Nutrition 👁
www.thebody.com/dietnut.html

> This page gives you links to articles compiled from resources such as POZ, AIDS Treatment News, Body Positive, Seattle Treatment Education Project, and many others.

The Body: Diet & Nutrition: Vitamins
www.thebody.com/dietnut/vitamins.html

> Thinking about supplementing your diet with vitamins, minerals, antioxidants, or phytochemicals? Here's a list of articles compiled from various sources to help you understand what they are and how to use them.

The Body: Forum On Wasting, Diet, Nutrition & Exercise
www.thebody.com/cgi/wastingans.html

> For people who live with HIV, diet, nutrition, and exercise play an extremely important role in maintaining quality of life. Here's a place to read answered questions, or to send in your own question. Three outstanding specialists with extensive experience in this field discuss your questions.

The Hacker's Diet 👁
www.fourmilab.ch/hackdiet/www/hackdiet.html

> John Walker, the founding engineer of Autodesk, Inc. wrote this interesting book from the perspective of an engineer. His often humorous account of his own weight problem and how he has approached it is based on simple logic and common sense. He approaches obesity as merely another problem that needs to be solved. He's a true engineer. Download it for free and read it before you spend big bucks elsewhere.

The Learn Education Center
www.learneducation.com/weight.htm

> Take the weight loss readiness test here to see if you're ready to lose weight. You can also calculate your BMI and estimate your daily caloric needs.

This Week's Carrot - Nutrition for Kids 👁
www.nutritionforkids.com/Carrots/Weekly_Carrot.htm

> Each week a new "carrot" is posted on this site with ideas, startling facts, or web site recommendations about kids and nutrition. Sometimes a book or an activity is suggested. There's good information for parents and teachers here. Check it out.

Thriveonline.com: Biking Tips ⚓👁
www.thriveonline.com/outdoors/bike/biketips/toc.mtbiking.html

> Want to know how to do it? Want to know what equipment you'll need? Need advice, recommended workouts? Need to fix a flat tire? Everything you've always wanted to know, but were afraid to ask.

Thriveonline.com: Fitness ⚓ 👁
www.thriveonline.com/fitness/index.html

> If you want tools, motivation, advice, all presented in a way to hold your attention, you've come to the right place. Activities range from biking to yoga, from backpacking to total body fitness. Plan on spending way too much time here before you choose an activity you might like to try. I lost an hour while slouching at my computer; go ahead, try it out.

Thriveonline.com: Hiking & Backpacking 👁

www.thriveonline.com/outdoors/hike/hikingindex.html

If you enjoy walking, try strapping on a pack and exploring further away from home. There's beginner help, a big table of contents, and they'll even tell you where to go. Need a backpack, tent, or boots? Suggestions and reviews on all kinds of stuff are here. Got a question? Ask Gordo.

Thriveonline.com: Running 👁

www.thriveonline.com/outdoors/run/runindex.html

If you like to run, jog, sprint, or log serious miles, the collection of tips and advice will help you run better, faster, and stronger. Use thriveonline's G.O. Guide to search any state for running trail reviews.

Thriveonline.com: The G.O. Guide 👁

www.thriveonline.com/outdoors/go-guide/goindex.html

Are you thinking of taking on a new outdoors sport for your fitness project? Start here, and work your way through the browsable list of activities. Then you'll find info on getting the right equipment, getting started, and there are message boards if you want to talk about it, get advice, or find a buddy to go with.

Top 10 Fad Diet Plans in the USA

www.dietnutrition.com/faddiets.html

Here they are: the 10 most popular fad diets. Click on any one of them and see the details.

Toppfast Diet Plan $

www.toppfast.com/toppfast/default.htm

A protein sparing, modified fast system, which recommends you undertake the program under your doctor's supervision.

TOPS

www.tops.org

TOPS is an international weight loss group that provides members with support, motivation, and fellowship in attaining and maintaining weight goals. It is the oldest major weight control group, and has 11,000 chapters nationwide. They sell nothing, and you work with your own physician to set goals. There is a nominal annual fee and small monthly dues.

Trans Fat Info Web: Introduction

www.enig.com/0001t10.html

Trans fats are so huge now that they have their own web site! Here you can get a primer on fatty acids, but dust off your high school biology books before you start.

Treating Diabetes With Good Nutrition

www.cyberdiet.com/modules/diabetes/outline.html

> This is Cyberdiet's starting point for management of diabetes. It starts as a primer on diabetes and advances to food management tools and skills. There are also resources to further your understanding. If you're new to diabetes, or curious, this is a good starting point.

Trichinosis

www.cdc.gov/ncidod/dpd/trichino.htm

> Remember when our moms would cook pork 'til it was done, well done, totally done? Now, legislation concerning feeding of raw meat garbage to hogs has slowed this bug down. Keep cooking your meat, though, and beware of wild game meat.

Tufts University Health & Nutrition Letter

http://healthletter.tufts.edu

> This publication comes from Tufts University Scholl of Nutrition Science and Policy, and all articles are researched by the department and the editorial staff. You'll need to subscribe to the full newsletter, but there are sample articles from the current issue posted, as well as indexes of articles that appeared in recent years.

Tufts University Nutrition Navigator ♀ ☜

www.navigator.tufts.edu

> Tufts University maintains a rating guide to nutrition web sites. It is presented by their Center on Nutrition Communication, School of Nutrition Science. If you are just beginning your search in nutrition, whether it is targeted toward children, seniors, special needs, this is THE place to start. There are areas for parents, educators, and health professionals as well. Each site is rated and reviewed in depth, and gives you a good idea if you even want to go there. The sites are visited quarterly, and reviews updated, so that the web sites you visit are not stale. Give it a try.

UCLA School of Medicine: University Obesity Center

www.ccon.com/uclarfo

> "Weight loss programs that work quickly, easily, safely, and permanently." If you live around this school, it sounds like a safe place to visit. Surely they won't just sell you a can of powder. They offer everything from low calorie diets to surgery.

UDSA: Glossary of the Nutrient Data Laboratory

www.nal.usda.gov/fnic/foodcomp/Bulletins/glossary.html

> Did you need to know what ARS, AMS, and CFR stand for? Then here's your page, complete with all the acronyms the NDL uses in their web site. (This must be a government page.)

Understanding Adult Obesity

www.niddk.nih.gov/health/nutrit/pubs/unders.htm

> This fact sheet provides basic information about obesity: what it is, what causes it, how to measure it. Companion fact sheets provide more in-depth information about some aspects addressed briefly here, such as health risks of obesity and treatment options for the condition.

Understanding Your Training Heart Rate

http://primusweb.com/fitnesspartner/library/activity/thr.htm

> Learn why your training heart rate zone is a critical element in your program. There's more to it than taking your pulse!

University Institute for the Surgery of Morbid Obesity

www.shedweight.com

> The University Institute for the Surgery of Morbid Obesity (UNISMO) is a state-of-the-art surgical therapy program dedicated to the care and treatment of patients with clinically severe (morbid) obesity refractory to non-operative treatment.

University Nutrition Sites in the United States

www.sfu.ca/~jfremont/university.html

> Jean Fremont has listed some of the better university nutrition sites to be found on the Web. You can link to them from here. She's organized!

University of Minnesota - Research Project Updates

http://www1.umn.edu/mnoc/topics/Updates.html

> This is an interesting update on where research on obesity is focusing and is fairly scientific in presentation. But if you are well versed in obesity, you can see what researchers are up to.

University of Texas Center for Alternative Medicine Research in Cancer

www.sph.uth.tmc.edu:8052/utcam

> UT-CAM is dedicated to investigating the effectiveness of alternative/complementary therapies used for cancer prevention and control. The Center's mission is to facilitate the scientific evaluations of biopharmacologic and herbal therapies as well as innovative approaches. If you are looking for alternative treatment or concurrent therapy, this is a really great web site to begin your search. It is written for the layman, but you can delve into the scientific research behind the story if you are so inclined.

University of Texas Center for Alternative Medicine Research in Cancer: Corilous Versicolor

www.sph.uth.tmc.edu:8052/utcam/summary/coriolus.htm

> Research shows that this mushroom has antiviral, antimicrobial, and antitumor properties. Here's a good scientific review in layman's terms about this fungus that's been in use for ages in the Orient. You'll also find out how to take it and where to get it. Be sure to let your healthcare provider know you'd like to give it a try, so you are all on the same page.

MUST SEE!	VIDEO	AUDIO	$ SELLS STUFF
CHAT ROOMS	MAILING LISTS	MESSAGE BOARDS	ADULT CONTENT
FREE REGISTRATION REQUIRED	MEMBERS ONLY CONTENT	SEARCHABLE	

University of Texas Center for
Alternative Medicine Research in Cancer: Gerson Program
www.sph.uth.tmc.edu:8052/utcam/summary/gerson.htm

> Max Gerson was a German physician who developed this nutritional approach to cancer treatment in the 1940's. You have to comply with a raw vegetarian diet for a lengthy time and take coffee enemas for detoxification. It doesn't say if you can use cream and sugar, or have it as a coolatta. (You have to remember what some of those Germans were up to around World War II before you jump into this one, I think.)

University of Texas Center for
Alternative Medicine Research in Cancer: Green Tea
www.sph.uth.tmc.edu:8052/utcam/summary/greentea.htm

> Green tea has been consumed by billions of people throughout the ages, and has served not only as a beverage, but also as an elixir for good health. It has been known to enhance the immune system, and to decrease the risk of certain cancers. Studies in animals are showing that green tea reduces the metastatic potential of cancer cells. After reading this, you'll be brewing yourself a "nice cup of tea."

University of Texas Center for
Alternative Medicine Research in Cancer: Hoxsey
www.sph.uth.tmc.edu:8052/utcam/summary/hoxsey.htm

> Harry Hoxsey developed a formula of herbs in the early 1900's for the treatment of cancer. It is currently given in Tijuana, Mexico, for about $3,500. Be sure to click on "scientific review" to find who to contact.

University of Texas Center for
Alternative Medicine Research in Cancer: Macrobiotics
www.sph.uth.tmc.edu:8052/utcam/therapies/macrobiotic.htm

> This page has an excellent overview of macrobiotics, and goes into the science and summary of the research. This is must reading before delving into this regimen.

University of Texas Center for
Alternative Medicine Research in Cancer: Mistletoe
www.sph.uth.tmc.edu:8052/utcam/summary/mistletoe.htm

> Merry Christmas! Mistletoe preparations are used to stimulate the immune system and to kill cancer cells. Find out how it's given, and where you can go for treatment. And yes, it still is considered highly toxic if little kids eat the berries, but kissing under mistletoe does not qualify as cancer treatment.

University of Texas Center for Alternative Medicine Research
in Cancer: Research in Progress
www.sph.uth.tmc.edu:8052/utcam/resact.htm

> Get the latest scoop on current trials underway involving melatonin, mistletoe, ginseng, and green tea. Some studies are on humans, others on animals, and still others are being done in the lab. You'll find very interesting stuff seemingly on the cutting edge.

University of Texas Center for Alternative Medicine Research in Cancer: Reviews of Therapies

www.sph.uth.tmc.edu:8052/utcam/therapy.htm

If you want to know anything about herbal therapies, biologic/organic, chemical, pharmacologic, or any special integratd regimens, look here because you'll find this much more helpful than the American Cancer Society Web Site. The Center is co-funded by the National Cancer Institute and was established by the National Center for Complementary and Alternative Medicine at the National Institutes of Health.

University-Based Adult Weight-Control Programs

www.niddk.nih.gov/health/nutrit/unversit/univpro.htm

Universities that have weight control programs for adults are listed by state.

University-Based Child/Adolescent Weight-Control Programs

www.niddk.nih.gov/health/nutrit/unversit/childho.htm

This is simply a list of university-based programs for kids.

US Pharmacopeia: Just Ask

www.usp.org/pubs/just_ask/vitamin.htm

Just Ask about the quality of your vitamin and mineral supplement products on this page. The USP answers questions about how to tell if vitamins and minerals meet acceptable standards.

USA Pears - PearBear Healthy Kids

www.usapears.com/pbnw-kids.html

Meet Pear Bear from the Pacific Northwest, and read stories, do activities as your kids learn about the importance of fruit (pears!) in their diet. Parents, you can order "The PearBear Chronicles," or even a commemorative plate.

USDA Food Safety & Inspection Service

www.fsis.usda.gov

This is the government agency that is responsible for ensuring that the nation's commercial supply of meat, poultry, and egg products is safe, wholesome, and correctly labeled and packaged, as required by the Federal Meat Inspection Act, the Poultry Products Inspection Act, and the Egg Products Inspection Act. Their web site is BIG, and here you'll find links to product recalls, what's new in food safety, and recent news releases pertaining to food safety.

USDA Food Safety & Inspection Service: Listeria Monocytogenes

www.fsis.usda.gov/OA/pubs/listeria.htm

What is it? How do you know if you have it? How can you get it? How can you prevent it? Easy to read information from the USDA's FSIS.

MUST SEE!	VIDEO	AUDIO	$ SELLS STUFF
CHAT ROOMS	MAILING LISTS	MESSAGE BOARDS	ADULT CONTENT
FREE REGISTRATION REQUIRED	MEMBERS ONLY CONTENT	SEARCHABLE	

USDA Foodborne Illness Education Information Center ⚲
www.nal.usda.gov/fnic/food-borne/wais.shtml

The Foodborne Illness Educational Materials Database is a compilation of consumer and food worker educational materials developed by universities; private industry; and local, state, and federal agencies. This includes computer software, audiovisuals, posters, games and teaching guides for elementary and secondary school education; training materials for the management and workers of retail food markets, food service establishments and institutions; educational research and more.

USDA/FSIS: Additives in Meat & Poultry Products
www.fda.gov/fdac/features/1998/398_rad.html

People have been using food additives for thousands of years. Today about 2,800 substances are used as food additives. Salt, sugar, and corn syrup are by far the most widely used additives in food in this country. This is a primer on additives from the Food Safety and Inspection Service, a branch of the Department of Agriculture.

USDA/FSIS: Cutting Board Safety
www.fsis.usda.gov/OA/pubs/cutboard.htm

Which is better, wooden or plastic cutting boards? Some 500 consumers have called the USDA's Meat and Poultry Hotline with this question since one study suggested that wooden cutting boards were better. Recent research has confirmed the conventional belief that plastic is safer than wood for cutting meat and poultry. Bottom line? Use a designated cutting board for meats, and wash thoroughly, sanitize, and replace if worn or porous. Do they make disposable cutting boards yet?

USDA/FSIS: Does Washing Food Promote Food Safety?
www.fsis.usda.gov/OA/pubs/washing.htm

Washing raw poultry, beef, pork, lamb, or veal before cooking it is not recommended. Have I wasted a lot of time in the kitchen, or what? The FSIS says all I've done is increase the chances of contaminating the kitchen sink, counter, towels, and sponges. Got to go wash my hands.

USDA/FSIS: Focus on Hot Dogs
www.fsis.usda.gov/OA/pubs/focushotdog.htm

"Advanced Meat Recovery," and "Mechanically Separated Meat" are processes used in making hot dogs. If you really want to know how it's done, and what other things on a hot dog package mean, check this site out.

USDA/FSIS: Food Safety for Persons With AIDS
www.fsis.usda.gov/OA/pubs/aids.htm

Persons with Acquired Immunodeficiency Syndrome (AIDS) are susceptible to many types of infection including illness from food-borne pathogens. They are at higher risk than are otherwise healthy individuals for severe illness or death. Affected persons must be especially vigilant when handling and cooking foods. The recommendations provided here are designed to help prevent bacterial food-borne illness.

USDA/FSIS: Food Safety Publications for Consumers
www.fsis.usda.gov/OA/pubs/consumerpubs.htm

Most publications can be found here online. Find out how to safely stuff a turkey so it doesn't kill you! (Hint: Make sure he's unarmed.)

USDA/FSIS: Foodborne Ilness Peaks in Summer--Why?
www.fsis.usda.gov/OA/pubs/illpeaks.htm

Year after year, we hear and read the same advice: Handle food carefully in the summer because food-borne illness -- also known as "food poisoning" -- is more prevalent in warmer weather. Find out if this is really true, and learn how to have a safer summer.

USDA/FSIS: Keeping Food Safe During a Power Outage
www.fsis.usda.gov/OA/pubs/pofeature.htm

Hurricanes, tornadoes, snowstorms, thunderstorms, or just a frying squirrel can ruin your day and give you one big tummy ache if you don't follow these guidelines for food safety when the power goes out. What to throw out, what to keep; it's all here.

USDA/FSIS: Microwave Food Safety
www.fsis.usda.gov/OA/pubs/cimwave.htm

There are traits unique to microwave cooking that affect how evenly and safely food is cooked. "Cold spots" can occur because of the irregular way the microwaves enter the oven and are absorbed by the food. If food doesn't cook evenly, bacteria may survive and cause food-borne illness. Simple techniques ensure that meat and poultry microwave safely. Safe defrosting, reheating, and cooking in your microwave are discussed here.

USDA/FSIS: Panic Button Food Safety Questions
www.fsis.usda.gov/OA/pubs/panicbut.htm

This is the "best of" the FSIS's hotline holiday questions. It's very informative, and the questions sound like they all came from my house. I guess I'm lucky to be alive! But you can call the hotline any time of the year, not just during the holidays. If you have other questions Hotline home economists and registered dietitians answer calls in person from 10 a.m. to 4 p.m. ET Monday through Friday year round. Callers can also select from a menu of recorded food safety messages 24-hours a day. If you have other questions about meat and poultry safety, call the USDA Meat and Poultry Hotline, at 1 (800) 535-4555. Washington, D.C. residents should call (202) 720-3333.

USDA/FSIS: The Facts About Ground Poultry
www.fsis.usda.gov/OA/pubs/grndpoul.htm

Ground turkey has been celebrated as the latest low-fat substitute for ground beef. Did you ever wonder what was in it? Or did you check and wish you never had? Time to bone up on your poultry, then you can tell your friends all about mechanically separated poultry.

USFDA: Center for Food Safety & Applied Nutrition
http://vm.cfsan.fda.gov

This is a big one; it's the United States Food and Drug Administration's Center of Food Safety and Applied Nutrition. It's also searchable which means you can enter the word or food or nutrient you're looking for. I typed in "olestra," and it returned 6 sites pertaining to fat substitutes. It'll search their database of food, nutrition, cosmetic and women's health topics. You can also choose to search all of the FDA.

 MUST SEE!   VIDEO   AUDIO $ SELLS STUFF

 CHAT ROOMS   MAILING LISTS   MESSAGE BOARDS   ADULT CONTENT

 FREE REGISTRATION REQUIRED   MEMBERS ONLY CONTENT   SEARCHABLE

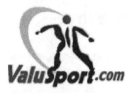

ValuSport.com $ ⅋

http://valusport.com/lib/nutrionline/index.html

Testosterone boosters, anabolic steroid alternatives, weight loss products, and exercise equipment are all available here.

Vega Study Center

www.vega.macrobiotic.net

Vega Study Center is America's premier macrobiotic residential school and the longest-running in the world. Famous for its friendly atmosphere, Vega allows each student to relax into their own understanding and pace of macrobiotic practice. It is located in Oroville, California.

Vegan Bikers

http://venus.nildram.co.uk/veganmc

Because being a vegan is kind to the environment, and riding a motorcycle is less polluting than driving a car, one can vastly improve his/her living standard by being a vegan biker. Click onto a short visit here; you may stay a while.

Vegan News

www.bury-rd.demon.co.uk

The Vegan News is a nonprofit Vegan newsletter coming from the UK. It is published monthly online, and you can visit back issues (to 1996). Each letter is filled with information on cooking, gardening, and product reviews.

Vegan Outreach

www.veganoutreach.org

Vegan Outreach is an organization dedicated to furthering education and understanding so that people may bring about fundamental change in their physical well-being, interaction with each other, and their environment. If you wonder why be a vegan, you can read their pamphlet, "Why Vegan?" online here.

Vegan Outreach: Forums ⬇

www.veganoutreach.org/forum/cgi-bin/Ultimate.cgi?action=intro

Here's a few vegan forums to check into where you can discuss, ask questions, or exchange recipes. They're quite active.

Vegan Outreach: Why Vegan?

www.veganoutreach.org/wv

If you've ever wondered why someone chooses a vegan lifestyle, this online pamphlet tells all. You can read text only, download (PDF), or order print copies.

Vegan Recipe Index
www.hut.fi/~jstalvio/cookbook1/Vegan-index.html

From the WWW Cookbook project comes this index of vegan recipes which are contributed from around the world.

Vegan Society: Teen Vegans
www.vegansociety.com/info/info07.html

From the Vegan Society in the UK comes a good primer for teens who are, or are considering a vegan lifestyle.

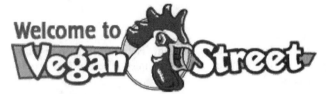

Vegan Street
www.veganstreet.com

Vegan Street's online newsletter was created to spread the message of veganism. There's a community center, a vegan living department, marketplace, calendar, links, and an "Activist's Handbook." For fun, check out the "Virtual Vegan World Quiz."

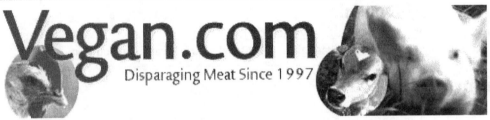

Vegan.com - Disparaging Meat Since 1997
www.vegan.com

There's lots of news and information on this web site. You'll find book reviews, animal rights news, nutrition information, and much more. The site is funded by sales of books through Amazon.com.

Veganet: The Centurion's Choice
http://library.advanced.org/20922/index.shtml

Here's a well-organized site that puts veganism, and all the questions anyone may have about this type of vegetarianism, in a logical sequence without the hype.

Veganism for the Over 60
www.vegansociety.com/info/info05.html

This is an informative page from the Vegan Society on the vegan lifestyle after the age of 60. It discusses key nutritional concerns of the older person.

  MUST SEE!   VIDEO   AUDIO   SELLS STUFF

  CHAT ROOMS   MAILING LISTS   MESSAGE BOARDS   ADULT CONTENT

  FREE REGISTRATION REQUIRED   MEMBERS ONLY CONTENT   SEARCHABLE

Vegetarian & Health Food Restaurants
www.ecomall.com/eat.htm

Click on a state or country of your choice and find a vegetarian restaurant.

Vegetarian Central: Nutrition & Health ♀
http://vegetariancentral.org/siteindex/Nutrition_and_Health

This site is basically a directory for virtually anything vegetarian. It's a great resource for both vegetarians and aspiring vegetarians.

Vegetarian Diet Pyramid
www.oldwayspt.org/html/p_veg.htm

Here's a healthy eating pyramid produced by Oldways jointly with the Harvard School of Public Health. Oldways is a young and growing non-profit organization with simple objectives: to promote healthy, clean foods and to encourage healthy eating.

Vegetarian Epicure
www.vegetarianepicure.com

Visit Anna Thomas's site and get a few sample recipes from her latest book. There's also a monthly letter that she posts. Her cookbooks have sold by the millions in many countries.

Vegetarian Food Pyramid
www.vegsource.com/nutrition/pyramid.htm

This pyramid contains dairy, but otherwise gives you a good view of vegetarian nutrition.

Vegetarian Journal
www.vrg.org/journal

This is the magazine "for those interested in vegetarian health, ecology, and ethics." Here, you can browse past articles on cooking, nutrition, travel, and science. The archives are a valuable resource for both vegetarians and veggie wannabes.

Vegetarian Journal: Subscribe $👁
www.vrg.org/journal/subscribe.htm

"The Vegetarian Journal is published by The Vegetarian Resource Group, a non-profit educational organization. The 36-page bi-monthly Journal contains informative articles, delicious recipes, book reviews, notices about vegetarian events, product evaluations, hints on where to find vegetarian products and services, travel tips, and more. All nutrition information in the Vegetarian Journal is based on scientific studies. Our health professionals evaluate the current scientific literature and present it in an easy and practical fashion to our readers so they can apply it to their own lives. In order to maintain an independent view, the Vegetarian Journal does not accept paid advertising." Subscribe here on their secure order form.

Vegetarian Nutrition for Teenagers
www.vrg.org/nutrition/teennutrition.htm

More and more teenagers are choosing vegetarianism, and face pressures from parents who are concerned about their health, and peer pressures as well. This is a good article that answers questions on teen nutrition and vegetarianism.

Vegetarian Pages
www.veg.org/veg

> Frequently asked questions are answered here, and a "mega-index" to vegetarian information can be found here.

Vegetarian Recipes Around the World
www.ivu.org/recipes

> There's over 1,600 recipes here from around the world. The site is sponsored by the International Vegetarian Union

Vegetarian Resource Group
www.vrg.org

> The VRG is a nonprofit organization dedicated to educating the public on vegetarianism, and the interrelated issues of health, nutrition, ecology, ethics, and world hunger. They are probably best known for publishing the Vegetarian Journal.

Vegetarian Resource Group: Choosing & Using a Dietician
www.vrg.org/journal/dietitian.htm

> Why use a dietician, especially since you'll probably hear the "variety, balance, and moderation" speech, and you want vegetarian help. This page will help you decide why you should find one, what to expect, what to ask. Always check those credentials.

Vegetarian Resource Group: The Vegetarian Game
www.vrg.org/game

> 20 questions for you to answer. I was awarded "intermediate vegetarian" for answering 15 correctly. Give it a try.

Vegetarian Resource Group:
Vegan Diet During Pregnancy & Lactation
www.vrg.org/nutrition/veganpregnancy.htm

> You're a pregnant vegan? Time to do a diet check. Make sure you're eating the right stuff. This is a good page brought to you by the Vegetarian Resource Group.

Vegetarian Resource Group: Vegetarianism in a Nutshell
www.vrg.org/nutshell/nutshell.htm

> Interested or just curious, there's a wealth of information at this site to answer any questions about vegetarians you may have. Sure you knew Paul McCartney is a vegetarian, but did you know that Mr. Rogers is also? It's a wonderful day in the neighborhood.

 MUST SEE!   VIDEO   AUDIO   SELLS STUFF

 CHAT ROOMS   MAILING LISTS   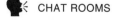 MESSAGE BOARDS   ADULT CONTENT

 FREE REGISTRATION REQUIRED   MEMBERS ONLY CONTENT   SEARCHABLE

Vegetarian Times' Virtual Vegetarian ⬇

www.vegetariantimes.com

Subscribe to Vegetarian Times here, or get a taste of what they have to offer, from recipes to brief articles. There's a message board as well as a links page.

Vegetarian Voice Online

www.cyberveg.org/navs/voice/voice.html

The Voice is the electronic counterpart of the Vegetarian Voice, the official quarterly newsmagazine of the North American Vegetarian Society. I saw a few articles on their "Vegetarian Express" program, which is designed to encourage fast food chains to offer more meatless choices; and there's a good section of book reviews.

Vegetarianism: Eat to Your Health

www.macalester.edu/~kwiik/Veggie/health.htm

Read some compelling reasons why vegetarianism is good for you. Eating a plant -based diet reduces the risk of heart disease, hypertension, and various forms of cancer. This page was constructed by two students from Macalster College who were taking a computer mediated communication class, and who are vegetarians themselves. The site is uncluttered and is presented persuasively and in a postive manner.

Vegetarianism: Glossary of Terms

www.macalester.edu/~kwiik/Veggie/terms.htm

If you thought that being a vegetarian meant not eating any meat, just look at the various kinds of vegetarianism there are.

Vegetarianism: Recipes

www.macalester.edu/~kwiik/Veggie/recipes.htm

Although only two recipes are listed here, they are meant to be served to someone who would not usually think of trying a vegetarian meal.

Vegetarianism: Vegetarian Fun Facts

www.macalester.edu/~kwiik/Veggie/funfact.htm

Light reading here which lists some trivial reasons over and above the dietary, moral, and intellectual arguments. For example, over 12 million Americans call themselves Vegetarians today!

Vegetarianism: Vegetarian Organizations

www.macalester.edu/~kwiik/Veggie/orgs.htm

Do you need help getting started, or do you need good information about vegetarianism? This site will put you in touch with organizations that lead you to your answers.

Veggie Kids

www.execpc.com/~veggie/tips.html

This site has several recipes with children in mind, and some ideas for you to get those five servings of fruit and vegetables into them.

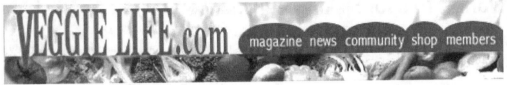

Veggie Life Magazine

`www.veggielife.com`

> *Veggie Life Magazine* is a comprehensive journal that covers the healthy lifestyle, from growing organically to cooking and eating to exercise, fitness, diet and nutrition. This is a nicely presented, uncluttered, and inviting web site. It's only downfall is that you can't take this magazine to the bathroom with you - unless you print it.

Veggies Anonymous:
Resources for Vegetarians, Vegans, & Other Non-Carnivores

`www.geocities.com/HotSprings/4664`

> Find information here on cooking, book lists, and other useful links. It is a nice resource page

Veggies Unite!

`http://vegweb.com`

> This web site claims to be "your on-line guide to vegetarianism, and it does a good job, too. It'll lead you to recipe exchanges, nutrition news, FAQs, and gardening info.

Vegging Out

`www.execpc.com/~veggie/index.html`

> Read excerpts from the USDA's 1995 "Dietary Guidelines for Americans," and you'll think that there may be a government conspiracy against the meat industry. The bottom line here is "Eat more vegetables, fruits, and grains!"

Vegie Info: Why Vegetarian?

`www.ozemail.com.au/~vego/whyveg.html`

> This page by Roger French lists a strong argument on why it makes such good sense to be a vegetarian. Not only does he list the health benefits, but he also writes about the differences between flesh and plant foods. It's a quick read, if you're in a hurry.

Vegie World: The Calcium Myth

`www.ozemail.com.au/~vego/calcium.html`

> Do you have concerns that a vegetarian diet is inadequate in calcium, iron, or protein? Read this page and you'll find out that in a recent study osteoporosis was far less prevalent in vegetarians than in omnivores.

	MUST SEE!		VIDEO	AUDIO	SELLS STUFF
CHAT ROOMS		MAILING LISTS		MESSAGE BOARDS	ADULT CONTENT
FREE REGISTRATION REQUIRED		MEMBERS ONLY CONTENT		SEARCHABLE	

Vegie World: Tips for Making the Change
www.ozemail.com.au/~vego/tips.html
> Whether you're going to a barbecue, taking a flight, or going to a fast food restaurant, you will have questions about continuing your new life as a vegetarian. Here's some tips to help you over the speed bumps.

Vegie World: Vegie Recipes ☜
www.ozemail.com.au/~vego/vegrecip.html
> WOW! Click on a flag of a country (13 are represented), and up comes vegetarian recipes for some awesome ethnic dishes. Here's an incredible mix of international flavors that include everything from appetizers to desserts.

Vegsource - Your Friendly Vegetarian Resource ☜
www.vegsource.com
> Here's a good stop for getting up to date health and diet information! A starting place for all things vegetarian!

Vegsource: Best of the Net Recipes ☜
www.vegsource.com/recipe
> This is cool. I scrolled down to desserts, clicked on brownies. Then about 12 different choices popped up, from high protein fudge brownies to raspberry brownies. When I clicked on fudge, I was linked right to the original site where it appeared. This is truly "Best of the Net." Although most recipes are vegan, they can be converted to lacto-ovo.

VegWeb - Recipe Directory ☜
www.vegweb.com/food
> Over 3,000 recipes are available here, and they are conveniently indexed. You can look something up by category or view the full listings. Find a recipe you like? You can then add the ingredients to a grocery list and take it to the store.

VegWeb - Vitamins & Minerals
www.vegweb.com/veginfo/vitamins.shtml
> Not only is this a list of your usual vitamins and minerals along with the recommended daily allowances, but it also lists vegetarian food sources for each.

Virginia Cooperative Extension: Food & Nutrition Newsletter
www.ext.vt.edu/news/periodicals/foods
> Virginia Tech's Department of Human Nutrition gives us information with links to many other sites. Articles are short, but there are lots of good links to lead you to more detailed info.

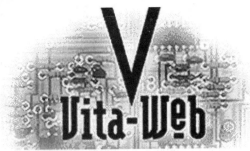

Vita-Web

www.vita-web.com

Roche laboratories proclaims this site as "The Internet's definitive source for the latest vitamin and nutritional information." It's divided into areas for the teacher and student, the professional, and the general public. It's a very "busy" web site, and if you like comic books, you'll like this page.

Vitamin Update ☞

http://bookman.com.au/vitamins

Vitamin Update informs you of the latest developments in vitamin and mineral research. Combined with comprehensive background information, their monthly updates will keep you informed of the very latest in a fast moving and often controversial area.

Viva Vegie Society

www.earthbase.org/vivavegie/home.html

The VivaVegie Society takes vegetarian advocacy to the streets. VivaVegie advocates confront Mr. and Ms. Pedestrian to get the facts out about their healthful, ethical and environmentally conscious vegetarian diet. They set up tables in busy pedestrian areas and distribute leaflets about vegetarianism.

Walking Connection

www.walkingconnection.com/index.html

Since 1989, the Walking Connection has been dedicated to providing people with information, new ideas, activities, products and services designed specifically for walkers. This free web site is committed to helping you get more from your walk -- whether it is on your treadmill at home, training to walk a marathon or ways to eat better and keep your feet healthier. You can sign up for free E-mail updates, too.

Walking Connection With Jo Ann Taylor

www.walkingconnection.com/Walking_Training.html

There's more to it than just putting one foot in front of the other, I guess. Find out what to do with your head, your arms, and below the belt!

 MUST SEE!   VIDEO   AUDIO   SELLS STUFF

 CHAT ROOMS   MAILING LISTS   MESSAGE BOARDS   ADULT CONTENT

 FREE REGISTRATION REQUIRED   MEMBERS ONLY CONTENT   SEARCHABLE

Walking For Exercise & Pleasure
www.hoptechno.com/book9.htm
> Hopkins Technology posted this reprint on walking from The President's Council on Physical Fitness & Sports.

Washington State Dairy Council: Take Aim
www.eatsmart.org/html/game.html
> Grab your bow and arrow, download Shockwave, and hit the falling categories. Then you answer nutrition questions while racing the clock. This one's great for adults, too, but you better know that sour cream and chives don't occur naturally in a baked potato.

Weight Commander Diet Program
www.interaccess.com/weightcmdr/dt.html
> Weight Commander will track your progress; just enter your weight every day and you'll see nifty charts and graphs. You can download a free trial version that's only 1.2MB in size and shouldn't take too long .

Weight Control Information Network
www.niddk.nih.gov/health/nutrit/win.htm
> WIN was established in 1994 to provide health professionals and consumers with science-based information on obesity, weight control, and nutrition. They produce, collect, and disseminate information on obesity, weight control, and nutrition.

Weight Management Centers
www.weightmanagement.com
> Located in Tampa, Florida, this physician practice has programs designed for nearly anyone serious about losing weight, from just 5 pounds to hundreds.

Weight Table Comparison Study
http://www1.mhv.net/~donn/wtabl.html
> Here's some weight tables from the 80's mostly which give acceptable weight based upon a person's height. Body Mass Index , the benchmark of the 90's, is not here but it is interesting to see that I am overweight no matter which table I use!

WeightLoss2000.com
http://WeightLoss2000.com

> WeightLoss2000.com is dedicated to providing practical, up-to-the-minute information about weight loss and obesity. This comprehensive site contains up-to-date news on obesity, drug and herbal remedies, as well as nutrition and support. It is published by NetHealth.

WeightLoss2000.com--A Little Exercise: Weight Loss Is Just One of Many Benefits
http://WeightLoss2000.com/health_library/exercise/exer_02_alittle.html
> Exercise: it isn't just for weight loss. Check out all the benefits associated with a program of regular, low-intensity workouts.

WeightLoss2000.com--Drug Therapies
http://WeightLoss2000.com/drug

Weight-loss drugs do not take the place of diet, exercise, patience, and perseverance. But in physician-supervised weight-loss programs, medication can enhance weight loss. Here's a list of over-the-counter, as well as prescription-only medications. Articles here describe how they work, and what the possible side effects can be.

WeightLoss2000.com--Easy Exercises
http://WeightLoss2000.com/exer

Here's a list of articles citing latest studies that you don't have to join a club or even indulge in sweaty workouts; all you have to do is incorporate a little more physical activity into your daily life.

WeightLoss2000.com--Herbal Therapies
http://WeightLoss2000.com/herbs

"Herbal weight-loss formulas won't rid you of major pounds overnight. But medicinal herbs can play a supporting role in medically responsible weight-loss programs." Serotonin-elevating, diuretic, and stimulant herbs among others are discussed. Many articles cite studies which may or may not support the successful use of herbal therapies.

WeightLoss2000.com--Latest News
http://WeightLoss2000.com/news

Abstracts from sources ranging from reputable medical journals to newspapers are printed here; they date as far back as 1997, and can be good starting points for further study.

WeightLoss2000.com--Walking: Getting Started
http://WeightLoss2000.com/health_library/exercise/exer_07_walkstart.html

I seriously doubt that you need a primer on how to walk. We all can get to the fridge, can't we? But you will get a few pointers on developing a regular program. But wait, you can't go out in your slippers.

WeightLoss2000.com--What's Stopping You?
http://WeightLoss2000.com/health_library/exercise/exer_03_whatsstop.html

"I don't want anybody to see me!" or "I don't have time!" These are only two common excuses we use. Bet we can add to this list.

WeightLoss2000.Com--How Fit Are You?
http://WeightLoss2000.com/health_library/exercise/exer_01_howfit.html

Go ahead, you only have to answer five easy questions. There's no measuring or inputting any embarrassing information. Besides, you probably already know the answer.

 MUST SEE!   VIDEO   AUDIO   SELLS STUFF

 CHAT ROOMS   MAILING LISTS   MESSAGE BOARDS   ADULT CONTENT

 FREE REGISTRATION REQUIRED   MEMBERS ONLY CONTENT   SEARCHABLE

Wellness MD - Cabbage/Chicken Soup Fat Burning Diet $

www.wellnessmd.com/fatburn.html

Here's the enhanced recipe from the wellness MD. Although he claims that you can lose 10-20 pounds in one to two weeks, you will put it back on - unless you buy their 30 day Maintenance Diet. Oh yeah, you should also buy a thermometer from them so you can take your temperature before meals to determine your metabolism. Just feel your forehead...

Wellness Web: Chromium Picolinate

www.wellweb.com/nutri/chromium_picolinate.htm

Recent studies show that claims about muscle gain and fat loss associated with use of chromium picolinate are unsubstantiated. Hold on to your credit card a little longer and read this before you think you've found the fountain of youth.

Wellness Web: Nutrition Tips For People Living With AIDS

www.wellweb.com/nutri/living_with_aids.htm

People who are living with AIDS are encouraged to eat a balanced diet high in protein and in calories. Your immune system needs both for peak performance, but what do you do when you're tired or nauseated or have mouth sores? You'll find many good tips here.

What's Your Excuse?

http://primusweb.com/fitnesspartner/library/activity/excuses.htm

25% of all adults don't exercise at all, and 60% don't do it very much. Because this epidemic of inactivity can lead to crippling diseases and premature deaths, it's time to pry ourselves out of the couch and put that remote away. Read on.

WHOLEFOODS.COM   Whole Foods. Whole People. Whole Planet.

WholeFoods.com 🔽$👤🔍👁

www.wholefoods.com

WholeFoods.com is like an old-fashioned neighborhood grocery store, an organic farmer's market, a European bakery, a New York deli, and a modern supermarket all rolled into one! They have stores in about 25 states under 6 different names: Whole Foods Market, Bread and Circus, Fresh Fields, Wellspring Grocery, Merchant of Vino, and Nature's Heartland. The company is committed to sustainable agriculture, to expanding the market for organic products, and donating 5% of after tax profits to a variety of community and non-profit organizations. And now you can shop with them on-line, or read their informative and pleasing to the eye E-Zine.

WholeFoods.com: Marketplace $

www.wholefoods.com/market/index.html

At WholeFoods.com Marketplace you can browse through or search their extensive inventory of groceries, health and body products, household, pet and garden, and even gifts. After you've roamed their "store," order on-line on their secure server and have it delivered to your door. Purchases are shipped via UPS.

WholeFoods.com: Whole Living Magazine
www.wholefoods.com/magazine/index.html

In one issue of *Whole Living Magazine* you could read about the "Joy of Soy," as well as the amazing artichoke. Discover phytochemicals, isoflavones, and phytoestrogen. And you thought you just had to watch your caloric and fat intake! There's a wealth of information in short articles, all in a format that's pleasing to the eye.

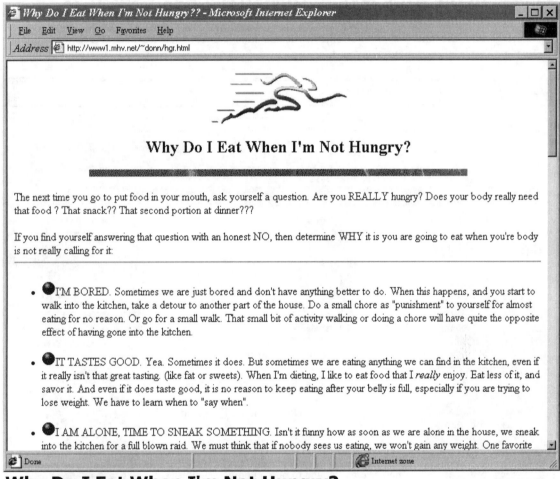

Why Do I Eat When I'm Not Hungry?? - Microsoft Internet Explorer

File   Edit   View   Go   Favorites   Help

Address   http://www1.mhv.net/~donn/hgr.html

Why Do I Eat When I'm Not Hungry?

The next time you go to put food in your mouth, ask yourself a question. Are you REALLY hungry? Does your body really need that food ? That snack?? That second portion at dinner???

If you find yourself answering that question with an honest NO, then determine WHY it is you are going to eat when you're body is not really calling for it:

- **I'M BORED.** Sometimes we are just bored and don't have anything better to do. When this happens, and you start to walk into the kitchen, take a detour to another part of the house. Do a small chore as "punishment" to yourself for almost eating for no reason. Or go for a small walk. That small bit of activity walking or doing a chore will have quite the opposite effect of having gone into the kitchen.

- **IT TASTES GOOD.** Yea. Sometimes it does. But sometimes we are eating anything we can find in the kitchen, even if it really isn't that great tasting. (like fat or sweets). When I'm dieting, I like to eat food that I *really* enjoy. Eat less of it, and savor it. And even if it does taste good, it is no reason to keep eating after your belly is full, especially if you are trying to lose weight. We have to learn when to "say when".

- **I AM ALONE, TIME TO SNEAK SOMETHING.** Isn't it funny how as soon as we are alone in the house, we sneak into the kitchen for a full blown raid. We must think that if nobody sees us eating, we won't gain any weight. One favorite

Done   Internet zone

Why Do I Eat When I'm Not Hungry?
http://www1.mhv.net/~donn/hgr.html

Here's a list of reasons why we eat when we're really not hungry. Reasons vary from "It's time!" to "I'm bored," to "I'm stressed!" Sounds familiar.

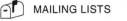 MUST SEE!   VIDEO   AUDIO   **$** SELLS STUFF

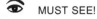 CHAT ROOMS   MAILING LISTS   MESSAGE BOARDS   ADULT CONTENT

 FREE REGISTRATION REQUIRED   MEMBERS ONLY CONTENT   SEARCHABLE

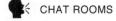

Women & Physical Activity: A Historical Journey
http://primusweb.com/fitnesspartner/library/activity/womenhistory
.htm

> Check out this enlightening and interactive look at the strides women have made throughout history to gain equality in physical activity and competitive sports as discussed in The Bodywise Woman.

Women of the Baby Boom: Time to Get Heart Smart 👁

http://primusweb.com/fitnesspartner/library/activity/femheart.htm

> Heart disease accounts for more women's deaths than cancer, diabetes and accidents combined. Reading this brief page may save your life.

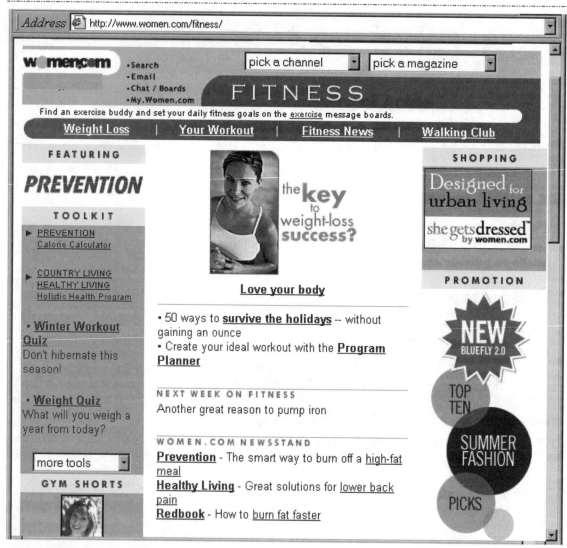

Women.com: Fitness 👁
www.women.com/fitness

> Check in with Fitness news, the Walking Club, Weight Loss, and Your Workout. Some stuff is gleaned from Prevention, Good Housekeeping, Cosmo, Country Living, and others in the Hearst Magazine family. There's lots to browse here.

World Guide to Vegetarianism
www.veg.org/veg/Guide

The World Guide to Vegetarianism is a listing of vegetarian and vegetarian-friendly restaurants, stores, organizations, services, etc. Just click on a country, and browse the listings.

World of Yoga
www.yogaworld.org

Here's an introduction to Yoga, and some info on the eight main Yogas.

Worldguide: Health & Fitness Forum
www.worldguide.com/home/dmg/Fitness/hf.html

This is a great place to start if you're trying to find some exercise and fitness ideas. Just click on strength training, cardiovascular, sports medicine or eating well for help.

WWW Cookbook
www.hut.fi/~jstalvio/cookbook1

The recipes are indexed by category, contributor, key word, or by recipe name. For instance, if you want to make something with potatoes just click on potato. All recipes are supposed to be fat-free, although I did not see nutritional analysis of any recipes.

Xenical
www.xenical.com/consumers/index.htm

From Roche Laboratories, this is the consumer information page for orlistat (generic name), the latest FDA approved oral prescription weight loss medication. What it is, who is a candidate, the probable side effects, how to take it, and all your questions are answered here.

Yoga For Busy People
www.indolink.com/Health/Yoga/yoga2.html

If you thought Yoga involved at least an hour of your time each day, go here to see how just fifteen minutes a day can help you.

Zone Home
www.zonehome.com/index.htm

This is self-admittedly the unauthorized source for Zone Diet information and more. John Weaver invites you to sit around his virtual campfire and interact in his "Paleo Zone." You'll find a multitude of topics on the message boards, and a library with useful documents to help you understand, and find, the Zone. Nothing is sold on this web site.

 MUST SEE!   VIDEO   AUDIO   SELLS STUFF

 CHAT ROOMS   MAILING LISTS   MESSAGE BOARDS   ADULT CONTENT

 FREE REGISTRATION REQUIRED   MEMBERS ONLY CONTENT   SEARCHABLE

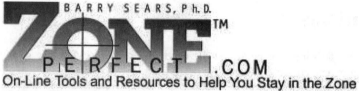

ZonePerfect.Com - The Official Home of the Zone Diet

www.enterthezone.com

If you've ever been browsing a diet section in a bookstore, you've seen the Zone books. Here's a very extensive web site that explains it all.

Have a Site You Think We Should Add?
Spotted a Change?

For review, e-mail details about the site (including its name and URL) to

mdauphin@gateway.net

Want to Find Out About
Other Titles in the
Incredible Internet Guide Series?

Visit us on the Web at

www.brbpub.com/iig

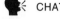 MUST SEE!　　 VIDEO　　 AUDIO　　 SELLS STUFF

 CHAT ROOMS　　 MAILING LISTS　　 MESSAGE BOARDS　　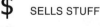 ADULT CONTENT

 FREE REGISTRATION REQUIRED　　 MEMBERS ONLY CONTENT　　 SEARCHABLE

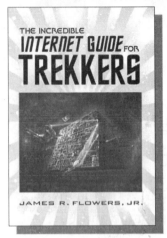
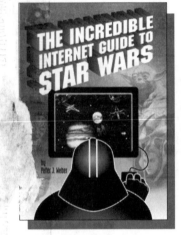
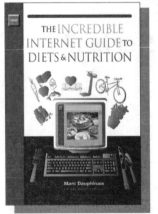